PEDIATRIC PHYSICAL EXAMINATION
An Illustrated Handbook

PEDIATRIC PHYSICAL EXAMINATION

An Illustrated Handbook

Karen G. Duderstadt

Clinical Professor
Department of Family Health Care Nursing
University of California at San Francisco
San Francisco, California

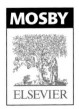

MOSBY

ELSEVIER

MOSBY
ELSEVIER

11830 Westline Industrial Drive
St. Louis, Missouri 63146

PEDIATRIC PHYSICAL EXAMINATION: AN ILLUSTRATED HANDBOOK   ISBN-13: 978-0-323-01904-0
                                                             ISBN-10: 0-323-01904-8
Copyright © 2006 by Mosby Inc.

Notice

Neither the Publisher nor the Author assumes any responsibility for any loss or injury and/or damage to persons or property arising out of or related to any use of the material contained in this book. It is the responsibility of the treating practitioner, relying on independent expertise and knowledge of the patient, to determine the best treatment and method of application for the patient.

ISBN-13: 978-0-323-01904-0
ISBN-10: 0-323-01904-8

Executive Publisher: Barbara Nelson Cullen
Acquisition Editor: Sandra Clark Brown
Senior Developmental Editor: Sophia Oh Gray
Publishing Services Manager: Deborah L. Vogel
Senior Project Manager: Ann E. Rogers
Book Design Manager: Bill Drone

Working together to grow
libraries in developing countries
www.elsevier.com | www.bookaid.org | www.sabre.org

Printed in China

Last digit is the print number: 9   8   7   6   5   4   3

ELSEVIER   BOOK AID International   Sabre Foundation

To
Richard Sanchez, M.D., F.A.A.P.,
who taught me everything about pediatrics.

CONTRIBUTORS

Patricia Jackson Allen, RN, MS, PNP, FAAN
Professor
Yale University
New Haven, Connecticut
12. Ears
13. Nose, Mouth, and Throat

Karen G. Duderstadt, RN, MS, PNP, PhD(c)
Clinical Professor
Department of Family Health Care Nursing
University of California at San Francisco
San Francisco, California
1. Approach to Child & Adolescent Assessment
2. Assessment Parameters
4. Comprehensive Information Gathering
5. Environmental Health History
9. Head and Neck
10. Lymphatic System
11. Eyes
15. Male Genitalia
18. Musculoskeletal System
19. Neurological System
20. Pediatric Health Visit Charting

Renee McLeod, DNSc, RN, CS, CPNP
Professor and Director
Pediatric Nurse Practitioner Program
Vanderbilt University School of Nursing
Nashville, Tennessee
6. Skin

Laura J. Ohara, RN, MS, PNP-CS, CNS
Pediatric Nurse Practitioner
Pediatric Gastroenterology Associates
San Jose, California;
Nurse Practitioner
Lucille Salter Packard Children's Hospital
Palo Alto, California
14. Abdomen

Naomi A. Schapiro, RN, MS, CPNP
Associate Clinical Professor
School of Nursing
University of California at San Francisco
San Francisco, California
4. Comprehensive Information Gathering
16. Male and Female Breast
17. Female Genitalia
18. Musculoskeletal System

Concettina Tolomeo, RN, MSN, APRN, BC, AE-C
Nurse Practitioner; Director,
Program Development
Pediatric Respiratory Medicine
Yale University School of Medicine
New Haven, Connecticut
8. Chest and Respiratory System

Elizabeth Tong, MS, RN, PCNS, FAAN
Clinical Research, Nurse Coordination
University of California at San Francisco
San Francisco, California
7. Heart and Vascular System

Andrea Windom, MSN, PNP, IBCLC
Pediatric Nurse Practitioner
Kaiser Permanente
Vallejo, California;
Assistant Clinical Professor
University of California at San Francisco
San Francisco, California
3. Developmental Parameters

REVIEWERS

Jane E. Anderson, MD
Clinical Professor
University of California at San Francisco
San Francisco, California

Daisy Ann Bennett, RN, MSN, BSN
School Nurse, Allied Health Instructor,
Pediatric Home Care Nurse
Administrator High School LPN Program
Scioto County Joint Vocational School
Lucasville, Ohio

Stephanie Bonney, MS, RN, CPNP
Pediatric Nurse Practitioner
Medical Services
St. Mary's Hospital for Children
Bayside, New York

Bill Campbell, MS, RN
Nursing Department
Salisbury State University
Salisbury, Maryland

Barbara A. Caton, RN, MSN
Southwest Missouri State University–
West Plains
West Plains, Missouri

Susan S. Cox, MSN, RN, CNS
Nursing Faculty
Huron School of Medicine
Cleveland Clinical Health System
Cleveland, Ohio

James E. Crawford, MD, FAAP
Medical Director
Center for Child Protection
Children's Hospital and Research Center at
Oakland
Oakland, California

Katy Garth, RN, MSN, FNP-BC
Senior Lecturer, Nursing
Murray State University
Murray, Kentucky

Rebecca Gesler, RN, MSN
Saint Catharine College
Saint Catharine, Kentucky

Amy Zlomek Hedden, RN, MS, NP
Instructor, Pediatric Content Expert
Department of Nursing
California State University
Bakersfield, California;
Advanced Practice Nurse
Bakersfield Family Medical Center
Department of Pediatrics
Bakersfield, California

Monica Kogan, MD
Children's Hospital Oakland
Oakland, California

Linda Mary Lockerbie, RN, BN, MN
Maternal Child Health Nurse Clinician
Pediatric/Obstetrics/Gynecologic/
Women's Health Program
Atlantic Health Sciences Corporation
Saint John, New Brunswick, Canada;
Clinical Instructor
Pediatrics
University of New Brunswick at Saint John
Saint John, New Brunswick, Canada

Kenneth J.A. Lown, RN, MSN, CPNP
Pediatric Neuro-oncology
Children's Hospital of Philadelphia
Philadelphia, Pennsylvania

Hiep T. Nguyen, MD
Assistant Professor
Urology and Pediatrics
University of California at San Francisco
San Francisco, California

David Paulk, MS, PA-C
Department of Medical Science and
Community Health
Arcadia University
Glenside, Pennsylvania

Kerry S. Risco, MSN, CPNP, RNCS
Assistant Professor
Slippery Rock University
Slippery Rock, Pennsylvania

Amy J. Sehnert, MD
Assistant Professor
Pediatric Cardiology
University of California at San Francisco
San Francisco, California

Lisa South, RN, DSN
University of Alabama at Huntsville
Huntsville, Alabama

Elizabeth Ann O'Rouke Sweet, BSN, MS, PNP
Pediatric Nurse Practitioner
Surgical Services
A.I. du Pont Hospital for Children
Wilmington, Delaware

Barbara William Taylor, RN, MSN
Nursing Instructor
Health Sciences
Chipola Junior College
Marianna, Florida

Deborah J. Throne, MSN, RN
Faculty Nursing Department
Lewis and Clark Community College
Godfrey, Illinois;
Staff Nurse
Emergency Department
Cardinal Glennon Children's Hospital
Godfrey, Illinois

Ruthanne Werner, RN, MSN, MED
Educational Nurse Specialist
Patient Services
Cincinnati Children's Hospital Medical Center
Cincinnati, Ohio

PREFACE

Pediatric Physical Examination: An Illustrated Handbook is intended, first and foremost, to be utilized in the education of the pediatric primary health care workforce, and second, to augment the skills of health care providers currently working with infants, children, and adolescents across pediatric practice settings. With the increasing pressures on the health care delivery system, primary health care providers need astute observation and assessment skills combined with quick references to assist them in caring for children and families. This first edition of *Pediatric Physical Examination: An Illustrated Handbook* will provide the novice or experienced provider with pediatric content from experts in the field, useful examination techniques from birth to adolescence, and clinical pearls not covered in other across-the-lifespan health assessment texts.

Chapter 1 begins with a helpful approach to the assessment of the pediatric age span and is followed by chapters on the important assessment parameters for growth and development. Chapter 4 includes a comprehensive section on history taking on infants as well as interviewing the adolescent. The reader will note that the text is not organized in a typical head-to-toe approach. A pediatric-oriented "quiet-to-active" format has been adopted to organize the systems chapters. Pediatric experts

consider this to be an effective approach to assessing children. This format begins with the "quieter" parts of the exam—cardiac and respiratory—which require astute listening skills and less active participation of the child. These "quiet" parts of the exam are followed by the more active parts that require more participation from the child, such as the eyes, ears, nose, and throat assessment. Chapter 16 presents male and female breast development, common adolescent breast conditions, as well as the female breast exam. The first gynecologic exam in adolescent females presented in Chapter 17 provides clinical pearls for preparing and working with the young adolescent. Chapter 18 includes a comprehensive assessment of the child and adolescent athlete for sports participation. Finally, Chapter 20 provides charting examples of the comprehensive, system-focused, and preparticipation sports physical examination.

Pediatric health care is a hopeful endeavor as it builds the foundation for health promotion and health protection throughout life. As a pediatric healthcare provider, you will have a key role in protecting and improving the health of the next generation. This text aids in the careful and comprehensive assessment of children to assist the practitioner in this most important endeavor.

ACKNOWLEDGMENTS

There are many to thank when the first edition of a textbook is finally published. This was a long and arduous process, and I am grateful for the support I received on the journey.

First, I need to thank Robin Carter, Executive Publisher at Elsevier, who was willing to support my idea for the text and invest in a new author and a *tabula rasa*. Second, I want to acknowledge my current and former pediatric faculty colleagues at the University of California at San Francisco. Patricia Jackson Allen, who I consulted when I was proposing the text, gave me the soundest advice, "Don't do it!" Her early contributions to the text and the contributions of other faculty members were key to getting the project off the ground. Danielle Rankin, my Administrative Assistant, deserves many thanks for helping me through the third revision of the chapters. This was a crucial point in the project and without her assistance, the text would not have moved forward.

I want to gratefully acknowledge the editors of the text: Sandra Brown, Editor, and Sophia Oh Gray, Senior Developmental Editor. Sandy encouraged me over and over with grace and patience, and faithfully believed in me when I had doubts. Sophia loyally mentored me throughout the writing of the text and shaped me as an author. Her mutual commitment to the project, endurance, willingness to assume many tasks, and frequent patient reminders made the text possible. Without her support, the project would never have been completed.

Finally, I would like to acknowledge my husband, Christopher, whose constant support of this project and willingness to assist me at every step along the way made it all possible. My hope is that the knowledge in the text will help to shape the next generation of pediatric health care providers.

Karen G. Duderstadt

CONTENTS

PEDIATRIC PHYSICAL EXAMINATION

An Illustrated Handbook

GENERAL ASSESSMENT

CHAPTER 1

APPROACH TO CHILD & ADOLESCENT ASSESSMENT

Karen G. Duderstadt

UNIQUE ROLE OF THE PEDIATRIC PROVIDER

The role of the pediatric provider is twofold: a collaborator with the parent and an advocate to protect and care for the child. Children have unique needs because of their long period of dependency and development, and this presents a unique challenge to the pediatric healthcare provider. Children's health and well-being depend greatly on the care received from their family units and the surrounding environment in which they live.[1] Addressing the needs of the parent while caring for the child and fostering a healthy relationship between the parent and child are the most important and difficult tasks in pediatrics.

ESTABLISHING A CARING RELATIONSHIP

Developing a caring relationship that delivers *contextual child health care*—care given within the context of the child's family and community—requires a personalized approach.[2] Several key components are involved in developing a successful, caring relationship with children and families in the pediatric setting.[2]

- Listen actively to the concerns of the family. A caring relationship is established by developing an understanding of the feelings and values within the family context.
- Understand the family expectations for the encounter. To successfully establish a caring relationship, the parent's agenda must be identified and addressed during the encounter.
- Ask open-ended questions, thereby allowing relevant data to unfold.
- Personalize your care. Taking the time to obtain relevant personal data on the child and family will build the caring relationship.
- Learn and understand the importance of cultural values in the family.
- Identify protective factors in the family that create a positive environment for the child. Social supports for the parents, involvement of relatives or extended family, shared family interest in activities such as sports, cultural events, or religious services often help to form a supportive and protective community for a child.

- Build a sense of confidence in parents by confirming and complimenting their strengths in caring for their child. This approach also builds a trusting relationship between the family and healthcare provider.

PARENT AND CHILD INTERACTION

One of the most important aspects of the health interview is eliciting and observing interaction between the parent and child or adolescent. Analyzing verbal responses and interactions during the encounter gives the healthcare provider an idea of how the parental relationship fosters child identity and child development. It also gives the healthcare provider a window into the child's world. Interactions between the parent/caretaker, the family members, and the healthcare provider reveal family dynamics, family authority, and the approach to problem solving.

Nonverbal cues provide the most revealing picture of the child's demeanor and of the parent/child relationship. Stop and observe these cues, and verbalize your concerns to the parent and child: "You look sad today. Can you tell me what that is about?" Ask yourself the following: Is the mother disengaged with the child or infant during the encounter? Does the mother or parent appear depressed or angry? Do the data from the health interview fit with the demeanor of the child during the encounter? The child or adolescent's nonverbal cues give the healthcare provider additional understanding of the *context* in which the child lives.

A child who is withdrawn, refusing to make eye contact, or who is consistently stressed when communicating with a parent is exhibiting signs of strain in her/his environment. This should alert the healthcare provider to communicate her/his concern to the family and provide support, counseling, and referral when indicated. Children often mirror the emotions of the adults around them. Families involved in conflict often cannot see their own interactions clearly or the impact their interactions have on the child. Early intervention by the healthcare provider in harmful or ineffective family communications is critical to the healthy psychosocial development of the child.

CULTURAL CONSIDERATIONS

The evaluation of cultural orientation is critical to the assessment of children and families. Cultural beliefs impact care-seeking behavior and affect the delivery of clinical care by healthcare providers. Exploration of cultural groups in the United States demonstrates differences *within* ethnic groups that are as great as the cultural differences *between* groups; therefore no valid assumptions can be made in health care on the basis of physical appearance or surname.[3] It is important to follow a model of care that incorporates sensitivity to cultural differences and enhances the protective factors of cultural practices within families. Ideally, delivery of healthcare services should occur in the first language of the client. When this is not possible, a model framework for the encounter between the healthcare provider, child, and family includes the following[4,5]:

- Recognizing language barriers and effectively using interpreters
- Exploring parental beliefs and their impact on the child
- Evaluating the cultural values and orientation of the family unit
- Recognizing folk illness, how it influences child health in the family, and the impact of folk beliefs on clinical care
- Understanding, as the healthcare provider, how your own personal values influence care delivery and impact health outcomes
- Altering care practices to eliminate health disparities related to race/ethnicity

Cultural competence is an essential component of responsible healthcare services for multicultural populations. Incorporating sensitive cultural understanding into the healthcare encounter will build honesty and trust in the caring relationship. Throughout the text, attention is given to how culture and ethnicity influence the assessment process in child health.

INTERVIEWING CHILDREN

Engaging children in the interview process can reveal their understanding of health, allow them to express misconceptions they may have, and provide insight into their social-emotional world.[4] Eye-level encounters are the most effective with young children and make the healthcare provider appear more approachable. The healthcare provider learns to make eye contact when the child is interested and to avoid it when the child is fearful. Initially directing attention to the parent or caretaker allows the infant or toddler time to adjust to the environment and interviewer.

Children are accepting of many different styles of interacting and will adapt to the practitioner who is at ease and competently structures the interview. Children are comfortable when they know what to expect in an environment. Therefore, "talking through" every step of the encounter decreases anxiety in the child and adolescent. Even busy practitioners

☞ Key Points

Children as young as 3 years of age can effectively participate in the health interview. Involving children at this age establishes the practitioner as an advocate for the child and gives voice to the concerns of the child in an objective manner. A recent study found that 84% of pediatric providers obtain part of the health history from preschool children.[6]

in time-pressured environments will find the child or adolescent to be a more willing participant when adding this *talk-through* format to the healthcare encounter.

Preschool children will commonly be asked about their activities, playmates, and school or childcare. It is important to engage children in discussion of health history issues, as well as topics such as daily routines and safety. Health education and anticipatory guidance can easily be offered following the child's responses when this interview technique is used.

School-age children can be directly interviewed and can participate in their health care. Healthcare providers can role model for parents as they engage the child in the health interview and teach aspects of health and safety education. This approach teaches children from a young age to understand and care about their health and establishes the importance of building healthy habits for life.

Adolescents should always be interviewed separately after inquiring about concerns from a parent or guardian. Allowing time to engage the adolescent independently will provide the best opening for discussion of personal or sensitive concerns that need to be voiced.

Effective Communication

Using the following clear communication techniques when interviewing will build a caring, trusting relationship with children/adolescents and their families.

- **Question indirectly** to encourage children and adolescents who are reluctant to discuss feelings. Engage the young child with, "I am going to tell you a story about a 5-year-old who lost his favorite pet. How do you think he feels?" or the adolescent with, "Some 15-year-olds have tried marijuana. Do you have any friends who smoke marijuana?"
- **Pose scenarios** to the child or adolescent. "What would you do if …?" is appropriate for the young child, in contrast to,

"How would you feel if …?" which is appropriate for the older school-age child and adolescent.

- **Begin with less threatening topics** and move slowly to topics more sensitive to the child or adolescent. "Tell me how things are going at school this year," in contrast to, "Has anyone ever hurt you?" or directed to the adolescent, "Has anyone forced you to have sex against your will?"
- **State your expectations clearly.** Say to the child, "I need for you to be very quiet now so I can listen to …" or to the adolescent, "To take care of you, I need for you to tell me …"
- **Do not offer a choice** to the child or adolescent when in reality there is no choice.
- **Use "I"** when speaking to the child or adolescent. "I need to ask you this question because I want to help you …" in contrast to, "You need to tell me what is going on." Avoid using the word "you," which creates a defensive atmosphere when interviewing children or adolescents.[5] This will provide positive role modeling for parents and also build the caring relationship between the healthcare provider, the child, and the parent.
- **Ask the preschool or young school-age child to draw a picture.** This captures the children's attention and establishes your interest in their abilities. Children often reveal feelings or communicate important issues through their art.[7]

"QUIET TO ACTIVE" APPROACH TO THE PHYSICAL EXAMINATION

"Quiet to active" is an important mantra that should be adopted by the healthcare provider who will be caring for infants and young children. It refers to the approach of beginning with the parts of the physical examination that require the child to be *quiet* or silent in order for the healthcare provider to differentiate physical findings. The "quiet" parts of the physical examination in infants and young children include pulse and respiratory rate, auscultation of cardiac sounds and respiratory sounds, and auscultation and assessment of the abdomen. Respiratory and cardiac sounds are subtle, and accurate assessment requires a relatively cooperative child. Therefore, approaching these areas first during the physical examination produces the best results. The assessment of the abdomen, genitalia, and cranial nerves in the young child can all be completed before the more invasive examination of the ears and mouth and measuring height, weight, and temperature. Varying the sequence of the physical examination to fit the temperament and activity level of the child is an essential part of pediatrics, but omitting an aspect of the exam is not serving the health needs of the child and risks a diagnosis made on an incomplete assessment.

Assessment Techniques

Inspection

Inspection is about *looking*, a skill developed by employing detailed and meticulous observation and learning to see the whole as well as the parts. It involves not only the sense of sight but also the senses of hearing and smell. Inspection requires good room lighting and complete visibility of the body part to be examined to accurately assess symmetry, shape, color, and odor. It is an essential skill for the pediatric healthcare provider, particularly when interacting with the nonverbal child, the young pediatric patient, or a child who is ill.

Palpation

Palpation is about *touching* and *feeling*, a skill used to discriminate temperature, vibration, position, and mobility of body parts. Palpation appreciates shape, pulsation, texture, and hydration of the skin and tenderness and discriminates differences in glands, vessels, organs, muscles, bones, and masses in all parts of the body. Various parts of the hand are used for palpation. Fingertips are most sensitive to tactile differences, the backs of the fingers are most sensitive to temperature, and flattened fingers and palm on the chest detect vibrations. The examiner's hands should move smoothly over the body without hesitation, first using light palpation, then followed by deep, firm pressure with palpation. It is important to know the distinction between palpation and massage. Massage incorporates *rubbing* in contrast to the technique of *palpation,* which is the movement of the fingers over an area for the purpose of identifying size, location, mobility, sensitivity, and temperature of lymph nodes, muscles, tissues, and body organs.

Percussion

Percussion requires using different parts of the examiner's hand to produce sounds on the area of the body being examined. The density of the body parts is determined by the sounds emitted when the examiner's finger strikes the middle finger of the opposite hand. The fingers produce sounds ranging from the least dense sound, *tympany* or *resonance,* as heard over the stomach or intestines, to the most dense sound, *dullness* or *flatness,* produced by striking over bone. Percussion is a helpful skill for mapping out the borders of the organs or sternum and for determining the presence of solid tumors. This technique can be useful when examining the abdomen to detect the size of an organ but is not generally useful in infants and young children when examining the chest for consolidations.

Auscultation

Auscultation is listening to body sounds transmitted through the stethoscope. With infants and small children, low-pitched cardiac sounds are heard best with the bell-shaped side of the stethoscope, and high-pitched lung and bowel sounds are best heard with the diaphragm, or flat portion, of the stethoscope. The bell shape is effective in isolating cardiac sounds from stomach sounds in the young infant. For children, it is essential to match the size of the

stethoscope head to the size of the child proportionately for the best results during the physical examination. A skill that is important to develop in performing pediatric auscultation is that of training the ear to screen out adventitious sounds that occur in infants and children when listening to lungs, heart, and stomach/abdomen. The close proximity of the organs requires the practitioner to screen out stomach sounds when listening to the heart and the respirations in the lung.

DEVELOPMENTAL APPROACH

Preterm Infants and Newborns

The hospital nursery setting provides a warming table for the initial newborn examination for the purposes of limiting body heat loss and stabilizing temperature. In the clinical setting, it is important to begin the physical assessment with the infant initially swaddled in the parent's arms or on the examining table to maintain body temperature. In this manner, auscultation of the cardiac and respiratory sounds can be accomplished before disturbing a sleeping infant. This is the most effective initial approach for the newborn. After the "quiet" parts of the examination are completed, transfer the infant to the examining table and begin a complete assessment with the infant wearing only a diaper. Observing the movements of the newborn for symmetry, strength, and coordination must be accomplished with the infant undressed. Assessment of overall appearance, skin color, breathing pattern, and degree of alertness or responsiveness should be noted. The healthcare provider should remain flexible in regard to the order of the exam throughout the encounter because often the physical examination is performed between the eating and sleeping cycles of the newborn.

Infants Up to 6 Months of Age

Until 4 months of age, infants are most effectively assessed on the examination table.

It provides a firm surface to support the infant's head during the physical exam and also provides a stable surface for the examination techniques required during a complete physical assessment. A calm, gentle approach works well and avoids possibly frightening the infant. The "quiet" parts of the exam may be accomplished with the infant in the parent's arms, but other parts of the physical exam are difficult to accomplish effectively in that position. Remember never to leave the examining table at any point when evaluating a young infant.

Infants and Toddlers

Inspection of infants and young children necessitates using a completely different social approach than with any other age-groups. When establishing a therapeutic relationship with an adult, etiquette requires immediate eye contact. With infants 6 to 9 months of age, a progression of eye contact is required because of the developmental phenomenon of stranger anxiety. First, observe the infant or toddler covertly while speaking with the parent or caretaker to allow the child to adjust to your presence in the environment. If the young child is looking at you and listening, then make a glancing eye contact. If you are not rejected, then speak to the young child and, finally, reach out to touch the child. This approach will produce the best results when establishing the caring relationship. Offering puppets or washable, small toys to the child or using dolls to demonstrate parts of the physical examination to the toddler also provides a calming effect at the beginning of the encounter.

Once the infant is able to sit stably, around 6 to 8 months of age, the examination can proceed with the child in the parent's lap to decrease fear and stranger anxiety. Clothing should be removed gradually as the physical exam progresses from "quiet" to "active." Optimum examination of the abdomen and genitalia occurs with the child on the examining table,

but in the fearful child, the exam may proceed with the child still in the parent's lap and with the examiner seated at the same level as the parent in a knee-to-knee position to create a surface for the child to lie on. With the young child's head and shoulder cradled on the parent or caretaker's lap, the examiner proceeds with assessment of the abdomen, genitalia, and hips, thereby avoiding the child's anxiety of being on the exam table. When the infant is old enough to begin walking, it is important to observe the infant toddling in only a diaper, at the end of the examination, to evaluate musculoskeletal coordination.

Preschoolers

By 3 years of age, most preschoolers, though still apprehensive, are able to make eye contact and separate briefly from the parent. Observe their ability to be comforted, evaluate their response to the environment, their level of social interaction, and their relationships with parents or caretakers and siblings, if present. How appropriate is their behavior in the setting? What is the quality and variety of their verbal responses? What is their level of activity and attention span? Young children, in general, respond best to a slow, even, steady voice.[8] Give the preschooler time to warm to the situation before undressing. Begin the assessment with the confident preschooler sitting on the examining table. The "quiet" to "active" approach is advisable with this age-group also, that is, beginning with the cardiac and respiratory examination. Give them clear directions, allow them to respond, and recognize success. Preschoolers particularly enjoy games, drawing, and role-playing the physical examination with dolls or stuffed animals (Figure 1-1). Modesty sets in during the preschool years, and healthcare providers need to be respectful and mindful of this developmental stage.

School-Age Children

School-age children benefit most from the talk-through approach to the physical exam.

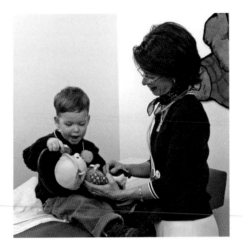

Figure 1-1 Use of play to decrease anxiety in preschooler.

Pediatric Pearls

Explain clearly to the child or adolescent exactly what you are going to assess during the physical exam to decrease anxiety and build trust. With each part of the exam, explain or "talk through" the assessment and the findings. Reassure the child or adolescent of your findings when normal and explain abnormal findings as appropriate for the child's age.

They are interested in learning about their bodies and are forming an image of themselves. They are becoming more independent from their parents, and this age-group gains the most from education concerning good health habits. Learning more about their bodies helps them connect their health with their health habits. Offer the school-age child choices about who will be present in the exam room, respect modesty, and allow the child to participate in all aspects of the exam. A "head-to-toe" assessment with the child on the examining table is effective during the school-age years.

Adolescents

The approach used with the adolescent during the healthcare encounter should be based on the developmental stage rather than the age of the client. This is true for all children, but particularly those in adolescence. Development during early, middle, and late adolescence proceeds unevenly and can vary widely among 12- to 18-year-olds. Respect and confidentiality are essential components of developing a trusting relationship with the adolescent. Parental input is important during the health encounter, but adolescents should be interviewed and examined separately from the parent or peers. Avoid power struggles and give the adolescent control whenever possible.[9] Involve adolescents in planning their health care and in establishing realistic health habits.

REFERENCES

1. Szilagyi PG et al: Evaluation of a state health insurance program for low-income children: implications for state child health insurance programs, *Pediatrics* 105(2):363-371, 2000.
2. Green M: The 10-minute visit: anything but routine, *Contemp Pediatr* 53-61, 1992.
3. Dana RH: Assessment of cultural orientation, *SPA Exchange* 2(2):14-15, 1992.
4. Dana RH: Culturally competent assessment practice in the United States, *J Personality Assess* 66:462-487, 1996.
5. Flores G: Culture and the patient-physician relationship: achieving cultural competency in health care, *J Pediatr* 136(1):14-23, 2000.
6. Mendelsohn JS, Quinn MT, McNabb WL: Interview strategies commonly used by pediatricians, *Arch Pediatr Adolesc Med* 153(2):154-157, 1999.

7. Dixon SD, Stein MT: *Encounters with children: pediatric development and behavior,* St Louis, 2000, Mosby.

8. Wong DL, Hockenberry-Eaton M, Wilson D et al: *Wong's essentials of pediatric nursing,* St Louis, 2001, Mosby.

9. Muscari ME: *Advanced pediatric clinical assessment: skills and procedures,* Philadelphia, 2001, Lippincott.

ASSESSMENT PARAMETERS

Karen G. Duderstadt

NORMAL GROWTH

Unique to children is the dynamic aspect of growth. Measurement of growth in the early years is a key indicator of health. Abnormal progression of growth and maturation is often the first indicator to the healthcare provider of abnormalities in the growing systems. Growth proceeds in a predictable pattern during childhood from *cephalocaudal* (head to tail) and from *proximodistal* (near to far). Plotting serial measurements regularly on a standardized, gender-specific growth curve chart is a reliable method of monitoring growth and is an essential component of comprehensive well child care (see Appendix A for gender- and age-specific growth charts).

GESTATIONAL AGE IN THE NEWBORN

The assessment of gestational age begins with the prenatal history. The prenatal assessment includes a maternal history of the last menstrual period, history of prenatal care, maternal weight gain during pregnancy, maternal infections, hypertension, history of toxemia, or history of substance abuse. Obtaining an accurate prenatal history can assist the healthcare provider in anticipating conditions associated with preterm birth.

The *Ballard scale* (Figure 2-1) is the tool most often used to evaluate the gestational age of newborn infants.[1] The scale accurately assesses extremely premature infants from 20 weeks of gestation to term infants from 40 to 44 weeks of gestation. The *Ballard scale* is a revision of the original *Dubowitz scale,* which may be used to determine gestational age of infants 35 to 42 weeks of age.[2] The *Ballard scale* consists of six physical and six neuromuscular criteria for assessing maturity. The criteria −1 and 0 assess the extremely preterm infant. Gestational age must be determined within 48 hours after birth except in the case of the extremely preterm infant, whose age should be determined within 12 hours of birth. Assessment of the neuromuscular maturity score should be repeated within the initial 48 hours after birth if neonatal asphyxia or maternal anesthesia may have affected initial assessments (Box 2-1).

The *Apgar scoring system* (Table 2-1) reflects the transition of the neonate to extrauterine life. The Apgar assessment performed at 1 minute and again at 5 minutes after birth reflects the heart rate, observation of respiratory effort, muscle tone, reflex irritability, and color of the newborn (Table 2-2). The Apgar score is not predictive of long term perinatal outcomes or neurological status.

ESTIMATION OF GESTATIONAL AGE BY MATURITY RATING

Neuromuscular Maturity

	−1	0	1	2	3	4	5
Posture							
Square Window (wrist)	> 90°	90°	60°	45°	30°	0°	
Arm Recoil		180°	140° - 180°	110° 140°	90° - 110°	< 90°	
Popliteal Angle	180°	160°	140°	120°	100°	90°	< 90°
Scarf Sign							
Heel to Ear							

Physical Maturity

Skin	sticky friable transparent	gelatinous red, translucent	smooth pink, visible veins	superficial peeling &/or rash, few veins	cracking pale areas rare veins	parchment deep cracking no vessels	leathery cracked wrinkled
Lanugo	none	sparse	abundant	thinning	bald areas	mostly bald	
Plantar Surface	heel-toe 40-50 mm: -1 <40 mm: -2	>50 mm no crease	faint red marks	anterior transverse crease only	creases ant. 2/3	creases over entire sole	
Breast	imperceptible	barely perceptible	flat areola no bud	stippled areola 1-2 mm bud	raised areola 3-4 mm bud	full areola 5-10 mm bud	
Eye/Ear	lids fused loosely: -1 tightly: -2	lids open pinna flat stays folded	sl. curved pinna; soft; slow recoil	well-curved pinna; soft but ready recoil	formed & firm instant recoil	thick cartilage, ear stiff	
Genitals (male)	scrotum flat, smooth	scrotum empty faint rugae	testes in upper canal rare rugae	testes descending few rugae	testes down good rugae	testes pendulous, deep rugae	
Genitals (female)	clitoris prominent labia flat	prominent clitoris, small labia minora	prominent clitoris enlarging minora	majora & minora equally prominent	majora large minora small	majora cover clitoris & minora	

Maturity Rating

score	weeks
-10	20
-5	22
0	24
5	26
10	28
15	30
20	32
25	34
30	36
35	38
40	40
45	42
50	44

Figure 2-1 Ballard scale. (From Ballard JL, Khoury JC, Wedig K et al: New Ballard score, expanded to include extremely premature infants, *J Pediatr* 119(3):418, 1991.)

DEVELOPMENTAL CONSIDERATIONS

Term Infants

Term infants are born between the 38th and 41st weeks of gestation and normally lose about 5% to 10% of their birth weight in the first 72 hours after birth. The average weight loss is 5% to 7% over 3 to 4 days.[3] A weight loss of >10% may indicate a poor feeding pattern or another more serious postnatal condition

| Box **2-1** | **Tests For Assessing Neuromuscular Maturity** |

Posture. With infant quiet and in supine position, observe degree of flexion in arms, legs. Muscle tone and degree of flexion increase with maturity. Full flexion of the arms, legs = 4.

Square window. With thumb supporting back of arm below wrist, apply gentle pressure with index and third fingers on dorsum of hand without rotating infant's wrist. Measure angle between base of thumb and forearm. Full flexion (hand lies flat on ventral surface of forearm) = 4.

Arm recoil. With infant supine, fully flex forearms on upper arms, hold for 5 seconds; pull down on hands to fully extend and rapidly release arms. Observe rapidity and intensity of recoil to state of flexion. A brisk return to full flexion = 4.

Popliteal angle. With infant supine and pelvis flat on firm surface, flex lower leg on thigh, then flex thigh on abdomen. While holding knee with thumb and index finger, extend lower leg with index finger of other hand. Measure degree of angle behind knee (popliteal angle). Angle of <90 degrees = 5.

Scarf sign. With infant supine, support head in midline with one hand; use other hand to pull infant's arm across shoulder so that infant's hand touches shoulder. Determine location of elbow in relation to midline. Elbow does not reach midline = 4.

Heel to ear. With infant supine and pelvis flat on firm surface, pull foot as far as possible toward ear on same side. Measure distance of foot from ear and degree of knee flexion (same as popliteal angle). Knees flexed with popliteal angle of <90 degrees = 4.

From Hockenberry M, Wilson D, Winkelstein ML: *Wong's essentials of pediatric nursing,* ed 7, St Louis, 2005, Mosby.

and requires thorough investigation and close follow-up. By 2 weeks of age, term infants have normally achieved their birth weight.

Preterm Infants

An infant is considered preterm when born before the end of the 37th week. The weight and gestational age of the infant together predict the relative risk of mortality.[4] During the first year of life, premature infants tend to grow more slowly than term infants even when using the growth curve standard for corrected age (see Preterm Growth Curve in Appendix A). Healthcare practitioners should

TABLE 2-1 APGAR SCORING SYSTEM

Sign	0	1	2
Heart rate	Absent	Slow <100	>100
Respiratory rate	Absent	Irregular, slow, weak cry	Good, strong cry
Muscle tone	Limp	Some flexion of extremities	Well flexed
Reflex irritability	No response	Grimace	Cry, sneeze
Color	Blue, pale	Body pink, extremities blue	Completely pink

Data from Apgar V: Evaluation of the newborn infant, second report, *JAMA* 168, 1985.

TABLE 2-2 INTERPRETATION OF APGAR SCORES

Total Score	Assessment
0-2	Severe asphyxia
3-4	Moderate asphyxia
5-7	Mild asphyxia
8-10	No asphyxia

Box 2-2 Maternal and Fetal Factors Impacting Intrauterine Growth*

PREGNANCY COMPLICATIONS

- Maternal hypertension
- Placental insufficiency
- Toxemia of pregnancy
- Intrauterine infection
- Multiple births
- Maternal hypoxia

MATERNAL SUBSTANCE ABUSE

- Alcoholism
- Tobacco use
- Elicit drug use
- Over-the-counter (OTC) drug use

CHRONIC ILLNESS IN THE MOTHER

- Tuberculosis
- Lupus erythematosus
- Epilepsy
- Insulin-dependent (type 1) diabetes under poor control or exacerbated during pregnancy

FETAL COMPLICATIONS

- Hypoxia
- Genetic abnormalities
- Congenital anomalies
- Environmental toxin exposure

*Data from Thureen PJ, Deacon J, O'Neill P, Hernandez J: *Assessment and care of the well newborn*, Philadelphia, 1999, Saunders; and Porth CM: *Pathophysiology: concepts of altered health status*, Philadelphia, 1998, Lippincott.

use the adjusted age standard when plotting the growth of the preterm infant until the infant is 2½ years old. At this point, the difference is no longer statistically significant.

Small for Gestational Age

Infants weighing less than 2500 grams (gm) at birth or who fall below the 10th percentile for age are considered small for gestational age (SGA). The head may be *microcephalic*, or small in proportion to the body, and below the 5th percentile for age. With adequate nutrition, SGA infants experience overall catch-up growth. However, 50% of SGA infants are below average weight at 3 years of age.[5] The mortality rate for the SGA infant is 5 times that of term infants. See Box 2-2 for factors impacting fetal growth.

Large for Gestational Age

Large for gestational age (LGA) is defined as birth weight >2 standard deviations (SD) above the mean for gestational age or above the 90th percentile for age. The overgrowth of the fetus can be related to a familial predisposition, an abnormal uterine environment, genetic aberration, or *maternal* hyperglycemia. Increased insulin levels increase fat deposits in the fetus and result in the large weight gain. Diabetic mothers who are insulin-dependent and in poor control of the condition during the early trimesters of pregnancy have characteristically large infants. LGA infants may experience trauma at birth, neonatal asphyxia, hypoglycemia, and polycythemia.

MEASUREMENT

Accurate assessment of growth begins in the newborn (using corrected gestational age) by evaluating progress on the growth curve and continues throughout childhood and adolescence by evaluating growth in relation to age. Employing the correct technique when gathering measurements is one of the significant challenges in pediatrics.

Head Circumference

Measurement of *head circumference* is a routine part of growth assessment in the first 2 years of life. Consistency and accuracy of the head circumference measurement is a critical part of the assessment of normal growth and development. Accurate measurement of the head is taken at the point of greatest circumference from the occipital protuberance above the base of the skull to the midforehead or point of greatest bossing of the frontal bone (Figure 2-2). If the initial measurement indicates a concern in the pattern of head growth, the practitioner must take a second measurement to ensure accuracy of head size. Plot the head circumference measurement on the growth curve specific for sex and age at each well child visit to determine whether the growth pattern is normal. Head circumference that plots 1 to 2 SD above height and weight on the growth curve or that is >95% or <5% for age should be evaluated. *Microcephaly* may be indicative of intrauterine growth retardation or premature closure of the

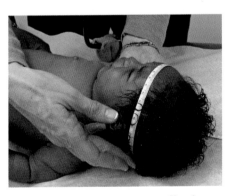

Figure **2-2** Accurate measurement of head circumference.

cranial sutures, termed *craniosynostosis*, which requires timely referral. *Macrocephaly,* large head in proportion to body, may indicate increased intracranial pressure or a familial variant.

Chest Circumference

The *chest circumference* is measured at the nipple line. The head circumference is normally 2 cm greater than the chest circumference in the first 6 months of life. Molding of the head in the term newborn may make it appear as though the measurements are equal. From 6 months to 2 years of age, the chest circumference should closely equal the head circumference. With the progression of growth, the chest circumference becomes larger than the head at about 2 years of age and continues to grow faster during childhood. Chest measurements are not routinely taken unless an infant has abnormal physical findings at birth or demonstrates abnormal growth.

Height

Height is almost entirely attributed to linear skeletal growth and is the most stable measurement of growth and maturation in childhood. Linear growth is genetically predetermined and, therefore, adult height generally occurs within a predictable range if accurate family history is available. Linear growth often occurs in spurts followed by long quiescent periods in which no growth occurs. Infants and young children may demonstrate an increase in appetite before a growth spurt, followed by an increased need for sleep.

For the infant or toddler, *recumbent* height is required for accurate measurement of linear growth. Place the infant supine on a flat surface or examination table equipped with a measuring device. Term newborns vary in height between 18 and 22 inches (45 to 55 cm) at birth, and height increases by 1 inch per month and doubles in the first year of life. Measurement also can be taken on the examination table by marking the position of the top of the head and the bottom of the foot on table paper and afterward determining length with a measuring tape.

After 2 years of age, transition to standing height is appropriate although recumbent height is often easier to obtain in the first part of the second year if the child is fearful. The increase in height averages 3 inches (7.5 cm) over the second and third years. Measurement is recorded to the nearest tenth of a centimeter (0.1 cm) or 0.25 inch without shoes. Standing height should be taken without shoes using a wall-mounted or portable *stadiometer* for accuracy. A stadiometer, an instrument used to obtain accurate height measurement, is available at medical suppliers. From the end of the third year through school age, the increase in height averages 2 inches (9.5 cm) per year (Box 2-3).

The periods of accelerated growth in height that occur in infancy level off in early childhood and remain relatively slow during the school-age years until early adolescence when the rapid increase in growth begins. Ideally, height in the preschool and school-age child should be measured in approximately 1-year intervals. Obese children are taller than children of average weight, often one standard deviation above their counterparts for age.[6] In adolescence, girls' growth potential is generally realized by 16 years of age, and boys' growth potential continues until 18 to 21 years of age. Linear growth ceases when the maturation of the skeleton is complete.

Familial short stature is often not recognized as the most likely assessment when parents are anxious for their child to achieve a socially acceptable height. Short stature also may be a key indicator in children with poor nutritional status or indicative of chronic conditions including cardiac and renal disease, fetal alcohol syndrome, methadone exposure, growth hormone deficiency, or congenital syndromes.[5]

Pediatric Pearls

Height at 2 years of age is approximately 50% of adult height. To estimate adult height, double the height at 2 years of age.

Arm Span

An adolescent male or female of tall stature should be evaluated for arm span measurement. An *arm span* measurement should be taken with the arms outstretched. Measure the distance from the tip of the middle finger across the crest of the shoulders to the other middle fingertip.

Box 2-3   Accurate Measurement of Height

BIRTH TO 24 MONTHS

- Infant's head must be held firm on flat surface against top of measuring bar.
- Push knees gently toward table while leg is extended. Bottom of foot is placed directly against footboard of measuring device.

24 TO 36 MONTHS

- Repeat above procedure for accurate measurement.

36 MONTHS THROUGH SCHOOL AGE

- For accurate height in the young child, maintain head erect by placing slight upward pressure under chin.
- Child should be standing erect with buttocks and back against stadiometer or wall.

The arm span measurement should equal the height. In *Marfan's syndrome*, the arm span measurement exceeds the height and is associated with a disproportionate appearance.

Weight

Birth weight is a more accurate reflection of intrauterine growth than is height (i.e., length) and, therefore, is more variable than height. The average birth weight in the term infant is 7 to 7.5 pounds (3175 to 3400 gm). The average range of weight in a healthy term newborn is from 5 pounds 8 ounces to 8 pounds 13 ounces (2500 to 4000 gm). Poor weight gain in early infancy is indicative of failure to thrive and may be caused by poor feeding patterns, malnutrition, neglect, cardiac or renal disease, chronic infection, or congenital anomalies.

Infants can be accurately weighed lying on an infant balance scale with a paper liner. Infants should be weighed in the sitting position only with extreme caution and only after they are able to sit without support. Weight is recorded to the nearest 0.5 ounce/10 gm.

After 2 years of age, standing weight should be recorded to the nearest 0.25 pound/100 gm (Box 2-4). If the toddler is very fearful or irritable, parent and child can be weighed together on standing scale; then parental weight is subtracted from total weight to obtain an *estimate* of child's weight. For children with special healthcare needs or disabilities, accommodations for wheelchair scales or special purpose scales should be made in the clinical setting.

CULTURAL VARIATIONS IN HEIGHT AND WEIGHT

Native-American and Latino children are smaller in height than African-American or Caucasian children at birth. Asian-American children are on average smaller than all other racial and ethnic groups and have a lower birth weight.[7] The incidence of low birth weight and extremely low birth weight is higher in African-American infants. Their birth weight averages 180 to 240 gm lower than other racial

---

Box **2-4**   Accurate Weighing

BIRTH TO 12 MONTHS

- Infant should be undressed (without diaper) or weighed consistently with clean, dry diaper.
- *Safety* is of primary concern. Examiner cannot leave infant unattended at any time.

12 TO 24 MONTHS

- Before 2 years of age, weight is measured most accurately on infant balance scale with dry diaper. *Exceptions:* when child is very large or more cooperative/stable on standing scale.

2 TO 6 YEARS OF AGE

- At 2 years, weight can be measured accurately on standing balance scale when child is cooperative.
- Weight should be measured with child in underwear consistently when using standing balance scale until 3 years of age.
- From 3 to 6 years children can be weighed in clothing without shoes.
  After completing the accurate measurement of height and weight, the measurements should be plotted on the growth curve appropriate for sex and age to determine the percentile and evaluate overall progression of growth.

and ethnic groups. Native-American newborns have the largest average birth weight of over 4000 gm, reflecting a higher incidence of gestational diabetes during pregnancy.

◎━╗ **Key Points**

African-American children have a more rapid growth and maturation rate than do Caucasian children and enter puberty at an earlier age.

Body Mass Index for Age in Children

Body mass index (kg/m^2), or BMI, provides a guideline for healthcare providers to use to determine the healthy weight of an individual based on height. The formula for determining BMI is weight in kilograms divided by height in meters squared. BMI is used to determine whether an individual is overweight or underweight, and interpretation of the BMI in children depends on age. As children grow, their composition of body fat changes over time, and the amount of body fat compared to height differs between boys and girls during maturation. Normally, the BMI decreases during the preschool years and begins to increase during the prepubertal years and continues to increase into early and middle adolescence. This is particularly true for pre-adolescent girls, who often will experience their peak weight gain before beginning peak increase in height. Children with BMIs that do not follow this pattern or who demonstrate an earlier increase in body fat are more likely to have an increased BMI as an adult (see BMI charts in Appendix A).

BMI charts are gender and age specific and indicate the healthy weight range. To plot BMI using the measurements of weight in kilograms and the height in meters, find the age on the horizontal scale and follow the vertical line to the BMI. BMI growth curves follow the normal growth pattern, which

TABLE 2-3 INTERPRETATION OF BMI STANDARDS

Weight	BMI for Age (percentile)
Underweight	<5th percentile
At risk of overweight	85th to 95th percentile
Overweight	>95th percentile

Data from National Center for Chronic Disease Prevention and Health; Centers for Disease Control and Prevention, 2002.

declines during the preschool years and increases in adolescence. Fluctuations up and down within the normal age range for children are very common and should not be overinterpreted unless they indicate trends above or below healthy body weight. BMI in children and adolescents compares well to laboratory measures of body fat and is strongly related to adult health risks.[8] Table 2-3 indicates the established percentiles for underweight and overweight.[6]

Overweight children are likely to become overweight adults.[9] In children and adolescents with a BMI for age >95th percentile, 60% have at least one risk factor for cardiovascular disease and 20% have two or more risk factors.[10] Calculating and plotting BMI during the routine health visit and discussing this information with parents is an important part of providing comprehensive health care to children. The BMI growth curve may be easier to use than traditional growth charts when the intent is to point out weight trends to parents before overweight becomes a problem.

VITAL SIGNS

Temperature

Measurement of temperature continues to be a dynamic process in the infant and young child. Much discussion has occurred on the accuracy of temperature measurement and the ideal instrument to use. Currently there is a range of acceptable methods for measuring temperature in the infant and young child. The tympanic membrane thermometer (TMT) measures internal body temperature with an ear probe placed in the external auditory canal. Using pediatric-size probes is essential for obtaining accurate temperature readings. Temperature readings obtained with TMTs may be higher on occasion than those obtained with other methods. If otitis media is present, it may alter the TMT temperature reading, and therefore alternate methods should be used. Electronic thermometers measure temperatures swiftly and accurately within 30 seconds. Probe covers are used when obtaining either oral or rectal temperatures, and the unit must be fully charged and calibrated.

Axillary temperature measurement is the most favored method for the healthy newborn. Place the thermometer under the arm at the base of the axilla for 3 to 5 minutes, and hold the arm firmly against the side of the body. Rectal temperature is most easily measured from early infancy to 8 to 9 months with the infant placed in the supine position on the examining table with knees flexed toward the abdomen. The infant can see the practitioner and be secured more easily in this position. Proper positioning prevents injury. In males, stimulation often elicits urination so the penis should be covered. A child from 9 months to 2 years of age can be placed in the parent's arms or laid supine on the parent's lap. Insert the lubricated tip of thermometer into the anal opening of the rectum a distance of 0.5 to 1 inch. Oral measurement is the preferred method for cooperative children over 4 years of age. Place the thermometer under

the tongue to the left or right of the frenulum in the posterior sublingual pocket.

Pulse

Pulses should be assessed for the quality of rate, rhythm, and volume. Children under 2 years of age require apical pulse (AP) measurements. Readings should be taken when the child is quiet. AP measurements are taken with the stethoscope held over the heart below the nipple at the apex. For children over 2 years of age, the radial pulse is a satisfactory measurement. Figure 2-3 illustrates the location of the pulses. Table 2-4 presents the grading of pulses used to evaluate strength and quality. In infants and young children, the pulse should be counted for a full minute to account for irregularities in rhythm. To detect any differences in circulation between the upper and lower extremities, the radial and femoral pulses should be evaluated and compared. Absent or weak pulse in the lower extremities compared to the upper extremities is diagnostic of *coarctation of the aorta*.

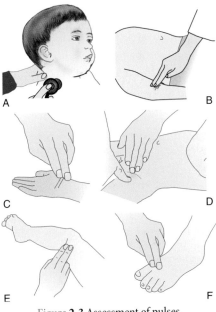

Figure **2-3** Assessment of pulses.

Key Points

Mercury presents an environmental hazard in the practice setting. Consequently, mercury thermometers are obsolete.

TABLE 2-4 STRENGTH AND QUALITY OF PULSES

Strength	Quality
0	Not palpable
1+	Difficult to palpate, thready, obliterated by pressure
2+	Weak, difficult to palpate, may obliterate with pressure
3+	Palpable, normal strength
4+	Strong, bounding, not affected by pressure

Respirations

Respirations should be assessed for rate and pattern. Readings should be taken when child is quiet in order to accurately assess the rate. In infants and young children, observe the abdominal movements to assess respirations. Infants are obligate nose breathers and respirations are primarily diaphragmatic. Respirations should be assessed for a full minute because of typical irregular respiratory rates in the newborn and very young infant. Table 2-5 shows the normal range for vital signs in children.

Oxygen Saturation

Measurement of *oxygen saturation* has become a standard in most clinical settings for respiratory assessment in the ill pediatric patient. *Pulse oximetry* is a noninvasive method of determining oxygen (O_2) saturation and should be part of the criteria for evaluating any child with respiratory distress or respiratory compromise. O_2 saturation should be kept >92%; it assists the practitioner in clinical decision-making when determining the need for prolonged observation or hospital admission.

Blood Pressure

Beginning at 3 years of age, blood pressure should be assessed at all routine well child visits. Infants and children younger than 3 years of age who are at risk or who have chronic conditions also should be evaluated. The size of the blood pressure cuff is critical to obtaining an accurate measurement. The blood pressure cuff should cover about two thirds of the upper arm and should encircle the arm once. A cuff that is too large will result in a low blood pressure reading. If the cuff is too small, the blood pressure reading may be too high. For obese children and adolescents, an extra-large adult cuff may need to be used to obtain an accurate measurement. Blood pressure readings can increase in children who are crying and in adolescents who are feeling anxious. Table 2-5 reviews the normal range of blood pressure at different ages. In a healthy child or adolescent, a blood pressure reading above the 95th percentile for age should be considered accurate after three independent readings are taken to confirm the diagnosis of *hypertension*.

Pain: The Fifth Vital Sign

The response to pain in infants and young children is developmental, and accurate assessment of the pain response requires strategies specific to the developmental level of the child. The use of the pain scale in children 3 years of age and older has greatly improved the ability of the healthcare practitioner to accurately assess and treat pain in the pediatric patient. Figure 2-4 presents the FACES pain rating scale used across most pediatric clinical settings.[2]

TABLE 2-5 EXPECTED RANGE OF VITAL SIGNS

	Temperature	Respirations	Heart Rate*	Blood Pressure
Newborn	36.5°-37° C clothed and swaddled	30-60 without signs of respiratory distress (grunting, flaring, retracting, stridor)	80-160 AP (range 80 when sleeping to 220 when active/crying)	65/41 mean 75/49 90th percentile 78/52 95th percentile
1 week to 3 months	37°-37.5° C average	30-50	100-220 AP (range 100 when sleeping to 220 with fever/crying)	87/52 mean 104/64 90th percentile 106/68 95th percentile
3 months to 2 years	37.4°-37.7° C	20-30	80-150 AP	95/58 mean 106/68 90th percentile 110/71 95th percentile
2 to 6 years	37°-37.2° C	20-28	75-120	101/57 mean 112/66 90th percentile 115/68 95th percentile
8 to 12 years	36.8°-37° C	16-20	70-110	112/73 mean 115/75 90th percentile 120/80 95th percentile
12 years to adult	36.6°-36.7° C	12-20	50-105	119/78 mean 132/85 90th percentile 138/87 95th percentile

*AP, Apical pulse rate taken in children younger than 2 years of age.

Figure 2-4 FACES pain rating scale.

Brief word instructions: Point to each face using the words to describe the pain intensity. Ask the child to choose face that best describes own pain, and record the appropriate number. NOTE: Use of these instructions is recommended. Rating scale can be used with people 3 years and older.

Original instructions: Explain to the person that each face is for a person who feels happy because he has no pain (hurt) or sad because he has some or a lot of pain. FACE 0 is very happy because he doesn't hurt at all. FACE 1 hurts just a little bit. FACE 2 hurts a little more. FACE 3 hurts even more. FACE 4 hurts a whole lot. FACE 5 hurts as much as you can imagine, although you don't have to be crying to feel this bad. Ask the person to choose face that best describes how much hurt he has. Record the number under the chosen face on the pain assessment record.

(From Wong DL, Hockenberry-Eaton M, Wilson D, Winkelstein ML, Schwartz P: *Wong's essentials of pediatric nursing,* ed 6, St Louis, 2001, p. 1301. Copyrighted by Mosby, Inc. Reprinted by permission.)

REFERENCES

1. Ballard JL, Khoury JC, Wedig K et al: New Ballard score, expanded to include extremely premature infants, *J Pediatr* 119(3):417-423, 1991.
2. Hockenberry M, Wilson D, Winkelstein ML: *Wong's essentials of pediatric nursing,* ed 7, St Louis, 2005, Mosby.
3. Thureen PJ, Hall D, Hernandez JA: *Assessment and care of the well newborn,* ed 2, Philadelphia, 2005, Saunders.
4. Muscari ME: *Advanced pediatric clinical assessment: skills and procedures,* Philadelphia, 2001, Lippincott.
5. Porth CM: *Pathophysiology: concepts of altered health status,* Philadelphia, 1998, Lippincott.
6. National Center for Chronic Disease Prevention and Health: *CDC growth chart: United States,* 2002, Centers for Disease Control and Prevention.
7. Andrews M, Boyle M: *Transcultural concepts in nursing care,* Philadelphia, 1999, Lippincott.
8. Pietrobelli A, Faith MS, Allison DB et al: Body mass index as a measure of adiposity among children and adolescents: a validation study, *J Pediatr* 132(2):204-210, 1998.
9. Whitaker RC, Pepe MS, Wright JA et al: Early adiposity rebound and the risk of adult obesity, *Pediatrics* 101(3):E5, 1998.
10. Freedman DS, Dietz WH, Srinivasan SR, Berenson GS: The relation of overweight to cardiovascular risk factors among children and adolescents: the Bogalusa Heart Study, *Pediatrics* 103(6 Pt 1):1175-1182, 1999.

CHAPTER 3

DEVELOPMENTAL PARAMETERS

Andrea Windom

Each child achieves developmental skills at a pace consistent with his or her genetic capabilities, temperamental style, and environmental opportunity. The sequence of developmental milestones is generally constant although the age at which a child achieves them is highly variable. Screening children for developmental delay and behavioral difficulties requires a skilled pediatric provider and is among the most critical aspects of well child care. Taking time to observe the child's developmental level and interaction with the parent or caretaker is key (Figure 3-1). This is especially true for infants, toddlers, and preschool-age children who may have limited contact with other knowledgeable professionals skilled at detecting developmental delays. While fully 16% of children suffer developmental delay, only half of these will be identified before school entry.[1] Timely identification and prompt referral for early intervention may prevent the negative consequences of developmental delay.

⚷ Key Points

The care environment vastly impacts the development of a child's full potential.

DEVELOPMENTAL ASSESSMENT

The components of language acquisition and developmental assessment are presented in Box 3-1 for infants to school-age children and incorporate literacy as a developmental task. The acquisition of language is a critical developmental skill, and pediatric healthcare providers can promote literacy as a component of screening for language deficits. Practitioners interested in establishing a pediatric literacy promotion program may contact the national *Reach Out and Read* office at www.reachoutandread.org. Children who participate in *Reach Out and Read* demonstrate increased receptive and expressive language in preschool and are less likely to suffer school failure.[2] Components of a developmental assessment include monitoring the child for appropriate progress of fine and gross motor skills (**M**); social skills and interaction (**S**); receptive and expressive language (**L**); cognitive achievements (**C**); and book use (**B**).

Development and Child Temperament

Development is significantly influenced by a child's temperament. *Temperament* is the inborn tendency to react to one's environment

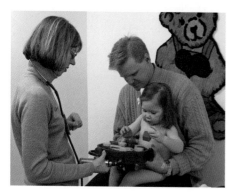

Figure **3-1** Developmental tasks for toddler.

in certain ways. Temperament is thought to be generally constant and at least partially genetically determined. The personality of an individual child reflects the interaction between the child's temperament and environment. Temperament can be measured by report, clinical observation, or a formal assessment tool. The term *"goodness of fit"* describes the

concept of how well the child's temperament meets the expectations of his or her parents and caretakers. This has a critical influence on each child's development, emotional well-being, and behavior. Table 3-1 identifies the nine characteristics of temperament.

Temperament characteristics identify differences in the personality of a child and provide noninflammatory language and a conceptual framework that can be used in discussions with parents. Understanding temperament characteristics removes judgment and blame, and assists parents in recognizing that some rules do not work equally well with all children. Some children are harder to manage than others, get into more mischief, and require more parental ingenuity. Temperament theory objectifies these differences. A comprehensive approach to assessing development includes understanding temperament. A temperament assessment tool for parents may be accessed online at "The Preventive Ounce," www.preventiveoz.org.

TABLE 3-1 TEMPERAMENT CHARACTERISTICS

Characteristics	Description
Activity	Amount of motor activity and proportion of active to inactive periods
Intensity	Amount of emotional energy released with responses
Sensitivity	Amount of sensory stimuli required to produce response
Approach/withdrawal	Nature of initial response to new stimuli
Adaptability	Ease of accepting new situation after initial response
Frustration tolerance	Length of time activity is pursued
Mood	Amount of pleasant versus unpleasant behavior child exhibits
Distractibility	Effectiveness of extraneous stimuli in altering direction of ongoing behavior
Regularity	Predictability of physiological functions such as hunger, sleep, elimination

Box 3-1 MSLCB Developmental Milestones

6 MONTHS

M Pulls to sit without head lag; bears weight, sits with support; feeds self crackers

S Can self-comfort

L Babbles, says, "dada/baba"

C May look after fallen object; may demonstrate stranger anxiety

B Excited by picture book, tries to touch, grab, mouth

12 MONTHS

M Cruises, may take steps alone; uses precise pincer grasp; feeds self

S Consolable; explores office from safety of parent's lap

L Says first word (*not* mama/dada); uses jargoning, waves bye-bye

C Looks for hidden object (object constancy)

B Holds book with help; turns several pages at a time

18 MONTHS

M Walks ups steps, walks backward; uses spoon, cup; scribbles

L Uses three to six words, *not* echolalia (repetition of another person's words); indicates desired objects with index finger (not whole hand); follows simple directions; points to at least one body part

C Works wind-up toys, on-off buttons (cause/effect)

B Points to pictures in book; may name objects

2 YEARS

M Goes up/down stairs one step at a time; kicks ball; stacks five or six blocks; makes circular stroke with crayon

S Interested in other children, but much of play is parallel

L Says two-word phrases, says at least 20 words, can follow two-step command

C Exhibits imitative play

B May carry book around house; "reads" to dolls

3 YEARS

M Broad jumps, copies O; rides tricycle

S Dresses self mostly, with supervision; achieves toilet training

L 3-4 word sentences; understands prepositions; speech at least 50% intelligible to examiner; knows name, age, and gender

C Early imaginative behavior

B Child wants same story repeatedly; explains story when asked "what" questions

4 YEARS

M Balances on 1 foot for 4-5 seconds, rides bike with training wheels, throws overhand; dresses with little help

S Understands taking turns; uses words, not hitting; establishes friendships

L Speech entirely intelligible, mostly correct grammar, asks questions

C Draws a person with 3 or more parts, knows at least 2-3 colors

B Turns pages one at a time, retells familiar story, pretends to read and write

5 YEARS

M Balances on one foot for 5 to 10 seconds; dresses self; may be able to skip

M Copies square, triangle; draws six-part person

S Plays well with group of children; dresses with little help; vulnerable in social relationships

L Has fluent use of language with correct use of *me, I, past tense, plurals*

C Can answer correctly: "If I cut an apple in half, how many pieces will I have?" "What do you do to make water boil?"

B Explains "What will happen next?" in stories; retains interest in 10- to 20-minute-long stories

Data from Reach Out and Read National Center: *Developmental milestones of early literacy,* available at www.reachoutandread.org.

Developmental Surveillance

Developmental screening identifies children who require more intensive evaluation and referral. All children must be routinely screened at periodic intervals, and it is an important method of detecting delays. The acquisition of speech and fine motor skills has significant prognostic value for later school success compared to the acquisition of gross motor skills. The acquisition of appropriate social behaviors in the young child is important in predicting future functioning as an emotionally healthy adult. Early identification of developmental and learning problems can lead to interventions that resolve or lessen the impact of a delay or disability on the functioning of the child and family.

Developmental surveillance is accomplished by comparing skill acquisition of the infant or child with the appropriate developmental milestones for age. In high-risk children, developmental surveillance includes (1) eliciting concerns from the child's parents, (2) obtaining a developmental history, (3) direct observation of child behavior, and (4) identification of developmental risk factors.

Pediatric Pearls

Parental concern regarding delays in fine and gross motor skills and language and social development are often highly accurate and always warrant in-depth analysis.

Developmental Risk Factors

Some factors increase the likelihood that a child will exhibit developmental delay. Factors that influence development include intrauterine exposure to maternal substance abuse, maternal infection, compromise resulting from chronic health conditions in the mother, neonatal history of prematurity with gestational age <33 weeks, birth weight <1500 gm, Apgar score <3 at 5 minutes, hyperbilirubinemia >20 mg/dL. A family history of congenital anomalies,

developmental delay, or maternal depression also impacts development. Environmental factors such as serum lead exposure level >19 mg/dL, lower socioeconomic status, poor social support, later birth order in a large family, and access to care also may contribute to developmental delays.

Children at risk require especially diligent developmental surveillance, including the routine use of formal developmental assessment tools and prompt referral to a pediatric neurologist or developmental specialist at the first sign of delay.

Developmental Red Flags

Even mildly abnormal findings during developmental surveillance warrant further investigation. Any loss of a previously acquired developmental milestone or an increase or decrease in normal muscle tone indicates the need for referral for specialty evaluation. Box 3-2 presents developmental red flags in infants and young children and language delays that warrant referral.

Developmental Assessment Tools

The Denver-II Developmental Screening Test (DDST-II) is the most widely used developmental screening tool. The DDST-II has only modest sensitivity and specificity and may result in over-referral, but this test is readily available and acceptable to pediatric providers. Reliability is enhanced by ensuring that the examiner has been adequately trained in the administration of the DDST-II and by rescreening any questionable results on another day. Furthermore, parents should be asked whether the child's performance was typical of his or her normal behavior, and results should be interpreted with an awareness of norms for subpopulations to determine whether delays may be attributable to sociocultural or environmental differences (see Appendix C).

The Parents' Evaluation of Developmental Status (PEDS) and the Ages and Stages Questionnaires use parental report as an

Box 3-2   Developmental Red Flags and Language Delays: Referral Warranted

3 MONTHS

Persistent fisting

Failure to alert to visual/auditory stimuli

4-6 MONTHS

Poor head control

Failure to reach for objects by 5 months

No social smile

6-12 MONTHS

Persistence of primitive reflexes after 6 months

No babbling by 6 months

No reciprocal vocalizations by 9 months

Inability to localize sound by 10 months

12-24 MONTHS

No consonant production by 15 months

No word other than mama/dada by 18 months

Hand dominance before 18 months

Not walking by 18 months

Inability to walk up/down stairs by 24 months

No two-word sentences by 24 months

Echolalia beyond 24 months

Unable to follow simple command by 24 months

Does not play with toys in functional way (such as push car to make it go by 24 months)

Cannot name one picture in book by 27 months

3 YEARS

Speech <75% intelligible

Lack of or inappropriate pronoun use

Sentences contain <3 to 4 words

Cannot feed independently with fork/spoon

4 YEARS

Speech <95% intelligible

Has not achieved independent daytime toileting

Cannot separate from parent without crying

Cannot balance on one foot for 2 seconds

Cannot copy circle or use mature pencil grasp

Unable to name two to three colors

Not able to take turns and share most of the time

Data from High PC, LaGasse L, Becker S, Ahlgren I, Gardner A: Literacy promotion in primary care pediatrics: can we make a difference? *Pediatrics* 105(4 Pt 2):927-934, 2000; Moses S: Developmental red flags, *Family practice notebook,* available at: www.fpnotebook.com/PED45.htm.

effective screening tool for developmental delay. Parental report of a child's current abilities can accurately predict developmental delays.[3] Table 3-2 presents options for developmental and psychosocial screening.

The Developmental Drawing Interview

Children's drawings are often a source of delight and insight for parents and pediatric providers. Most importantly, children's drawings offer insights into their neuromotor performance and mental status. Beginning at the age of 18 months, children should be familiar with crayons or markers (Figure 3-2). By presenting these things to the child, the provider capitalizes on the opportunity to reinforce the value of this activity for even very young children. Incorporating children's drawings into pediatric care may help build rapport with the child, occupy the young child during parental interviews, and relieve some of the anxiety associated with physical assessment or medical treatments.

Drawing milestones to assess during the well child exam include the following:

- 18 months: scribbles
- 3-3½ years of age: imitates a circle; picks longer of 3 lines
- 3½-4½ years of age: draws a cross and a three-part person

TABLE 3-2   PEDIATRIC DEVELOPMENTAL ASSESSMENT TOOLS

Assessment Tool	Age Range	Time to Administer	Description
Parent's Evaluation of Developmental Status (PEDS) Ellsworth and Vandemeer Press, Ltd. P.O. Box 68164 Nashville, TN 37206 615-226-4460; www.pedstest.com	0-8 years	2 minutes	10 questions elicit parent's concerns. Available in English or Spanish at 5th grade reading level
Ages and Stages Questionnaires Paul H. Brooks Publishers P.O. Box 10624 Baltimore, MD 21285 (800) 638-3775; www.pbrookes.com	0-4 years	5 minutes	10-15 items for each age range available in multiple languages and using simple drawing directions
Denver Developmental Materials, Inc. P.O. Box 371075 Denver, CO 80237-5075 (800) 419-4729; www.denverii.com/ DenverII.html	0-6 years	20 minutes	Provider assesses development in gross motor, language, fine motor/adaptive, personal/social realms by eliciting behavior or parental report on approximately 20 items
Bayley Infant Neurodevelopmental Screener (BINS) www.harcourtassessment.com	3-24 months	10-15 minutes	Trained examiner uses 10-13 directly elicited items to assess neurological processes, neurodevelopmental skills, developmental achievements

TABLE 3-2   PEDIATRIC DEVELOPMENTAL ASSESSMENT TOOLS—CONT'D

Assessment Tool	Age Range	Time to Administer	Description
Draw-A-Person (DAP) Test Psychological Corporation 555 Academic Ct. San Antonio, TX 78204-2498 (800) 228-0752	3-10 years		Assigns 1 point for each of 64 items present in drawing; standardizes drawing interview, estimates approximate mental age of child, minimizes cultural basis of 64 items present in a drawing; standardizes the estimates and approximate mental age for the child; minimizes cultural bias
Pediatric Symptom Checklist (PSC) http://psc.partners.org	6-16 years	7 minutes	35 questions elicit parental response on short statements about problem behaviors including conduct, depression, anxiety, adjustment

Data from High PC, LaGasse L, Becker S, Ahlgren I, Gardner A: Literacy promotion in primary care pediatrics: can we make a difference? *Pediatrics* 105(4 Pt 2): 927-934, 2000; Romeo S: To know what is before you: developmental screening in children, *Adv Nurse Pract* 10(2):55-58, 2002.

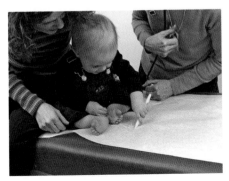

Figure **3-2** Scribbling to assess handedness.

- 4½-5½ years of age: draws a square and a six-part person
- 7½ years of age: draws a diamond

Dixon and Stein have identified characteristics of preschool drawings that raise concerns regarding school readiness: poor integration of torso, absence of eyes or ears, unusual placements or size distortions, wobbly lines with overcorrections or undercorrections, reversals, and difficulty sustaining effort, which results in the initial aspects of the drawing being much better than the last.[4]

ABNORMAL CONDITIONS

Learning Differences and Disabilities

Approximately 6% to 7% of all school-age children are identified as learning disabled. *Learning disability* refers to difficulty in acquiring and using basic reading skills, reading comprehension, oral expression, listening comprehension, mathematical reasoning, and mathematical comprehension that occurs without an environmental precipitant in otherwise normally intelligent children. The definition requires at least a 2-year discrepancy between the child's expected level of achievement and his or her performance. These disorders are assumed to be due to central nervous system dysfunction and persist into adulthood. Twice as many boys as girls are affected. Pediatric primary care providers assist with the diagnosis of learning disabilities by performing an initial thorough history and physical examination including a complete neurological examination and an evaluation of school performance. Confirmation of learning disabilities includes referral for neuropsychometric testing and evaluation by a licensed psychologist.

ADHD

Attention deficit hyperactivity disorder (ADHD) is a cluster of behaviors that appear early in a child's life and persist throughout childhood and adolescence. ADHD occurs in 3% to 5% of the pediatric population, with males outnumbering females 3:1 to 6:1. The diagnosis of ADHD is based on a characteristic clinical presentation and observable behaviors. The problematic behaviors include inattention, hyperactivity, and impulsivity. The practitioner must rule out the possibility that such behaviors merely represent variations in normal development or temperament, and that they are not attributable to environmental factors such as a poor fit with the teacher and/or classroom. Furthermore, ADHD may coexist with other disorders or conditions that must be addressed before an appropriate diagnosis can be given. Between 10% and 40% of children with ADHD have learning disabilities. Schools are federally mandated to perform appropriate evaluations if a child is suspected of having a disability, such as ADHD. Parents should be assisted in obtaining such an evaluation. An evaluation for ADHD includes a comprehensive history, with careful attention given to developmental level; complete physical examination, including neurological exam; vision and hearing screening; consideration of lead and hematocrit levels in preschool children; input elicited from teachers; initiation of an individual education plan coordinated with the child's school; and referral to a developmental-behavioral specialist, pediatric neurologist, or mental health professional.

Autism

Autism is a neurobiological disorder with an onset before the age of 3 years. It is characterized by delays in language and social skills and unusual or restricted interests or play. It is viewed as a subcategory under the broader diagnostic umbrella of pervasive developmental disorders as detailed in the American Psychiatric Association's *Diagnostic and Statistical Manual of Mental Disorders (DSM-IV)*. Approximately 75% of autistic children also suffer other cognitive deficits. Careful attention given to screening for language and social delays assists in early identification. Autism is at least partially genetically determined, though no single gene abnormality or mode of inheritance has been identified. The recent increased prevalence of autism (10 to 20 per 10,000) has been attributed to an increased awareness of this disorder and a broadened definition, but may also represent a true increase in incidence. Immunizations have not been proven to increase the incidence of autism.

CHARTING

Documentation of a developmental assessment serves as a record of the child's neuromaturational progress over time.

 CHARTING

A Healthy 9-Month-Old Infant

Mother without concerns regarding child's development or behavior, states she reads to child daily. Infant initially exhibits stranger anxiety, consolable by mother. Creeps, pulls to stand, bangs two cubes, thumb-finger grasp. Jargons and plays peek-a-boo. Plays "pat-a-cake" per parental report. Passes DDST-II.

REFERENCES

1. American Academy of Pediatrics: Developmental surveillance and screening of infants and young children, *Pediatrics* 108(1):192-196, 2001.

2. High PC, LaGasse L, Becker S, Ahlgren I, Garnder A: Literacy promotion in primary care pediatrics: can we make a difference? *Pediatrics* 105(4 Pt 2): 927-934, 2000.

3. Glascoe FP, Macias MM: How can you implement the AAP's new policy on developmental and behavioral screening? *Contemp Pediatr* 20(4):85-102, 2003.

4. Dixon SD, Stein MT: *Encounters with children: pediatric development and behavior,* St Louis, 2000, Mosby.

CHAPTER 4

COMPREHENSIVE INFORMATION GATHERING

Karen G. Duderstadt and Naomi A. Schapiro

The skill of obtaining a comprehensive and holistic health history remains the most important clinical tool for the pediatric provider. Despite the high tech world of health care, expert assessment is still mostly about observing, listening, and thinking critically in a clinical setting. Recognizing patterns of health and illness in infants, children, and adolescents requires obtaining relevant pieces of data from the health history, thinking about their meaning, and explaining them logically. Taking a comprehensive history with families not only develops a profile to guide physical assessment, diagnosis, and treatment but also contributes to the development of a continuity relationship between the family and healthcare provider that promotes responsible health behaviors. When collecting the history, it is important to talk to children and adolescents about the amount of physical activity they engage in and their dietary habits. Equally important is the need to assess behavioral and psychosocial issues facing children and families.

CULTURAL CONSIDERATIONS

A *cultural assessment* should be included in every family evaluation, and gathering information on family culture begins with the interview questions. The interview process should include the family's perception of the child's health and their belief about the origin of wellness or illness. Integrating respect for culture is a continuing process in the provider/family relationship.

The following are interview questions aimed at developing a cultural understanding[1]:

1. Where was the child born? *If an immigrant:* How long has the child lived in this country?
2. What is the child's ethnic affiliation and how strong is the family's ethnic identity? Does the child live in an ethnic community?
3. What are the child's primary and secondary languages? What is the family's speaking and reading ability of the primary language in the home?

4. What is the family's religion, and do they practice their religion daily or weekly?
5. Are the family's food preferences linked to cultural or religious preferences?
6. What are the health and illness beliefs and practices of the family?
7. *If interviewing an adolescent:* Are there conflicts with parents concerning cultural norms or customs?

THE GENETIC FAMILY HISTORY

With the advent of the Human Genome Project, genetic mapping has become a key component of the comprehensive family history. It is the primary tool used to understand and apply genetic concepts and lays the foundation for accurate risk assessment. The *genetic family history* establishes a *family pedigree.* Healthcare providers should gather the health information on family members from a reliable family source. Family history and pedigree facts to include in the interview are as follows[2]:

- Age/year of birth
- Status: alive or deceased
- Cause of death
- Offspring: include stillbirths and miscarriage
- Infertility vs. no children by choice
- Current health risks (obese, hypertension, diabetes)
- Ethnicity
- Blood relationship (consanguinity)

This information is then expressed graphically in a *genogram* or *family pedigree.* This approach leads to insights in patterns of inheritance across generations, and targets children and families at high risk for preventable conditions and conditions requiring referral to specialty care.[3] Figure 4-1 is an example of a family pedigree with a multigenerational inheritance of cardiovascular disease.

FAMILY-CENTERED HISTORY

Pediatric healthcare providers are uniquely suited to assess children from a family-centered perspective (Box 4-1). Families hold trust in

the pediatric provider and their relationship is based on the knowledge, understanding, respect, and care the pediatric provider demonstrates during the encounter with their child. Stressors affecting the child can be identified most effectively within the family and social context, as well as emotional or behavioral problems that result from the parent-child relationship (Figure 4-2).

Pediatric Pearls

The *ripple effect:* everything that happens to a child occurs, at some level, within a family and affects the whole family. Everything that affects the family affects the child. It is like the ripple effect of a pebble tossed into a pond.[4]

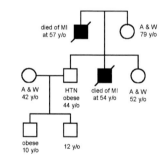

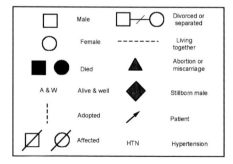

Figure **4-1** Family pedigree. (Data from Bennet RL: *The practical guide to the genetic family history,* New York, 1999, Wiley-Liss, Inc; Engel J: *Pocket guide to pediatric assessment,* St Louis, 2002, Mosby.)

Box **4-1**	The Three Levels of the Family-Centered Approach

LEVEL 1
The *child* (elements of physical, developmental, behavioral, emotional health)

LEVEL 2
The *family* (parental/caretaker physical and mental health, emotional stability, temperament, style of parenting, significant relationship [marriage/partner/extended family])

LEVEL 3
The *child and family social context*
(family income, housing, social supports [friends/extended family], neighborhood/community, access to health care)

Data from Coleman WL: *Family-focused behavioral pediatrics*, Philadelphia, 2001, Lippincott Williams & Wilkins.

COMPONENTS OF INFORMATION GATHERING

The information gathered during an encounter reflects the parent or caretaker's opinion and experience and, therefore, needs to be viewed as subjective. The information guides the objective findings of the physical assessment and assists the healthcare provider in evaluating the family functioning, their approach to health and illness, and the reliability of the parent or caretaker.

INFORMATION GATHERING OF SUBJECTIVE DATA

Child Profile

Evaluate identification information
- Child's name and parent's or step-parent's name(s)
- Birth date and age
- Birthplace
- Home and caretaker's contact information
- Home phone number and/or cellular phone number
- Date of last well child visit? Previous healthcare provider?

The Open-Ended Question

Beginning the interview with an open-ended question such as "What brings you here today?"

allows the family to tell their story in their own words. Summarizing a list of the parental concerns establishes the basis of the *family-centered interview*. Clarifying the expectations of the child and family for the encounter and negotiating a plan are important to establishing trust in a provider/parent relationship.

Present Concern

After summarizing the initial interview, transition to the *provider-centered interview* to complete information gathering on the presenting concern. Include information in the following areas to clarify or to gather information the family has not addressed:
- When did you first notice the symptoms? or date/time child was last well?
- Character of symptoms (time of day, location, intensity, duration, quality)?
- Progression of symptoms (How is she doing now?)
- Associated symptoms (fever, rash, etc.) (Anything else bothering her?)
- Changes in activity (school/daycare attendance, play at home?)
- Home management (What has the family tried? What has helped?)
- Medications taken (dosage, time, date)?

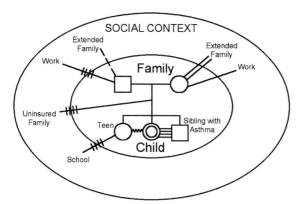

Figure **4-2** Family-centered ecomap. (Data from Engel J: *Pocket guide to pediatric assessment,* St Louis, 2002, Mosby; Coleman WL: *Family-focused behavioral pediatrics,* Philadelphia, 2001, Lippincott Williams & Wilkins.)

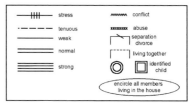

- Exposure to others who have been ill?
- Pertinent family medical history? (Is anyone in the family immunosuppressed or does anyone have a chronic illness?)
- What changes have occurred in the family as a result of this illness (effects or secondary gain)? Has the family seen other providers for the concern?

For a *symptom-focused* encounter, the healthcare provider should include only pertinent parts of the comprehensive history presented below.

Prenatal and Birth History

The initial history of the child is important in relation to the first 2 years of life and particularly relevant for infants and children with developmental delays or neurological impairments.

Prenatal History

- Maternal and paternal age, month prenatal care started, planned pregnancy?

- Length of pregnancy, weight gain.
- Maternal health before and during pregnancy—substance use or abuse; prescription drug use; smoking; injuries or exposure to abuse; hypertension; infectious diseases, including TB and HIV status.
- Hospitalizations.
- GTPAL (Gravidity, number of pregnancies; Term deliveries; Premature deliveries; Abortions, spontaneous or induced; Living children).

Birth and Neonatal History

- Location of birth, nature of labor—how long? cesarean or vaginal delivery? anesthesia? forceps? unusual presentation?
- Birth weight?
- Apgar score, breathing problems?
- Who was present at delivery, how soon after birth did parent(s) touch or hold baby?
- Problems in nursery—feeding, jaundice, elimination, irritability?
- Length of hospitalization?

Past Medical History

It is important to review the past medical history from birth to adolescence during a comprehensive visit.

- **Childhood conditions:** Frequent upper respiratory infections (URIs), ear infections, sore throats; wheezing; viral, streptococcal, or bacterial infections; skin problems.
- **Chronic conditions:** Seasonal or household allergies, asthma; diabetes; frequent otitis; bedwetting; HIV or immunodeficiency; other conditions? Year of diagnosis of chronic condition?
- **Hospitalizations:** Date and reason for hospitalization, history of surgery, length of stay, problems after hospitalization.
- **Unintentional injuries:** Falls, motor vehicle accidents, nature of injury, age of child when injury occurred, problems after injury
- **Intentional injuries:** History of family violence, physical abuse or domestic violence; ask about verbal abuse of family members? Child interview should include the following questions: Has anyone hurt you? Have you felt afraid someone would harm you?
- **Immunization:** Review immunization dates and current status; ask parent/caretaker about reactions to vaccines; date of last TB skin testing and result.
- **Allergies:** Allergic to medications or antibiotics or foods? What type of reaction occurred? Severity of the reaction? Was an epinephrine pen recommended? Reaction to insect bites? Pets in home? Environmental triggers?
- **Medications:** Is child taking vitamins, fluoride, or medications regularly? Type of medication? Use of over-the-counter (OTC) medications? Use of herbs or native medicines? Cultural healing practices?
- **Laboratory tests:** Review of neonatal screen? Lead screening? Hemoglobin or hematocrit screening for anemia?

Sexual History

Sexually Active Female

History of abortions, pregnancies? last Pap smear? (See Chapter 17 for detailed history.)

Sexually Active Male or Female

Gonorrhea/chlamydia screen (urine or genital probe), other sexually transmitted infection (STI) screens (syphilis, HIV, hepatitis)?

Activities of Daily Living

- **Nutrition and feeding:** For all ages: Is there a usual time daily when the family has a meal? Are there usual family eating patterns? Who does the food shopping and meal preparation? Are there any special cultural or religious food preferences? Does the family participate in any food programs? WIC (Women, Infants, and Children Nutrition program)? Obtain a 24-hour dietary recall from every child and adolescent. (See age-specific content on nutrition and feeding below.)
- **Elimination:** *<2 years of age*—stool pattern, frequency, and consistency. *>2 years of age*—plans for toilet training; difficulties with bowel or bladder control; age bowel and bladder control attained, occurrence of wetting, parental attitudes toward wetting incidents, history of encopresis or enuresis?
- **Sleep:** Sleep patterns and amount of sleep day and night, bedtime routines, where does the child sleep? Always sleeps in same household? Concerns about nightmares, night terrors, night waking, somnambulism (sleepwalking)?
- **Dentition:** Number of teeth? Tooth loss pattern? Pattern of teeth brushing? Use of night bottle? Use of sugary foods/sodas/juices? Has child seen dentist? Last dental appointment?

School

- **2- to 5-year-old child:** What is your child's school experience? Daycare, nursery school, or kindergarten experience? How well did your child adjust to school entry?

- **School-age child or adolescent:** Likes school? Number of missed school days? Reason for school absence? School performance? Teacher or school concerns? Attends special classes?

Interests/Hobbies/Sports

- Number of hours of TV or video games or computer use daily?
- After-school activities?
- Sports participation?
- Exercise routine?

Safety

- Car seat, seat belt use?
- House childproofing, poison control?
- Stranger safety taught?
- Presence of gun in home? loaded/unloaded, how stored?
- Bicycle safety practiced? sports safety equipment used?

Developmental History

Developmental Milestones

Note the ages at which the child attained key milestones. This information is particularly important during infancy and early childhood and when there are concerns about delayed physical growth or delayed psychomotor or intellectual development.

- **Personal/social:** Smiles, feeds self, separates from mother, dresses without help, peer interaction.
- **Language:** First word, combination of words. Do you have any concerns about your child's speech? Do you understand your child's speech/do others? Does child follow directions? Does child get confused, stutter, repeat words?
- **Fine motor:** Manual dexterity, handedness, drawing, writing, dressing, tying shoes
- **Gross motor:** Holds head up while prone; rolls over; sits with support and alone;

crawls; has begun standing and walking, exhibits balance and coordination, climbs stairs, rides tricycle or bicycle; plays in schoolyard. (See Chapter 3 for complete developmental screening.)

- **Sexual development:** Normal self-pleasure exploration in infant and masturbation in preschooler, parental comfort with answering child's questions; sex education provided in the home and school.
- **Preadolescent/adolescent interview:** Menstruation, nocturnal emissions, peer relations, sexual debut. (See adolescent-specific content below.)
- **Temperament/personality:** Degree of independence; relationships with parents, siblings, and peers; congeniality; self-image; adaptability to change, moods; activity level; attention span; consolability.
- **Habits:** Thumb sucking, nail biting, tics, rocking, ritualistic behavior.
- **Discipline:** What type of discipline do you use when your child misbehaves? When do you use it? Is discipline effective? Consistent parenting styles? Does child live at more than one home? Behavior issues at home or at school?

Family History

- **Family health history:** Diabetes, epilepsy, hypertension, sickle cell anemia, stroke, tuberculosis, mental problems, alcoholism, cancer, heart disease, asthma, allergy, eczema, mental retardation, migraine, congenital anomalies, kidney disease, learning problems, STIs, death in first year of life, history of substance abuse, HIV+, early death from any cause.
- **Socioeconomic background:** Employment status, education, parents' occupations, medical insurance, religious background (if pertinent), cultural or ethnic identity. (See Cultural Considerations.)
- **Home situation:** Who is the primary caretaker? Type of home or dwelling? Is it temporary or permanent? Number of people

living in home? Housing problems? Is the neighborhood safe? Parents' or caretakers' work schedules? Sleeping arrangements?

- **Support systems:** Relatives living near or in home? Help caring for child? Supportive family/friends? With whom do you talk when you have a problem? Who is your chief critic?

Review of Systems

Information gathering for each system is found in the chapters that follow.

🔑 Key Points

Describe the quality of interaction between parent/caretaker and child: Is it appropriate and comforting? Was there warmth of interaction? Did you observe age-appropriate limit setting? Does parent encourage independence as age-appropriate or is supervision inappropriate?

AGE-SPECIFIC NUTRITIONAL INFORMATION GATHERING

Infant

Nutrition is critically important in the first 2 years of life—a period of rapid growth and development. With a thorough dietary history, problems of undernutrition or overnutrition can be recognized early. Dietary history for the first year of life includes the following:

- **Breastfeeding**—Frequency and duration of infant feeds; use of supplemental formula feedings or water; difficulties with nippling or feeding patterns? Concern about infant weight gain? Mother's diet or dietary restrictions? Father's participation in feeding routines? Mother receiving adequate rest? Experiencing nipple soreness? Plans for return to work? Plan for expression of breast milk or weaning?
- **Formula feeding**—Type of infant formula, how is formula stored and prepared?

Concentrated formula or powdered formula? Amount and frequency of feeds? Concern about infant weight gain? Bottle-feeding at night? How often? Difficulty feeding? or slow feeder? Plans for bottle weaning and transition to cup?

- **Juice**—Drinking juice? Type of juice? Any reactions? Drinking juice in cup or bottle? Amount of juice daily?
- **Solid foods**—Age at introduction of solid foods; types and amounts of baby foods, spoon use; introduction of table foods; feeding finger foods? Cup drinking? Any concerns about your child's eating? Document sources of protein, iron, vitamin C, calcium (Ca^{++}). A 24-hour dietary history can be very informative.

Toddler and Preschooler

During the toddler years, it is particularly important to establish weaning. Persistent bottle-feeding may be associated with iron deficiency anemia and early childhood caries; therefore, determining the amount of milk intake is key to understanding overall nutrition and oral health. Eating habits are established during the early years and a balanced diet is important to maintain a healthy weight and for optimum growth and development. Dietary history for the toddler includes the following:

- Food likes and dislikes?
- Meal habits or snacks?
- Parental attitude toward eating?
- Any concerns about appetite or overeating? Document sources of protein, iron, vitamin C, Ca^{++} (milk intake) in the diet with a 24-hour dietary recall.

Psychosocial adjustment of the toddler and preschooler includes gathering information about tempter tantrums and parental reaction. Breath-holding spells also can occur during the toddler period, and the healthcare provider should explore parental concerns around temperament and behavior. Habits such as thumb sucking and ritualistic behavior are common and should be explored with this age-group.

School-Age Child

About 11% of children and adolescents are currently classified as overweight, with a body mass index (BMI) greater than the 95th percentile, and an additional 14% of children and adolescents have a BMI between the 85th and 95th percentiles.[4] Overweight children and adolescents have a 70% chance of becoming overweight or obese adults. Therefore, during the interview with the school-age child and parent, it is important to discuss the importance of healthy eating habits. Determine whether the parent uses food as a reward or punishment and what the parental attitude is toward the weight of the child. Dietary history for the school-age child should include the following:

- Daily meal pattern and snack habits, amount of soda and fast foods, daily quantity of juice and water, amount of high-fat, salty foods and sugary sweets in the diet. A 24-hour dietary history is the best method for evaluating a balanced diet.
- Does child contribute to preparation or planning of family meals? Does the child have any interest in cooking?

Evaluation of the psychosocial adjustment for the school-age child includes school adaptation and performance, peer interactions with classmates, current grades, relationship with teacher, and developing interests. Habits such as nail biting and tics should be explored.

Adolescent

"Disordered eating" is unfortunately the norm for many adolescents who do not necessarily have an eating disorder. In a recent survey, 28% reported inadequate fruit intake, 36% reported inadequate vegetable intake, and 13% of young women reported less than adequate daily intake of dairy products. Of even more concern, among young women, 12% report chronic dieting, 30% report binge eating, 12% report self-induced vomiting, and 2% report use of diuretics or laxatives.[4] Teens often skip breakfast, either because of lack of time, lack

of available food, or the misconception that skipping breakfast will aid in weight loss. Although a vegetarian diet is often a healthy choice for adults or for children who have been raised as vegetarians, in teens a sudden switch to a vegetarian diet may actually be a red flag for a developing eating disorder.[5] Even though eating disorders are more common among adolescent girls, boys are also at risk. A 24- or 48-hour diet recall can be quite helpful in evaluating nutrition status.

When asking adolescents about body image, the provider should avoid the assumptions that an adolescent with a low BMI for age is satisfied with his or her weight, or that

---

Box **4-2**   **Body Image and Dieting Behavior in the Adolescent**

Ask the following questions to gather nutritional information when assessing an adolescent.

SATISFACTION WITH WEIGHT

- Is adolescent happy with weight?
- What has he or she done to gain/lose weight?
- Exercise history?

DIET AND DIETING HISTORY

- Number of diets in past year? Does adolescent feel he or she should be dieting? Dissatisfaction with body size?
- Is adolescent eating in secret? Using supplements, laxatives, or diuretics?

SELF IMAGE

- How much does weight affect how adolescent feels about herself or himself?
- Has a specific binge/purge cycle been established?

Data from Anstine D, Grinenko D: Rapid screening for disordered eating in college-aged females in the primary care setting, *J Adolesc Health* 26(5):338-342, 2000.

an adolescent with a high BMI wants to lose weight (Box 4-2).

ADOLESCENT PSYCHOSOCIAL HISTORY AND CONFIDENTIALITY

The most important caveat of the adolescent psychosocial history is that it should be conducted without the parent or guardian in the room. A review of studies on adolescent access to healthcare services shows that a perceived lack of confidentiality is a barrier to care, and only a minority of adolescents have ever discussed confidentiality of the health visit with a healthcare provider.[6-9] Although the explicit laws vary from state to state, all 50 states have laws allowing adolescents to consent to some confidential services, including confidential discussions, related to sexuality, reproduction, mental health and drug and alcohol use.[10] In all 50 states, there are some limitations to confidentiality. Providers are generally required to notify parents and/or police or child protective services if an adolescent under 18 years of age expresses a desire to harm himself or herself or others, or if an adolescent has been abused or neglected. In addition, some states have mandatory reporting laws about consensual sexual activity, depending on the age and age discrepancy of the teen and the sexual partner; other states encourage reporting, but give the provider some discretion.[11]

Current federal regulations, which are required under the 1996 Health Insurance Portability and Accountability Act (HIPAA), sever the longstanding link between the right to consent to confidential services and the right to control medical records related to those services, but state laws that are more specific about privacy of medical records take precedence.[12] It is crucial for the provider to become familiar with the specific state laws pertaining to adolescent consent, confidentiality, privacy, child abuse reporting, and the amount of control the adolescent has over the release of medical records related to confidential services.

HEADSSS Assessment

The HEADSSS psychosocial history (Box 4-3) is a key part of a comprehensive adolescent assessment.[13] The order of questioning, in general, proceeds from less private and sensitive questions to more sensitive, giving the provider and adolescent a chance to establish some rapport. It can be tailored to early, middle, or late adolescents by modifying the questions. Remember that early and sometimes middle adolescents can have concrete thinking[14] and younger teens, in particular, may wonder why the provider is asking such unusual questions. It helps to explain first that you ask all teens the same questions and to start the interview by asking about the activities of acquaintances and friends before asking about the teen directly. Avoid medical jargon and try to use the teen's own terminology without sounding as though you are trying to talk like a teen. Remember that adolescents tend to be oriented in the here and now: A "long time ago" may refer to years or months ago or as little as a few weeks ago.

Begin the interview with an opening such as "I'm going to ask you questions about sex, drugs, and feelings. What you tell me is private, unless you tell me that you have been hurt by someone else, that you are thinking of hurting yourself, or thinking of hurting someone else." Questions are asked in as neutral and nonjudgmental a manner as possible to avoid making assumptions about the family structure, kinds of sexual activity, or sexual orientation of the adolescent. Asking open-ended questions such as, "How are things at home?" sets a neutral tone.

Ricciardi[15] extends the emphasis on psychosocial issues of violence in the lives of adolescents with another adaptation of the HEADSSS assessment. The 'HEADSSS is *Very Good*' adolescent interview model expands the original elements to include violence and gangs.

HEADSSS Assessment for Adolescence[13]

(H) Home: Problems at home, with family

(E) Education: Connection to or disconnection from school

(A) Activities: Sports, school activities (school connection), hobbies, church involvement, youth groups, jobs, and hours per week for each

(D) Drug, alcohol, tobacco experimentation and abuse

(S) Sexual activity and history of sexual abuse; issues about sexuality

(S) Safety issues: Guns in home, neighborhood safety, seat belts, bicycle/skateboard helmet use

(S) Suicidal ideation/depression

(V) Violence: Witnessed violence at school, in home

(G) Gangs: Gangs at school, involvement in gangs

Box **4-3**   **HEADSSS Adolescent History**

HOME

- Who lives with you? (One or both parents, grandparents, aunts/uncles, adult siblings, group home, foster care?) Do you live with boyfriend/girlfriend and family? Immigrant teens may live with adult siblings/extended family while parents live in home country.
- Have you lived with… your whole life? (Changes because of divorce or death of parent? separation/reunification with parents resulting from immigration? conflict with parents/guardians? illness, incarceration, homelessness of family members?)
- How do you get along with…?

EDUCATION

- Are you in school? (Regular or continuation? English learner/bilingual? Special education/504 Plans?) Attend regularly? Suspensions?
- Favorite/most difficult subjects?
- What are your grades/GPA?
  - Low: Recent if changes in GPA? Is work too difficult? Not doing work?
  - High: Any stress about college goals or grades?
- Plans after high school graduation? (Realistic? Is teen taking right courses/activities? Taking SATs, sending college applications on time? Taking vocational training?) If no specific plans, end of high school can be scary, vulnerable time.

ACTIVITIES

- How do you spend free time? What do you do for fun? Sports/other extracurricular activities? (Measure of connection to school, extra motivation for attendance/grades) Exercise? Hobbies? Church or community activities?
- Jobs? (Number of hours/week, schedule, location, hazards?)
- Names of friends, best friend?

DRUGS/ALCOHOL/TOBACCO

Introduce the subject gently, especially with young teens

- Does anyone at your school…? Do any of your friends…? Then, have you…? If yes, use CRAFFT questions (Box 4-4).
- Attempts to quit?
- Family members using drugs/alcohol/tobacco?

Box **4-3**   **HEADSSS Adolescent History—cont'd**

SEXUALITY AND SEXUAL ABUSE

Warn the teen of limits of confidentiality

- "Have you ever had sex or ever come close to having sex?"
  - "Come close to" covers a broad range, includes oral/anal sex, which teens often do not define as sex. For teens with the intention to initiate sexual activity, it is important to explore choice and decisions about sex in relationship. Important to elicit history before discussing safer sex, contraception, need for pelvic exam.
- "Are your partners girls, boys, or both?" or "Are you attracted to girls, boys, or both?" Ask of everyone. Be sensitive to teens engaging in same-sex activities.
- Condom/barrier: "At what point in encounter do you use condoms?" ("late use" problem) Condom education in school? Knowledge of other barriers (gloves, dental dams)? Difficulties in negotiating condom use with partner. Teens with less formal education may lack awareness of anatomy/ physiology of genitals, reproductive organs.
- "Has anyone ever touched you sexually without permission or tried to force you to have sex?" *If yes*, history of childhood sexual abuse? Acquaintance or date rape? Stranger assault?

SUICIDE AND DEPRESSION

- Present/past suicidal ideation, attempts? Suicide gesture vs. self-cutting without suicidal intent. Suicidal gestures/attempts may be impulsive acts after disagreement with parents, peers—teen may not self-identify as depressed.
- Depression: Changes in energy, appetite, weight? Sleep disturbances, difficulty concentrating? Irritability is hallmark of depression in teens. Difficulty with homework, school?
- Warn parent/guardian if teen contemplating suicide, even if not at immediate risk.

SAFETY ISSUES

- Guns in home: Feel safe at school?
- Physical fighting/abuse in home (between siblings, parents, parent-child)?
- Teen involved in physical fights at home, neighborhood, school?

VIOLENCE

- How are conflicts handled at home? (i.e., late for curfew?) At school? At work?
- Do you carry weapons? Start fights?

GANGS

- Are gangs present in high school? How many?
- Friends in gangs? Have you ever been a member? Do you have any gang clothing or insignias? Teen, peers, siblings/cousins involved in gangs? May be reluctant to disclose neighborhood vs. regional gang.

Data from Seidel HM, Ball JW, Dains JE, Benedict GW: *Mosby's guide to physical examination*, ed 5, St Louis, 2003, Mosby; Ricciardi R. First pelvic examination in the adolescent, *Nurse Pract Forum* 11(3):161-169, 2000; Zayas LH, Kaplan C, Turner S et al: Understanding suicide attempts by adolescent Hispanic females, *Soc Work* 45(1):53-63, 2000; Knight JR, Shrier LA, Bravender TD et al: A new brief screen for adolescent substance abuse, *Arch Pediatr Adolesc Med* 153(6):591-596, 1999.

Box 4-4   CRAFFT Substance Abuse Screening Test

The **CRAFFT** test is intended specifically for adolescents. It draws upon adult screening instruments, covers alcohol and other drugs, and calls upon situations that are suited to adolescents.

	Yes	No

1. Have you ever ridden in a **C**ar driven by someone (including yourself) who was high or had been using alcohol or drugs?

2. Do you ever use alcohol or drugs to **R**elax, feel better about yourself, or fit in?

3. Do you ever use alcohol or drugs while you are **A**lone?

4. Do you ever **F**orget things you did while using alcohol or drugs?

5. Do your **F**amily or Friends ever tell you that you should cut down on your drinking or drug use?

6. Have you ever gotten into **T**rouble while you were using alcohol or drugs?

SCORING: 2 or more positive items indicate the need for further assessment.

From Knight JR, Sherritt L, Shrier LA, Harris SK, Chang G: Validity of the CRAFFT substance abuse screening test among adolescent clinic patients, *Arch Pediatr Adolescent* 156(6):607-614, 2002. Reprinted here with permission from Center for Adolescent Substance Abuse Research at Children's Hospital, Boston.

REFERENCES

1. Lipson JG, Dibble SL: *Culture and clinical care,* San Francisco, 2005, University of California, San Francisco School of Nursing.
2. Bennet RL: *The practical guide to the genetic family history,* New York, 1999, Wiley-Liss, Inc.
3. Hunt SC, Gwinn M, Adams TD: Family history assessment: strategies for prevention of cardiovascular disease, *Am J Prev Med* 24(2): 136-142, 2003.
4. Neumark-Sztainer D, Story M, Resnick MD et al: Lessons learned about adolescent nutrition from the Minnesota Adolescent Health Survey, *J Am Diet Assoc* 98(12):1449-1456, 1998.
5. Perry CL, McGuire MT, Neumark-Sztainer D et al: Characteristics of vegetarian adolescents in a multiethnic urban population, *J Adolesc Health* 29(6):406-416, 2001.
6. Allen LB, Glicken AD, Beach RK et al: Adolescent health care experiences of gay, lesbian and bisexual young adults, *J Adolesc Health* 23:212-220, 1998.
7. Kapphahn CJ, Wilson KM, Klein JD: Adolescent girls' and boys' preferences for provider gender and confidentiality in their health care, *J Adolesc Health* 25(2):131-142, 1999.
8. Klein JD, Wilson KM, McNulty M et al: Access to medical care for adolescents: results from the 1997 Commonwealth Fund Survey of the Health of Adolescent Girls, *J Adolesc Health* 25(2):120-130, 1999.
9. Thrall JS, McCloskey L, Ettner SL et al: Confidentiality and adolescents' use of providers for health information and for pelvic examinations, *Arch Pediatr Adolesc Med* 154(9):885-892, 2000.

10. Maradiegue A: Minor's rights versus parental rights: review of legal issues in adolescent health care, *J Midwif Women's Health* 48(3):170-177, 2003.

11. Madison AB, Feldman-Winter L, Finkel M, McAbee GN: Consensual adolescent sexual activity with adult partners: conflict between confidentiality and physician reporting requirements under child abuse laws, *Pediatrics* 107(2):E16, 2001; available: http://pediatrics. aappublications.org; accessed 3/7/05.

12. Dailard C: New medical records privacy rule: the interface with teen access to confidential care, *Guttmacher Report on Public Policy* 6(1),

March 2003; available: www.agiusa.org/pubs/ tgr/06/1/gr060106.html; accessed 3/7/05.

13. Goldenring JM, Rosen D: Getting into adolescent heads: an essential update, *Contemp Pediatr* 21:64-80, 2004.

14. Radzik M, Sherer S, Neinstein, LS: Psychosocial development in normal adolescents. In Neinstein LS, editor: *Adolescent health care: a practical guide,* Philadelphia, 2000, Lippincott, Williams & Wilkins.

15. Ricciardi R: First pelvic examination in the adolescent, *Nurse Pract Forum* 11(3):161-169, 2000.

CHAPTER 5

ENVIRONMENTAL HEALTH HISTORY

Karen G. Duderstadt

Children are unique from adults in relation to environmental exposures. Young children breathe more air and drink more water per pound of body weight than adults. Children are at higher risk for toxins in the environment because they absorb toxic substances at a rate 5 to 1 times that of an adult.[1] The respiratory tract, gastrointestinal tract, and the skin are particularly vulnerable and absorb substances more readily and efficiently than in the adult. Children also live and play closer to environmental hazards on the ground, which increases their concentrations of inhaled toxic substances.[2]

Environmental health is defined as "freedom from illness or injury related to exposure to toxic agents and other environmental conditions encountered in the home, workplace, and community environments that are potentially detrimental to human health."[3] The *dose-response* rate in children for exposure to *environmental hazards* is more rapid than in adults. It is critically important for healthcare providers to understand the impact of environmental hazards and exposures on the healthy growth and development of infants, children, and adolescents and to develop knowledge about the risks present in the child's environment and in his/her community.

 Key Points

Toxicant refers to an environmental hazard from chemical pollutants, and *toxin* refers to hazards from a biological source.

ENVIRONMENTAL RISK FACTORS

Children can encounter environmental hazards and be exposed to many different toxic substances in the home, car, school, childcare setting, and play environments (Box 5-1). This includes physical agents: sun, water, air temperatures, and noise; chemical agents such as outdoor and indoor air contaminants, water and soil or dust contaminants; and biological irritants, allergens, toxins, and infectious agents.[4]

DEVELOPMENTAL APPROACH TO ENVIRONMENTAL RISKS

All children should be considered at risk for exposures. However, different developmental stages put children at risk for types of exposure to environmental hazards. Prenatal exposure of the fetus to maternal smoking, substance use, and chemical or biological agents increases risk of absorption of toxicants and toxins.

Box **5-1** **Risk Categories of Environmental Hazards**

INDOOR AIR POLLUTANTS AND HOUSEHOLD EXPOSURES

- Mold spores
- Animal dander
- Carbon monoxide
- Tobacco smoke
- Mercury vapors
- Radon
- Smoke from wood-burning stoves
- Lead

OUTDOOR AIR POLLUTANTS

- Air particulates
- Ozone
- Nitrogen dioxide

SCHOOL OR DAYCARE EXPOSURES

- Polychlorinated biphenyls (PCBs)
- Arsenic from pesticide-treated wood
- Pesticides
- Friable asbestos

COMMUNITY EXPOSURES

- Insecticides
- Herbicides

WATER POLLUTANTS

- Bacteria
- Parasites

FOOD CONTAMINANTS

- Mercury
- Pesticides

UNINTENTIONAL INGESTIONS OR POISONINGS

PARENT'S OCCUPATION/HOBBIES

- House painters
- Smelters
- Car mechanics
- Farm workers

From Etzel RA: Indoor air pollutants in homes and schools, *Pediatr Clin North Am* 48(5):1153-1165, 2001.

In the newborn, particular attention should be given to toxicants in breast milk or preparation of infant formula, dermal contacts, and parental occupations. The infant and toddler have expanded mobility giving them increased exposure to their environment. They are particularly vulnerable to oral exposures because of their hand-to-mouth activity and inhaled substances within the physical zone they occupy near the ground. Preschool and school-age children become susceptible to toxicants in the school, childcare setting, or playground environments.[5] Occupational hazards are of particular concern in adolescents, as well as harmful exposures that occur through experimentation with illicit drugs, alcohol, and intentional inhalation of leaded gasoline, known as *huffing*.

WHAT PLACES CHILDREN AT RISK?

Children are at risk for toxic environmental sources: lead paint chips (pre-1970 housing), lead-contaminated soil and dust in homes from paint or soil, industrial toxicant in or near neighborhoods, landfill sites or waste treatment sites, charcoal mills, pre-1989 plumbing suggesting presence of lead pipes or lead solder, well water or contaminated tap water, drinking water contaminated with lead, and playing near high-traffic areas with old deposits from leaded gasoline.

Children are at risk for indoor air pollutants: environmental tobacco smoke, mold, or pesticides in the home or school; products containing lead, such as leaded candle wicks, pottery with lead glaze, and other imported products containing lead. Poor childhood nutrition puts children at risk for iron or calcium deficiency, which enhances lead toxicity in the body. Food contaminants are also a significant risk including contaminated breast milk. Children of farm workers are particularly vulnerable to pesticide exposure. Exposure to toxins through contact with a parent's workplace or work clothes; hobbies such as soldering stained glass or refinishing old painted furniture can put children at risk.

Adolescents are at particular risk for exposure to workplace hazards, alcohol ingestion, substance abuse or inhalation of toxic substances or leaded gasoline, called *huffing*, or excessive exposure to the sun and ultraviolet radiation (UVR).

RISK COMMUNICATION

The concept of risk communication is particularly important to assessing environmental health in children and is part of a holistic approach to working with families in the clinical setting (Box 5-2). *Health risk communication* requires active listening to identify a parent's concern or a child or adolescent's fear.[1] It requires a determination of the presence of an environmental hazard, assessment of the risk, the severity of the dose, acceptability of the risk, the impact on the health of the child or adolescent, and communicating the risk effectively to the family.[6]

ENVIRONMENTAL HEALTH HISTORY

All healthy children and adolescents should have an environmental health screening history at their routine well-care visit to establish risk of exposures.[6] An environmental health screening establishes known school or community environmental health risks and/or a history of exposure in a sibling or parent.[7] Box 5-3 assesses risk for lead toxicity. Table 5-1 presents an environmental health screening to use in establishing a risk profile for exposure to pesticides, poor indoor or outdoor air quality, contaminated drinking water, or chemical *toxicants.*

CLINICAL FINDINGS

Children with excess lead levels usually show no unique features on physical examination. Environmental exposures are often insidious and affect the internal organs and brain. Children with lead toxicity may present with one or more of the following symptoms: fatigue, malaise, abdominal pain, loss of appetite,

---

Box **5-2**   **Why Take an Environmental Health History?**

1. Providers should obtain basic environmental health history from parent/patient:
   - To identify environmental health risks that may lead to harmful exposure in infants, children, adolescents.
   - To establish possible cause/effect relationship between exposure to environmental health risks and symptoms
2. Providers have professional responsibility to obtain knowledge:
   - About environmental risks present in community in which they practice
   - To access available risk data from community surveillance programs
   - To report exposures to appropriate local/state authorities
   - To advocate for change to protect infants, children, adolescents from toxic environmental exposures
3. Providers are mandated to:
   - Conduct appropriate screening tests
   - Educate parents/patients about all health risks including toxic environmental health risks
   - Guide parents/patients on primary prevention of toxic environmental exposures

---

Data from National Environmental Education and Training Foundation: *Pesticides and National strategies for health care providers,* Washington, DC, 2002, The National Environmental Education & Training Foundation, United States Environmental Protection Agency.

Box 5-3   Quick Lead Screening Questionnaire for Children

1. Within the last 6 months, has your child lived in or regularly visited a house, apartment, or school built before 1960? Are there paint surfaces that are peeling or chipped in the home or school?
2. Does your child live in or regularly visit a house or school built before 1960 that is undergoing renovation or has been recently renovated?
3. Have you ever seen your child eating paint chips or other non-food substances such as paper?
4. Has your child ever taken home remedies such as *azarcon, pay-loo-ah, carol, ghasard, kohl, greta, bala goli, shurma,* or *rueda*?
5. Do you use ceramic pottery from Mexico, Central America, South America, or Asia for cooking, serving, or storing food or beverages?
6. Have you ever been told that your child has an elevated blood lead?

Data from Centers for Disease Control and Prevention: Childhood Lead Poisoning Prevention Program, *Healthy Families, 2001*, 2003, CDC; available at http://www.cdc.gov/nceh/lead/lead.htm.

TABLE 5-1   QUICK ENVIRONMENTAL SCREENING QUESTIONNAIRE

Where does your child spend time during the day?

Source	Exposure
HOME	
Do you have a basement where children sleep or play?	Asbestos, radon
Do you have water damage or visible mold in home?	Indoor air pollutants
Do you use pesticides in lawn/garden area or in home?	Pesticide
Do you have a gas stove or wall heater?	Carbon monoxide
Do you live near a freeway, industrial area, or polluted site?	Outdoor air/water pollutants
SMOKING	
Does anyone smoke in the home environment?	Tobacco smoke (ETS)
FOOD AND WATER	
Do you use tap water or well water? Do you wash fresh fruits/vegetables?	Pesticides, nitrates, lead, biological agents
WORKPLACE	
What do teens or adults in the household do for a living? Are you involved in a hobby at home?	Chemical, physical, and biological agents
SUN EXPOSURE	
Do you use sun protection for your child?	UV index

Data from Etzel RA, Balk SJ, editors: *Handbook of pediatric environmental health*, Elk Grove Village, Ill, 1999, American Academy of Pediatrics Committee on Environmental Health.

constipation, irritability, headache, weakness, or clumsiness. Any signs of developmental delay, neurobehavioral disorders such as tics, persistent hand-to-mouth activity such as pica, unexplained seizures, anemia, chronic abdominal pain, learning difficulties, or attention deficit disorder warrant an in-depth environmental health history to relate positive history to exposure to environmental hazards. Figure 5-1 illustrates the primary organs and body systems affected by exposure to environmental hazards.

to test for exposure, and how to assess and manage clinical cases of exposures (Box 5-4). Having access to evidence-based research and resources on environmental health is key to responsible risk communication. Policy statements by the American Academy of Pediatrics (AAP) are important guides to environmental hazards such as ultraviolet light, contaminants in breast milk, environmental tobacco smoke, and *thimerosal* (the mercury-containing preservative in vaccines).[8] The Centers for Disease Control and Prevention (CDC) (2001) published "reference ranges" for many common environmental

Pediatric Pearls

Children exposed to folk remedies such as azarcon, pay-loo-ah, carol, ghasard, kohl, greta, and bala goli are at increased risk for lead exposure. Children's toys manufactured outside of the United States also may contain lead.

RESOURCES

A number of resources are available to providers, including information about contaminants, ways

 CHARTING

Environmental Exposure History on a 5-Year-Old

5-year-old healthy-appearing male who lives on a farm where pesticides are used seasonally on crops. Father works part-time as a crop duster. House built before 1950 with some restoration underway in the family living area. House is partially heated with wood stove. Parents refinish old furniture as a hobby in garage area adjacent to house. Well water is primary source of drinking water for family.

 CHARTING

Environmental Exposure History on a 2½-Year-Old

2½-year-old healthy-appearing female living in subsidized housing built before 1978. Mother gives history of obvious mold on the bedroom and bathroom walls. The building has water damage on the walls that has not been repaired over the past 2 years. The building overlooks a large gas station, a high-traffic area adjacent to the freeway.

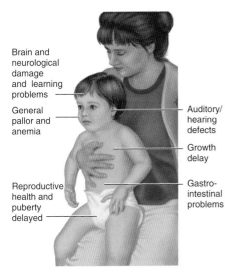

Brain and neurological damage and learning problems

General pallor and anemia

Reproductive health and puberty delayed

Auditory/hearing defects

Growth delay

Gastro-intestinal problems

Figure 5-1 Effects of lead exposure on a child's body.

Box 5-4 Environmental Health Web Sites

Children's Environmental Health Network
www.cehn.org

National Center for Environmental Health
www.cdc.gov/nceh

Center for Health, Environment and Justice
www.chej.org

Columbia University's Center for Children's Environmental Health
www.ccceh.org

The National Environmental Education & Training Foundation: Pesticide Resource Library
www.neetf.org/health/pestlibrary.htm

Health Schools Network, Inc.
www.healthyschools.org

US Environmental Protection Agency: Ground Water and Drinking Water Topics
www.epa.gov/safewater/topics.html

Data from Burns C, Dunn AM, Sattler B: Resources for environmental health problems, *J Pediatr Health Care* 16(3):138-142, 2002.

chemicals for children. A total of 27 environmental hazards have been studied including chemical pollutants, lead, mercury, pesticide metabolites, and nicotine exposure.[9] Blood metabolite levels were studied in children from 1 year of age, and urine metabolites were studied in children from 6 years of age. Exposure to significant levels of toxicants should be reported to local, state, and federal authorities.

REFERENCES

1. National Environmental Education and Training Foundation: *Pesticides and National strategies for health care providers,* Washington, DC, 2002, The National Environmental Education & Training Foundation, United States Environmental Protection Agency.
2. Shea KM: Pediatric exposure and potential toxicity of phthalate plasticizers, *Pediatrics* 111(6):1467-1474, 2003.
3. Pope AM, Snyder MA, Mood LH: *Nursing, health, and the environment,* Washington, DC, 1995, Institute of Medicine.
4. Schneider D, Freeman N: *Children's environmental health: reducing risk in a dangerous world,* Washington, DC, 2000, American Public Health Association.
5. Gitterman BA, Bearer CF: A developmental approach to pediatric environmental health, *Pediatr Clin North Am* 48(5):1071-1083, 2001.
6. Etzel RA, Balk SJ, editors: *Handbook of pediatric environmental health,* Elk Grove Village, Ill, 1999, American Academy of Pediatrics Committee on Environmental Health.
7. Abelsohn A, Sanform M: *International Joint Commission: Environmental health in family medicine,* Ontario, 2001, Ontario College of Family Physicians.
8. Balk SJ: Resources for pediatricians: How do I answer questions from parents, patients, teachers, and others? *Pediatr Clin North Am* 48(5):1099-1111, 2001.
9. Centers for Disease Control and Prevention: *National report on human exposure to environmental chemicals,* Atlanta, 2001, Centers for Disease Control and Prevention.

System-Specific Assessment

CHAPTER 6

SKIN

Renee McLeod

Careful examination of the skin gives the examiner insight into the overall health of the child. Examination of the skin, hair, and nails provides clues to the nutritional and hydration status of the child and any underlying disease pathology. The skin of an infant, child, and adult shares similarities in structure and function, but the skin reacts differently to the unique environmental demands of each age-group. For example, an infant's diaper area is a challenging environment for the skin because of the intermittent contact with urine and feces and the variety of materials used to diaper. The recent addition of petrolatum-based emollients to some diapering products has added both more occlusion and more protection.[1] All skin, regardless of age, is affected by seasonal factors such as the heat and humidity of summer or the dryness and low humidity of winter, but the differences in an infant's skin and ability to sweat compared with an adult's can create many more problems associated with these seasonal changes.

The skin is the largest organ in the body and has five distinct functions. The skin controls fluids, regulates temperature, protects against invasion from microbial and foreign bodies, and protects against damage from the ultraviolet (UV) rays of the sun. Finally, our skin is an organ of communication. Touch and skin-to-skin contact is one of the ways we bond with our mothers and families at birth and later bond with our sexual partners. Research conducted over the past 50 years has proven that touch is more important to humans than food in regard to optimal development.[2-5] Having a disease of the skin, hair, or nails that prevents or decreases human touch can be devastating to a child's self esteem.

ANATOMY AND PHYSIOLOGY

The skin consists of three layers: the *epidermis*, the *dermis*, and the *subcutaneous layer* (Figure 6-1). The *epidermis* is the outermost layer of the skin and consists of two main layers: the *stratum corneum*, and the *cellular stratum*. The *stratum corneum* is the very top layer of the skin and is composed of stacked, overlapping nonnucleated keratinized cells called *corneocytes*. The thickness of this layer depends on the region of the body, being thinnest on the face and thickest over the soles of the feet.[1] This layer forms the protective barrier of the skin and contains the waterproofing protein *keratin,* which restricts water loss and penetration of a variety of substances through the skin. The innermost layer of the

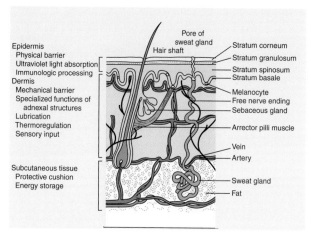

Figure **6-1** Anatomy of the skin. (From Cohen BA: *Pediatric dermatology,* ed 2, St Louis, 1999, Mosby.)

epidermis consists of a single row of columnar cells called *basal cells,* which reside in the *stratum basale.* These cells divide to form the *keratinocytes* that move to the surface through the *stratum spinosum, stratum granulosum,* and *stratum lucidum* to replace the cells that are sloughed off every day in the stratum corneum.[6] The stratum basale also contains *melanocytes,* which synthesize melanin to provide color and protect the skin from damage by the UV rays of the sun. The dermal-epidermal junction lies beneath the stratum basale and is an important site of attachment in the skin. This junction allows nutrients to pass through the dermis to the avascular epidermis.

The *dermis* is a richly vascular layer consisting largely of fibroblasts and collagen. Its collagen matrix supports and separates the epidermis from the subcutaneous fat layer. Papillae project up into the epidermis to provide nourishment to the living epidermal cells. In addition, the dermis contains a large network of sensory nerve fibers. These fibers provide sensations of pain, itch, and temperature. *Meissner's corpuscles* are encapsulated end organs of touch found in the dermal papillae

close to the epidermis. They are most numerous in hairless portions of the skin such as the volar surfaces of the hands, fingers, feet, toes, lips, eyelids, nipples, and tip of the tongue. The dermis also contains autonomic nerve fibers that innervate blood vessels, the *arrectores pilorum* muscles, the sweat glands, sebaceous glands, hair, and nails.

The *sweat glands* in the dermis control thermoregulation by releasing water through the skin. The *eccrine sweat glands* are distributed throughout the body except for the lip margins, eardrums, nail beds, inner surface of the prepuce, and the glans penis.[7] The *apocrine sweat glands* are larger and deeper than the eccrine glands and secrete an odorless white fluid (sweat) in response to emotional or physical stimuli. They are located in the axillae, around the nipples, areolae, anogenital area, eyelids, and external ears. Body odor in adolescence comes from bacterial decomposition of the sweat produced by these glands; activation of these glands earlier than adolescence should be investigated.

The *sebaceous glands* arise from the hair follicles deep within the dermis. The oil produced by these glands is called *sebum,* a lipid-rich substance that helps lubricate the skin and hair. The level of oil produced is related to hormonal levels in the bloodstream (primarily testosterone) and therefore varies throughout the life span. In the newborn, the production of sebum is accelerated while still under the influence of maternal hormones, and the glands themselves become hyperplastic until maternal hormones wane in the infant's body. This stimulated activity results in skin conditions in the newborn such as neonatal acne and tinea versicolor, conditions that appear again in adolescence.

The nail bed starts to keratinze to form a hard, protective plate around 8 to 10 weeks of gestation. It sits on a highly vascular bed that gives each nail its color. The *cuticle,* or *eponychium,* the white crescent-shaped area at the end of the nail matrix, is the root and site of nail growth. It is covered by a layer of stratum corneum that pushes up and over the lower part of the nail body. The paronychium is the soft tissue that surrounds the nail border on each digit.

The *subcutaneous* layer of the skin is composed of adipose tissue. This layer connects the dermis to underlying organs and provides insulation and shock absorption and generates heat for the body. It also provides a reserve of calories for use by the body.

DEVELOPMENT

Hair and nails are part of the anatomical structure of the skin. Hair is formed by epidermal cells that go deep into the dermal layer of the skin and consists of a *root,* a *shaft,* and a *follicle.* The loop of capillaries at the base of the follicle, known as the *papilla,* supplies nourishment to the hair to promote growth. *Melanocytes,* which lie in the hair shaft, supply color to the hair. In the newborn, all the hair on the body consists of fine *lanugo* hair—all of the hair is in the same phase of growth. As the lanugo is shed, it is replaced by hair that is increased in diameter and coarseness; the first

to form are *vellus* hairs, which are short, fine, soft, and nonpigmented hairs on the body, and then adult-type *terminal* hairs, which are coarse, thick, longer, and pigmented, and grow on the scalp and eyebrows. During adolescence, vellus hairs located in androgen-sensitive areas (pubic area, axillae, and the face in males) undergo a similar transition to terminal hairs.

PHYSIOLOGIC VARIATIONS

The stratum corneum does not develop until between 23 and 25 weeks of gestation. Extremely premature infants are born without this critical top layer of skin and, therefore, have no protective barrier and are not able to control water loss. They need protection from the environment and can tolerate only the least amount of touching. The term newborn has a fully functional stratum corneum, but it is only about 60% the thickness of adult skin depending on the location. A thin stratum corneum with the larger body surface area-to-weight ratio of the newborn may allow substances placed on the skin to pass more easily through to the bloodstream.[1]

The blood vessels continue to mature into a more adult pattern until 3 months after birth. The nerves in the skin are small and poorly myelinated at birth. The growth and myelination of the nerve fibers continue on into puberty (Table 6-1).

SYSTEM-SPECIFIC HISTORY

A careful age-appropriate history is critical to making an accurate assessment of the skin (Table 6-2). The healthcare provider needs to gather data related to current skin problems, any significant past medical history, and family history of similar problems. Skin care routines and any recent changes in skin, hair, or nail care habits should be addressed. Sun exposure habits and application of sunscreens are also important considerations.

TABLE 6-1 STRUCTURAL AND FUNCTIONAL DIFFERENCES OF SKIN

Structure	Preterm Infant	Term Newborn Infant	Child	Adolescent	Significance/Implications
Epidermis	Thinner Cells more compressed Fewer layers of stratum corneum Increased transepidermal water loss	Stratum corneum appears as adherent cell layer Greater absorption because higher skin surface to body weight ratio	Stratum is getting thicker, starts to appear as separate sheet of cells	Stratum corneum appears as separate sheet of cells Adult-like pattern	Thin skin of infant and child allows for easy absorption of products placed on skin Apply thin layer of topical medications
Dermis	Less cohesion between layers Fewer, immature elastin fibers Thinner than in older infants	Fewer immature elastin fibers Thinner than adult	Elastin fibers are maturing	Full complement of elastin fibers	Decreased elasticity Increased tendency to blister
Melanosomes	Melanin production low	Melanin production low Final overall skin tone is shown in genitalia where the scrotum, labia have darker pigment	Melanin production after 6 months of age like adult	Adult pattern of melanin production	Infants, young children need sunscreen/complete sun block because can sunburn easily

Eccrine sweat glands	May be more typical of fetus than adult Ducts are patent but do not produce sweat	Equivalent in structure to adult Dense distribution due to body surface area	Distribution starts becoming less dense as child grows, but has decreased neurological control until 2-3 years old	Distribution is less dense than in infant, child	Reduced sweating capability, especially first 13-24 days of life Decreased response to thermal stress
Apocrine sweat glands	Not present	Small, nonfunctional Devoid of secretory granules	Start to appear but generally nonfunctional in childhood	Apocrine sweating in response to mechanical, pharmacological stimuli	Secrete oily substance in adolescent
Sebaceous glands	Large and active	Large and active but diminish rapidly in size and activity several weeks after birth	Decreased activity throughout childhood	Large, active, produce sebum in large amounts	Infants get acne as do teens because of hormone activity and large active sebaceous glands

Continued

TABLE 6-1   STRUCTURAL AND FUNCTIONAL DIFFERENCES OF SKIN—CONT'D

Structure	Preterm Infant	Term Newborn Infant	Child	Adolescent	Significance/Implications
Nervous and vascular systems	Vascular system not fully organized Most nerves are small in diameter Sensory and autonomic nerves are unmyelinated, typically fetal in structure Meissner's touch receptors* not fully formed	Vascular system fully organized after 3 months Most nerves are small in diameter Sensory autonomic nerves are unmyelinated Cutaneous nerve network not fully developed Meissner's touch receptors not fully formed	Cutaneous network continuing to develop	Cutaneous network of nerves may continue to develop into adolescence Rest of nervous, vascular systems are in adult pattern	
Hair	Lanugo may be present Hair growth is synchronous	Lanugo covering body often shed within 10-14 days Vellus and terminal hairs appear quickly after birth Hair growth is synchronous	Vellus and terminal hairs present Hair growth is asynchronous	Vellus and terminal hairs present Hair growth is asynchronous	Dry, dull, and brittle hair may indicate protein-calorie malnutrition

*Meissner's touch receptors are encapsulated end organs of touch found in dermal papillae close to epidermis.

TABLE 6-2 INFORMATION GATHERING AT KEY DEVELOPMENTAL STAGES

Age	Questions to Ask
Newborn	*At birth*: History of skin trauma at birth or significant bruises to face/body? Presence of skin tags, dimples, cysts? Any extra digits? Moles or nevus? Hair or nail variations present at birth?
Infant	*Diaper history:* Type of disposable wipes used? *Skin care history:* Types of soap, moisturizing/cleansing lotion, other lotions, emollients, creams, oils? *Dress habits:* Amounts/types of clothing in relation to environmental temperature, how clothing is washed, use of detergents, fabric softeners, dryer sheets? *Home environment:* Temperature, humidity, type of home heating? Air conditioning? *Feeding history:* Breast or bottle, type of formula, what foods introduced and when?
Toddler	History of eating large amounts of yellow fruits, vegetables? History of prolonged crawling on hands, knees without protective clothing? History of rubbing head against furniture/walls?
Preschooler	Eating habits/types of food? History of exposure to communicable diseases? Pets/animal exposure? History of dry skin, eczema, urticaria, pruritus, nasal allergy, asthma? History of nail biting, hair twisting?
School-age child	History of skin injuries: cuts, falls, fractures, need for sutures? Any unexplained scarring? Outdoor exposure to plants during hiking, camping, picnics? Bee stings, contact with plants resulting in allergic reactions, dog bite?
Adolescent	History of skin/hair changes, acne? Acne treatments used? Sports-related injuries? Body tattooing, ritual scarring, piercing? Were they done professionally using sterile techniques/supplies? Problems/infections related to these practices?
Environmental risks	Exposure to tobacco smoke? Contact with chemical cleaning agents/other chemicals at home, school, work? Exposure to chemicals, toxins from parent's work?

Preterm Infant Skin History

The preterm infant's skin is particularly vulnerable to insult. Information gathering for this age group includes the following questions: Any history of wounds from line placement (i.e., subclavian, jugular) or chest tubes in the neonatal intensive care unit (NICU)? History of umbilical or radial artery catheterization? History of prolonged phototherapy or infiltrated IVs? Thermal burns from exposure to heated water bed, radiant warmer, transcutaneous oxygen monitor, or heated humidified air in an isolette? History of repeated heel sticks, reaction to adhesive tape removers, or solutions containing topical iodophor (i.e., Betadine or benzoin) from removal of endotracheal or nasotracheal tubes or monitor leads in the NICU?

General Information Gathering for Skin Conditions

Recent changes in skin, hair, or nails including dryness, pruritus, sores, rashes, lumps, color, texture, odor? What signs or symptoms are present (itching, pain, exudates, bleeding, color changes)? Where is the problem located? When did it start, sequence of occurrence, rapidity of onset, date of recurrence? Recent exposure to drugs, environmental or occupational toxins, or person with similar condition? History of recent travel? What has been done to treat the problem, including medications (over-the-counter [OTC] or prescription) and/or lotions or other emollients applied? Did the problem get better or worse?

PHYSICAL ASSESSMENT

The skin is one of the most accessible and easily examined organs of the body and is often the organ of most concern to children, adolescents, and parents. A complete examination of the skin using a consistent, systematic approach will increase the likelihood that important findings critical to making a diagnosis will not be missed. Be deliberate and methodical. Avoid making a quick diagnosis after only a brief observation of the skin. Dermatology has its own language. Using the correct terminology facilitates accurate description of skin lesions. A *skin lesion* refers to any variations or skin change. If the inspection and palpation of the skin reveal a lesion, more examination is necessary. Skin lesions may be *primary* or *secondary* (Tables 6-3 and 6-4).

Rashes cannot be diagnosed over the phone, and as simple as it sounds, it is important to conduct a complete skin examination before making a diagnosis. It is usually very easy to do a complete exam on a naked newborn, but there may be a great deal of resistance from many adolescents to the idea of a complete skin exam. When the child or adolescent is uncomfortable being completely undressed because of developmental stage or cultural belief, then the exam must be conducted using a systematic approach that divides the skin into areas that are sequentially uncovered and examined and then re-covered before going on to the next area. In younger children, this may prevent unnecessary cooling of the skin.

Inspection

Inspection of the skin is best conducted using natural light. A magnifying glass and a measuring tool such as a flat, clear ruler will be helpful for examining small skin lesions and moles. It may be necessary to follow a lesion's progress for several weeks. A light for transillumination of lesions or for closer inspection also may be helpful.

Pediatric Pearls

Transparent paper tape is very useful for recording the size and shape of a lesion. Place the tape on skin lesion and draw around the perimeter of the lesion on the tape. Then tape can be placed in the chart and referred to during each subsequent visit to see whether the lesion is growing or responding to treatment.

Nails should be examined for shape, color, and texture. Nail changes may be an early sign of systemic disease. Artificial nails or nail polish can interfere with the assessment. Inspect the curvature of the nail for clubbing

TABLE 6-3 PRIMARY LESIONS

Name	Photo	Description	Examples of Conditions
Macule/ patch		Flat, circumscribed lesion of any size, <1 cm is macule; >1 cm is patch; lesions usually rounded but may be oval, can be vascular, hyperpigmented, or hypopigmented	Freckle, café au lait spots, vitiligo, flat mole (nevus), blue-gray macules of the neonate (Mongolian spots), port-wine stain
Papule		Circumscribed elevated lesions <1 cm	Molluscum contagiosum, papular urticaria, elevated moles, wart
Plaque		Circumscribed elevated disc-shaped lesion >1 cm; commonly formed by confluence of papules	Atopic dermatitis, lichen simplex chronicus (neurodermatitis), tinea corporis
Nodule		Circumscribed, elevated, usually solid lesion that measures 0.5-2 cm; may be in epidermis or extend deeper	Fibromas, neurofibromas, intradermal nevi, erythema nodosum, hemangioma, pyogenic granuloma
Cyst*		Elevated, circumscribed, encapsulated lesion in dermis or subcutaneous layer filled with liquid/ semisolid material	Sebaceous cyst, cystic acne
Vesicle		Sharply circumscribed, elevated, fluid-containing lesion that measures ≤0.5 cm	Herpes simplex, varicella, insect bite

Continued

TABLE 6-3 PRIMARY LESIONS—CONT'D

Name	Photo	Description	Examples of Conditions
Bulla		Sharply circumscribed, elevated, fluid-containing lesion that measures ≥1 cm	Contact dermatitis, epidermolysis bullosa, pemphigus vulgaris, burn, bullous impetigo
Wheal		Distinctive type of solid elevation formed by local, superficial, transient edema; white to pink-pale red in color; blanches with pressure, varies in size, shape	Urticaria, insect bite, dermographia, erythema multiforme
Comedones		Plugged secretions of horny material retained within pilosebaceous follicle; may be flesh-colored, closed (whiteheads); brown/black, open (blackheads)	Acne
Burrows		Linear lesion produced by tunneling of animal parasite in stratum corneum	Scabies, cutaneous larva migrans (creeping eruption)
Telangiectasia*		Fine, irregular, red lines produced by capillary dilation	Rosacea

*Cyst, comedones, telangiectasia images are from Habif T: *Clinical dermatology: a color guide to diagnosis and therapy,* St Louis, 2004, Mosby.

or spooning and feel the surface for ridges. Changes in coloration or splinter hemorrhages should be noted. Finally, check the periungual tissue and note any redness, edema, induration, or tenderness. Absence or atrophy of the nails in the newborn period may indicate a congenital syndrome and should be evaluated further.

Hair should be examined carefully. Be sure to assess terminal and vellus hairs for changes. Note distribution, color, and quantity. If there are areas of hair loss, determine whether the hair is broken or burned off or whether the hair is absent. Check for any lesions, dryness, oiliness, scaling, or infestation on the scalp.

TABLE 6-4 SECONDARY LESIONS

Name	Photo	Description	Example of Diseases
Scale		Formed by accumulation of compact desquamation of stratum corneum layers; may be greasy, yellowish in color; silvery, fine, barely visible or large, adherent, and lamellar	Seborrheic dermatitis Psoriasis Pityriasis alba Tinea versicolor Ichthyosis
Fissure		Dry, moist, linear, often painful, cleavage from epidermis to dermis that results from marked drying; long-standing inflammation, thickening, loss of elasticity of integument	Chronic dermatoses Intertrigo Atopic dermatitis Ichthyosis
Lichenif- ication		Rough, thickened epidermis secondary to persistent rubbing, itching, or skin irritation; often involves flexor surface of extremity	Atopic dermatitis Chronic dermatitis
Scar		Permanent fibrotic skin changes that develop following damage to dermis; initially pink/ violet in color, fading to white, shiny, sclerotic area *Keloid:* pink, smooth, rubbery; often traversed by telangiectatic vessels; increases in size long after healing of lesion; differentiated from hypertropic scars because surface of keloid scar tends to be beyond original wound area	Surgery Healed wound Stretch marks Keloid Herpes zoster Burn

Continued

TABLE 6-4 SECONDARY LESIONS—CONT'D

Name	Photo	Description	Example of Diseases
Erosions		Moist, slightly depressed vesicular lesion in which all or part of epidermis has been lost; heals without scarring	Impetigo Eczematous diseases Intertrigo Candidiasis
Purpura		Flat lesion; petechiae if pinpoint; does not blanch to pressure; larger areas of bruising may be present	Henoch-Schönlein Purpura fulminans

Data from Eichenfield L, Frieden I, Esterly NB: *Textbook of neonatal dermatology,* Philadelphia, 2001, Saunders; Seidel HM, Ball JW, Dains JE, Benedict GW: *Mosby's guide to physical examination,* ed 5, St Louis, 2003, Mosby; Infoderm.com, Galderma Laboratories, LP, 2002.

Palpation

Palpation of the skin should be done with warm hands. Use gloves if you think the child or adolescent may have an infectious lesion. Palpate skin temperature using the back of your hand, and compare the temperature of one area of skin to another area of skin using both hands. Temperature cannot be assessed accurately through gloves, and presence of a fever should always be checked using a thermometer. Check for *skin turgor* (resiliency or elasticity) by gently pinching a fold of the child's skin over the abdomen between your thumb and forefinger, then release it. *Skin turgor* can give important clues to the hydration and nutritional status of a child. How long the skin remains tented after it is released will provide clues to the degree of dehydration (Table 6-5).

CULTURAL CONSIDERATIONS

In dark-skinned individuals, color variations may be difficult to determine. Looking at the sclerae, conjunctivae, buccal mucosa, lips, tongue, and/or nail beds will assist with identifying color hue in very dark-skinned individuals. Variations of skin coloring are normal in persons with pigmented skin, including lighter pigment on palms, soles of

TABLE 6-5 ESTIMATING DEHYDRATION IN AN INFANT OR YOUNG CHILD

Return to Normal After the Pinch	Degree of Dehydration
<2 seconds	<5% loss of body weight
2-3 seconds	5%-8% loss of body weight
3-4 seconds	9%-10% loss of body weight
>4 seconds	>10% loss of body weight

Data from Seidel HM, Ball JW, Dains JE, Benedict GW: *Mosby's guide to physical examination,* ed 5, St Louis, 2003, Mosby.

feet, and nail beds. Freckling of the buccal cavity, gums, and tongue is also common. Areas that get regular exposure to the sun may be pigmented much darker.

Hair, skin, and nail care practices vary widely from culture to culture. Timing of a child's first hair cut is one such cultural variation. In many Asian and Latin cultures, it is common to shave the infant's head at 3 to 9 months of age in the belief the hair will grow in thick and long. In some cultures, shaving of the head is part of a religious ceremony. Some African-American communities believe an infant's hair should not be cut until he or she begins walking. Preference for skin, hair, and nail care products varies both culturally and in accordance with the type of skin and hair. The healthcare provider should support cultural practices that are not harmful and do not cause a skin problem for the child or adolescent.

ABNORMAL CONDITIONS

Skin Lesions

The *morphology* or characteristic form and structure of skin lesions should be identified when any condition is noted during the assessment of the skin. Attention to the distribution and pattern of lesions will assist in making a diagnosis. The *distribution* refers to the location of skin findings, whereas *pattern* refers to the specific anatomical or physiological arrangement of the lesions. Note the shape of skin lesions and whether they are clustered together or scattered. The border or margin, any associated findings such as central clearing, and the pigmentation of the lesion also should be identified. Find and study the

primary lesion and examine the distribution of any skin lesions or skin variations. Skin lesions also should be classified as primary or secondary (see Tables 6-4 and 6-5). Common newborn and infant skin conditions are presented in Table 6-6.

⌐⊙═ Key Points

Accurate charting using the correct terminology allows other healthcare practitioners to "visualize" the skin lesions and provide the necessary follow-up to evaluate whether there is change or improvement in lesions. Avoid the use of a specific diagnosis (e.g., diaper rash, candidiasis) when describing a lesion in the objective physical findings.

⬚ CHARTING

14-Month-Old With Candidial Diaper Rash

Skin: discrete, red papules and pustules over the perineum with satellite lesions over the legs and abdomen; otherwise skin lightly pigmented and clear.

⬚ CHARTING

15-Year-Old With Moderate Acne Vulgaris

Skin: moderate comedones over nose and cheeks, pustular lesions on forehead, no nodules or cyst noted. Skin oily with moderate papular, erythematous lesions over upper back.

TABLE 6-6   COMMON CONDITIONS IN NEWBORN AND INFANT SKIN

Condition	Photo	Description	Significance/ Treatment
Acrocyanosis		Bluish coloration of hands and feet present at birth; may persist up to 24 hours; circumoral cyanosis also may be present	Benign color variation in newborn; no treatment needed if gone after 24 hours
Accessory tragi		Pedunculated, flesh-colored, soft, round papules usually arising on or near the tragus	May occur anywhere from corner of ear to mouth and require removal by careful surgical dissection; do not confuse with skin tags, do not tie off with suture
Jaundice		Yellow coloration of skin and sclera caused by deposition of bile pigment resulting from hyperbilirubinemia	Color variation should be noted; bilirubin level should be drawn to determine level of jaundice
Cutis marmorata		Reddish-blue mottling or marbling of skin in response to changes in temperature; caused by dilation of capillaries and venules	Benign color variation; no treatment needed unless it does not disappear with skin warming

TABLE 6-6 COMMON CONDITIONS IN NEWBORN AND INFANT SKIN—CONT'D

Condition	Photo	Description	Significance/ Treatment
Erythema toxicum		Small white to yellow papules, vesicles with erythematous base; occurs in response to rubbing; starts as early as 24 hours of life, may continue until 2 weeks old	Common benign skin lesion in newborn; eosinophils in smear from papule confirms diagnosis
Miliaria rubra, m. crystallina, m. pustulosa		Clear, thin vesicles or discrete erythematous papules seen primarily over forehead, neck, in creases, or groin; occurs as a result of obstructed sweat glands in humid environment	Benign skin lesion in newborn; can be treated by eliminating precipitating factors such as heat, humidity, too many clothes
Transient neonatal pustular melanosis		Vesicles that rupture leaving collaret of scale and pigmented macule; macules may remain for up to 3 months after birth	Benign skin lesion requiring no treatment
Impetigo		Contagious infection of skin caused by staphylococcal or streptococcal bacterial invasion of epidermis; begins as small erythematous macule that changes to vesicle or bulla and often ruptures leaving honey-colored crust	Abnormal skin condition that can occur anywhere on body; correct diagnosis, treatment with appropriate antibiotics is important to limit contagion

Jaundice photo from Chaudhry B, Harvey D: *Mosby's color atlas and text of pediatrics and child health*, St Louis, 2001, Mosby.

REFERENCES

1. Eichenfield L, Frieden I, Esterly NB: *Textbook of neonatal dermatology,* Philadelphia, 2001, Saunders.
2. Bowlby J: Nature of a child's tie to his mother, *Intern J Psychoanal* 39:350-373, 1958.
3. Bowlby J: *Attachment and loss,* New York, 1969, Basic Books.
4. Klaus M, Kennell J: *Maternal infant bonding,* St Louis, 1976, Mosby.
5. Spitz RA, Cobliner WG: *The first year of life,* New York, 1965, International Universities.
6. Habif TP: *Clinical dermatology: a color guide to diagnosis and therapy,* St Louis, 2004, Mosby.
7. Seidel HM, Ball JW, Dains JE, Benedict GW: *Mosby's guide to physical examination,* ed 5, St Louis, 2003, Mosby.

CHAPTER 7

HEART AND VASCULAR SYSTEM

Elizabeth Tong

DEVELOPMENT

The heart begins to form in the fetus by the end of the third week after conception. A crescent-shaped structure is formed that fuses at the midline to create a single linear heart tube (Figure 7-1). As the primitive heart tube elongates, it differentiates into the *atria, ventricles, bulbus cordis,* and *truncus arteriosus.* The conduction system also begins to form during this time, and by day 23 after conception the heart begins to beat. Valve formation begins around the fourth to fifth week after conception, and the formation of the heart is complete by the eighth week after conception. Any early changes in this process caused by genetic, maternal, or external environmental factors can lead to structural malformations of the heart.

During fetal life, the lung sacs are collapsed and blood is oxygenated through the placenta. Oxygenated blood travels from the placenta to the heart via the umbilical veins and *ductus venosus* to the *inferior vena cava* (IVC) and into the *right atrium* (RA). Blood then streams to the *left atrium* (LA) through a *patent foramen ovale* (PFO) and into the *left ventricle* (LV), which pumps it out the *aorta* (Figure 7-2). The less saturated venous blood traveling from the

superior vena cava (SVC), and *coronary sinus* also flows to the right atrium, but is directed toward the *right ventricle* (RV) and *pulmonary artery* (PA). High pulmonary vascular resistance limits blood flow into the lungs and redirects it through the *patent ductus arteriosus* (PDA) to the descending aorta and lower body. The right ventricle is the dominant ventricle in the fetus because it ejects 55% of the cardiac output.[1]

With a baby's first breaths, pulmonary vascular resistance falls, causing a dramatic increase in pulmonary blood flow. The ensuing increase in pulmonary venous return to the heart raises LA pressure, causing closure of the PFO. Arterial oxygen saturation increases as a result of improved oxygenation by the lungs. This higher saturation promotes functional closure of the PDA by 10 to 15 hours after birth, with complete anatomical closure occurring by 2 weeks of age.[2]

ANATOMY AND PHYSIOLOGY

Anatomy of the Postnatal Heart

The heart is composed of four chambers. The upper chambers (atria) are low-pressure

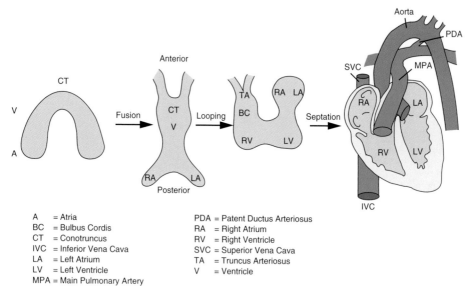

A = Atria
BC = Bulbus Cordis
CT = Conotruncus
IVC = Inferior Vena Cava
LA = Left Atrium
LV = Left Ventricle
MPA = Main Pulmonary Artery

PDA = Patent Ductus Arteriosus
RA = Right Atrium
RV = Right Ventricle
SVC = Superior Vena Cava
TA = Truncus Arteriosus
V = Ventricle

Figure 7-1 Fetal development of the heart.

receiving chambers, and the lower chambers, (ventricles), are high-pressure pumping chambers. The heart is further divided into right and left sides. The RA receives deoxygenated blood from the body, and the RV pumps it out the pulmonary artery to the lungs to become oxygenated. The LA receives oxygenated blood from the lungs, and the LV pumps it out the aorta to the body (Figure 7-3). The LV operates at a higher pressure than the RV. This normal circulation occurs in series, and there is no mixing of deoxygenated and oxygenated blood.

There are four valves in the heart that regulate blood flow between the atria and ventricles (atrioventricular, or AV, valves) and between the ventricles and great vessels (semilunar valves). The *tricuspid valve* on the right and the *mitral valve* on the left are the AV valves (Figure 7-3). The *pulmonic valve,* located at the base of the pulmonary artery between the right ventricle and the pulmonary artery, and the *aortic valve,* located at the base of the aorta between the aorta and left ventricle, are the semilunar valves. Closure of

these valves produces the heart sounds commonly referred to as "lub-dub" (S_1, S_2).

Physiological Variations

In preterm infants, the ductus arteriosus can remain open for several weeks after birth, causing hemodynamic instability. Medical intervention with the drug *indomethacin* or surgical ligation of the ductus is often required to stabilize the infant.

System-Specific History

Comprehensive information gathering at key developmental stages is an important part of a comprehensive cardiac evaluation.

Prenatal History

Maternal infections such as rubella, coxsackie, and other viruses contracted during pregnancy can be associated with congenital heart disease (CHD) or myocarditis. Medications, as well as alcohol and other drugs, also may act as teratogens on the developing fetus. For example, patients on lithium therapy have an increased

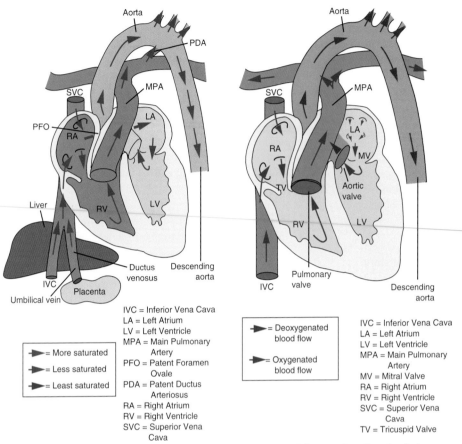

Figure **7-2** Fetal cardiac circulation.

Figure **7-3** Postnatal cardiac circulation.

risk of having a baby with Ebstein's anomaly of the tricuspid valve. There is also an increased risk of premature ductal closure if a mother takes nonsteroidal anti-inflammatory drugs (NSAIDs) and aspirin regularly during pregnancy.[3] NSAIDs and aspirin also have been shown to increase the risk for persistent pulmonary hypertension of the newborn (PPHN).[4]

Maternal medical conditions associated with an increased risk of the fetus developing CHD include diabetes mellitus that can cause cardiomyopathy, transposition of the great arteries (TGA), ventricular septal defect (VSD), patent ductus arteriosus (PDA), and systemic lupus erythematosus, which can be associated with congenital heart block.

Birth History

Apgar scores for children with CHD are usually within normal range, although points may be taken off for color if the child has cyanotic heart disease.

Children with CHD usually have a birth weight within normal range; however, infants with TGA and infants born of diabetic mothers often can be large for gestational age.

Circumstances surrounding labor and delivery, such as premature rupture of membranes, traumatic birth, or meconium aspiration should be elicited to help distinguish whether specific symptoms of lethargy or respiratory distress are due to heart disease, neurological disease, pulmonary disease, or infection.

⌐═ Key Points

Babies with CHD may have tachypnea (rapid, shallow breathing) and tachycardia but typically do not present in respiratory distress (i.e., retractions, grunting, nasal flaring) unless there is a significant increase in pulmonary blood flow or poor systemic output with acidosis.

Postnatal History

Abnormalities in color, feeding patterns, weight gain, activity level, and an increased frequency of respiratory infections all give clues to the possibility of CHD in an infant. Symptoms of CHD often show up with the first feeding because the increased work of feeding raises oxygen consumption and requires a greater cardiac output. Children experiencing congestive heart failure (CHF) may appear pale and sweaty (particularly on the forehead), and they may have an increased respiratory rate, decreased feeding tolerance, and failure to thrive. Children with cyanotic heart disease often turn dark blue or ruddy in color when they cry because the prolonged expiratory phase increases right-to-left shunting. Hypercyanotic spells can occur in infants and children with cyanotic heart disease, most often those with tetralogy of Fallot. Hypercyanotic spells in infants are often described by parents as staring spells or periods of extreme irritability. The infant's color is dark blue and respirations are rapid, deep, and occasionally labored.[1] Older children may squat or assume a knee-chest position, which increases systemic vascular resistance and promotes blood flow to the lungs. Breath-holding spells in young children often can be confused with hypercyanotic spells because both can cause

children to become quite cyanotic. Thus eliciting details about the events leading up to a spell and a description of chest movement and respiratory effort are important pieces of information that can help in distinguishing between the two events.[1]

Infants and children with left-to-right shunting lesions such as VSD, AV canal, PDA, or unobstructed total anomalous pulmonary venous return (TAPVR) often have a history of frequent respiratory infections and failure to thrive resulting from the increased blood flow to the lungs. CHD also can cause a decrease in exercise tolerance. **An important piece of history to obtain is whether the child can keep up with other children of the same age or requires frequent periods of rest.**

It is also important to document any history of acquired heart disease such as *rheumatic heart disease* from untreated streptococcal infections, or *Kawasaki's disease* with resulting coronary artery aneurysms. Symptoms of Kawasaki's disease include a sudden high fever of 5 days duration; bright red lips and a strawberry-colored tongue; bilateral nonexudative conjunctivitis; edema and erythema of the palms and soles of the feet; enlarged lymph nodes; and a rash resulting in postinflammatory coronary artery aneurysms.[1]

Family History

Most congenital heart disease (CHD) is due to a combination of genetic, maternal, and environmental factors. The incidence of CHD in the general population is 0.8%, but after one child with CHD has been born into a family, the risk for recurrence in future children increases to about 2% to 3%.[2] Therefore, it is important to elicit a history of any previous children born with CHD, as well as any history of miscarriages or known fetal CHD. Recurrence risks are greatest for those lesions that are most common in the general population (VSD, atrial septal defect [ASD], and PDA). If either parent has CHD themselves, the risk for having an affected child ranges from 2% to

15% depending on the lesion. This also is true if the underlying cause is unknown. However, if a transmissible genetic cause is identified, then the risk for recurrence can be as high as 50% as in inheritance of autosomal dominant transmission such as Marfan's syndrome.

A family history of sudden death, syncope (passing out), or arrhythmias provides important clues in the diagnosis of long QT syndrome and hypertrophic cardiomyopathy (HCM). Many congenital syndromes also have an association with CHD, such as Marfan's syndrome, Noonan's syndrome, DiGeorge syndrome, and Down syndrome. It is important to ask whether there is a family history of any of these syndromes and to refer any child with a confirmed diagnosis to a cardiologist for evaluation.

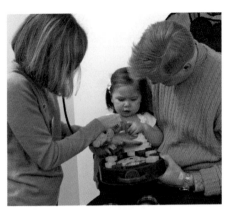

Figure **7-5** Decreasing fear of the cardiac examination through play.

PHYSICAL ASSESSMENT

The cardiac examination must be systematic and tailored to the child's developmental level (Figures 7-4 and 7-5). In addition, **findings should not be taken in isolation. A complete evaluation must be done before any conclusions can be made about the significance of any single abnormality** (Table 7-1).

It is important to consistently plot height, weight, and head circumference in children under 2 years of age to evaluate whether the

growth rate is proportional.[1] Temperature, heart rate, and respiratory rate should be measured and assessed. Fever and respiratory distress both can elevate heart rate. Blood pressure should be routinely measured throughout infancy, childhood, and adolescence. *Coarctation of the aorta* and systemic *hypertension* can go undetected if blood pressure measurements are omitted during well-child visits. Blood pressure in infants should be measured in all four extremities, or at a minimum in the right arm and in one leg to detect a coarctation of the aorta. In children, simultaneous palpation of the radial and femoral pulses is also important in assessing whether a coarctation may be present.

Inspection

Note general appearance and activity and whether the child is active, alert, lethargic, or acutely ill. Note nutritional status and body size with regard to the proportion of weight to length or height and head size. Also, note whether any unusual facial or other external features are present that may indicate the presence of a syndrome or chromosomal anomaly, and note any surgical scars on the anterior sternum or lateral thorax and chest. An incision on the sternum usually indicates a previous open-heart procedure. A right thoracotomy

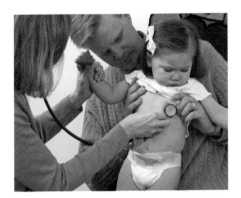

Figure **7-4** Cardiac examination of the toddler.

TABLE 7-1   ASSESSMENT AND RANGE OF FINDINGS OF THE CARDIOVASCULAR EXAMINATION

Assessment	Range of Findings
Height	Normal vs. abnormal for age, proportional for weight
Weight	Normal vs. abnormal for age, proportional for height
VITAL SIGNS	
Temperature	Normal, high, low
Heart rate	Normal for age, fast, slow, regular, irregular
Respiratory rate	Normal for age, fast, slow, any signs of distress NOTE: *retractions, grunting, nasal flaring*
Blood pressure	Normal for age, high, low, pressure differential between right arm and lower leg
Oxygen saturation	Normal for cardiac physiology NOTE: *75%-85% is normal with a right-to-left shunt*
Activity level	Active, alert, lethargic
Color	Pink, cyanotic, pale, mottled
Perfusion	Warm, cool, brisk vs. slow capillary refill time, finger clubbing
Pulses	Equal, full, bounding, faint, thready
Liver edge	1-2 cm below right costal margin is normal in infants At right costal margin in children and adolescents
Precordium	Quiet, active, any heaves, thrills, sternal or thoracic scars
AUSCULTATION	
Lungs	Clear, wheezing, grunting, rales
Heart	Normal S_1, normal S_2, any abnormal splitting, any extra heart sounds, murmurs

is often a sign of a previous Blalock-Taussig (BT) shunt and a left thoracotomy may indicate a previous coarctation repair, or PDA ligation.

Color

Note whether the child is pale or cyanotic; view under natural light if possible. Cyanosis indicative of CHD is due to arterial desaturation

and may not be visible unless the oxygen saturation is 85% or less.[1,5] Arterial desaturation or *central cyanosis* is best detected in the perioral area, the mucous membranes of the mouth, the lips, and the gums. *Central cyanosis* should be distinguished from *peripheral cyanosis,* which can occur in a cold environment, and *acrocyanosis,* which in newborns is due to sluggish circulation in the fingers and toes.[1] The intensity of cyanosis is dependent on the concentration of desaturated hemoglobin and not on the actual arterial oxygen saturation. Thus an infant who has *polycythemia,* an abnormal increase in circulating erythrocytes, will appear more cyanotic than an infant who is anemic in the presence of the same degree of arterial desaturation. Therefore, it is important to follow a cyanotic infant's hemoglobin and hematocrit levels, particularly at 2 to 3 months of age, the time of normal physiological anemia. Pallor can occur in infants who are anemic or who have vasoconstriction due to *congestive heart failure* (CHF).

Clubbing

Clubbing occurs when arterial desaturation has been present for at least 6 months or longer. The fingers and toes become red and shiny, and progress to wide, thick digits with eventual loss of the normal angle between the nails and the nail beds[1] (Figure 7-6).

Palpation

Pulses need to be evaluated for their presence or absence, intensity, timing, symmetry, and whether the pulse is regular or irregular, weak or bounding. A comparison also should be made as to right and left symmetry and quality of pulses in the upper and lower extremities. Absence or a weaker pulse in the lower extremities compared to the upper extremities

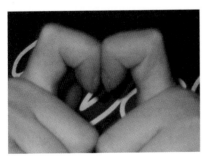

Figure **7-6** Clubbing of nails resulting from arterial desaturation.

is diagnostic of *coarctation of the aorta.* A strong pedal pulse is a good indication that there is no coarctation. Irregular pulses may be due to an *arrhythmia.* Weak and thready pulses may indicate poor perfusion or shock, whereas bounding pulses are usually noted with aortic run-off lesions such as a PDA, AV malformation, or aortic insufficiency.[1] *Peripheral perfusion* is also important to assess, especially in infants. Normally, extremities should be warm to the touch and have a brisk capillary refill time (CRT), a quick measure of cardiac output. One should be aware that older children with cardiac conditions may not have good distal pulses on one side or the other because of previous cardiac catheterizations or cardiac surgeries.

Pediatric Pearls

It is not unusual to feel bounding pulses in premature infants because of their lack of subcutaneous fat and the higher incidence of a patent ductus arteriosus in this population.[5]

Normal liver size is usually 1 to 2 cm below the right costal margin. In conditions of abnormal cardiac position, or situs (positional abnormalities), the liver edge is midline or on the left side of the abdomen. When *hepatomegaly* or liver engorgement occurs, it is a consistent indicator of right heart failure.

⊙━ਜ਼ **Key Points**

Palpation of the liver for position and size is a critical indicator of cardiac output and overall fluid status in infants and children with heart failure.

The precordium should be palpated to determine the location of the *point of maximal impulse,* or PMI. The PMI is important in determining ventricular overload, cardiomegaly, and the presence or absence of thrills. Normally, the PMI is felt at the apex in the left midclavicular line, indicating LV dominance. However, it is normal for newborns and infants to have a greater RV impulse, with the PMI felt at the left lower sternal border. A PMI that is diffuse and rises slowly is called a *heave,* and a PMI that is sharp and well localized is known as a *tap.*[1]

A *thrill* indicates turbulent blood flow and is never normal.[2] It is felt as a vibratory sensation, and should be examined not only on the precordium but also in the suprasternal notch and over the carotid arteries. Precordial thrills are best felt with the palm of the hand, whereas thrills in the suprasternal notch and over the carotid arteries are best felt with the fingertips.[1]

Auscultation

Auscultation of heart sounds in children should be done in a stepwise fashion and with both the diaphragm and the bell of a stethoscope to elicit both high (diaphragm) and low (bell) frequency sounds (Figure 7-7). Most children have a thin chest wall and heart sounds are louder than in adults. However, the faster heart rate can make it difficult to accurately distinguish the heart sounds from each other.[2] Thus it is recommended that the individual heart sounds be identified and analyzed first before identifying murmurs.[1] It may be helpful to feel the wrist pulse while listening to the heart.

The *first heart sound* is called S_1 and is created by the closure of the tricuspid and mitral valves. It is usually heard best at the left lower sternal border or at the apex. A split S_1 can be a normal finding in children, but if it is abnormally wide, it may indicate a right bundle branch block, or *Ebstein's anomaly.*

The *second heart* sound is called S_2 and is created by the closure of the aortic and pulmonic valves. It is usually heard best at the left upper sternal border. Evaluation of S_2 is critical in children because it provides important clues as to the presence of structural defects and to the pressures in the heart. S_2 normally varies with respiration—split with inspiration and single or narrowly split in expiration. A fixed split, single S_2, or loud S_2 warrants further evaluation by a cardiologist. Abnormal splitting of the S_2, may indicate increased pulmonary blood flow, pulmonary valve abnormality, or a cyanotic heart condition. A loud single S_2 may indicate pulmonary hypertension or malposition of the great arteries.[2,5]

A *third heart sound* (S_3) can be a common finding in children and young adults. S_3 can be heard at the apex and is caused by vibrations in the ventricle as it fills rapidly during diastole.

A *fourth heart sound* $(S_4$ or gallop rhythm) is rare in infants and children. An S_4 is an abnormal finding and suggests decreased ventricular compliance and could indicate CHF or restrictive cardiomyopathy.[2]

Ejection clicks are extra heart sounds that occur between S_1 and S_2. When heard, they suggest a bicuspid aortic valve, pulmonary valve stenosis, truncus arteriosus, or Ebstein's anomaly. Midsystolic ejection clicks are characteristic of mitral valve prolapse.

Murmurs

Murmurs are produced when blood flows across an area that has a pressure difference and causes turbulence or disturbed flow. Murmurs should be assessed and evaluated according to their timing in the cardiac cycle, location, transmission, intensity, frequency, and quality. It is always important to note whether or not a murmur radiates to the lung fields, axilla, clavicles, or neck. A normal grading scale is used to describe a murmur's intensity (Table 7-2).

Pediatric Pearls

Murmurs are a common finding in infants and children and do not always signify heart disease.

Non-pathologic murmurs are often referred to as *physiologic murmurs,* and are influenced by increased cardiac output, and are not present

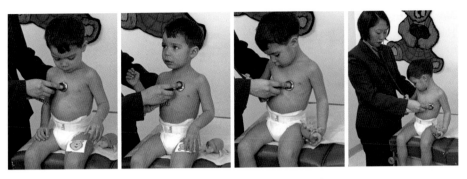

Figure **7-7** Auscultation of the heart sounds.

TABLE 7-2 GRADING SCALE FOR CARDIAC MURMURS

Grade	Sound
1	Barely audible and softer than usual heart sounds
2	Still soft, but about as loud as usual heart sounds
3	Louder than usual heart sounds, but without a thrill
4	Louder than usual heart sounds, and with a thrill
5	Can be heard with stethoscope barely on chest (rare)
6	Can be heard with stethoscope off chest, or with naked ear (extremely rare)

Data from Brook MM, Moore P, Van Hare G. In Rudolph AM, Kamei R, Overby K, editors: *Rudolph's fundamentals of pediatrics,* New York, 2002, McGraw-Hill; Park M: *Pediatric cardiology for practitioners,* ed 4, St Louis, 2002, Mosby.

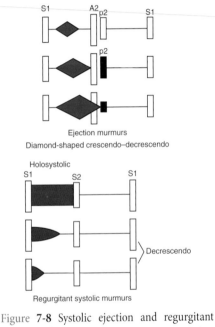

Figure **7-8** Systolic ejection and regurgitant murmurs. (Adapted from Park M: *Pediatric cardiology for practitioners,* ed 4, St Louis, 2002, Mosby, p. 24.)

at rest. Murmurs may develop or appear louder during exercise, periods of stress, or when a child is anemic or has a fever.[1]

Murmurs are described in relation to their timing during the cardiac cycle—systolic, diastolic, or continuous. Systolic murmurs occur between S_1 and S_2, and diastolic murmurs are heard after S_2. Systolic murmurs are further described as *ejection* crescendo-decrescendo or *regurgitant* long systolic-decrescendo. Figure 7-8 illustrates the difference between ejection and regurgitant murmurs in relation to when they occur in the cardiac cycle. Systolic ejection murmurs begin shortly after the first heart sound, are due to semilunar valve or great vessel stenosis, usually vary in intensity, and are diamond-shaped. They can be short or long in duration, but usually end before S_2. Regurgitant murmurs typically begin with S_1, although they usually do not obscure it, are the result of mitral or tricuspid valve insufficiency, can be long or short in duration, and are graded as mild, moderate, or severe. Holosystolic murmurs obscure S_1 at their maximal or loudest point and are usually caused by a ventricular septal defect (VSD).

Diastolic murmurs occur between S_2 and S_1 and are described as early, mid, or late. Diastolic murmurs are usually caused by aortic or pulmonic regurgitation or mitral stenosis and are never normal.

Continuous murmurs begin in systole and continue without interruption through S_2 and into diastole. They are usually caused by conditions in which vascular shunting occurs throughout the cardiac cycle, such as in PDA or a surgical aortopulmonary shunt. A continuous murmur from a PDA has a machinery-like quality, is best heard in the left clavicular area or back, and has a crescendo-decrescendo shape.[1]

The origin of a murmur provides valuable information regarding specific diagnoses and is usually found at the point where the murmur is heard the loudest. If a murmur is heard throughout the chest, the area of highest frequency will define its origin. Certain diagnoses produce murmurs that have a consistent pattern of radiation. For example, a systolic ejection murmur that radiates to the axillae and back is usually pulmonary in origin, and one that radiates to the neck and carotid arteries is typically aortic in origin. The frequency or pitch of a murmur is a good indicator of the pressure gradient across a valve or septal defect. The higher the pressure gradient, the higher the frequency of the murmur.

Physiologic vs. Pathologic Murmurs. Finally, it is important to distinguish physiologic, or innocent, murmurs from pathologic ones (Table 7-3). Innocent murmurs occur in 30% to 50% of children.[2] They are

systolic ejection murmurs that are usually heard best at the left lower sternal border (LLSB) and have a vibratory or musical quality (Figure 7-9). They tend to be short and well located. They are usually no louder than grade 2 to 3 in intensity, and are often accentuated during high output states such as exercise, stress, anemia, or febrile illness. Innocent murmurs are never purely diastolic, and usually are not associated with a diastolic murmur, except in the case of a venous hum which is a continuous murmur, a thrill, abnormal EKG or chest x-ray, cyanosis, or other symptoms of heart disease. Although they are heard most often in childhood, usually beginning around 3 to 4 years of age, innocent murmurs also may be heard in the newborn period. If a murmur is heard in the first 24 hours of life, there is a 1:12 risk of congenital heart disease being present. This decreases to 1:50 if the murmur is first noted at 1 year of age. However, if a murmur is first heard in the newborn period and persists for 12 months, then the risk for congenital heart disease increases to 3:5.[2]

DIAGNOSTIC PROCEDURES

Noninvasive Procedures

Pulse Oximetry

Pulse oximetry should be performed to verify and document the degree of central cyanosis and is an accurate way to assess arterial oxygen saturation, especially in infants. Measurements are taken from the right hand and a lower extremity to ascertain information about flow patterns through a PDA. Ideally, these measurements should be done simultaneously with two oximetry machines. After initial evaluation, the probes should then be switched and measurements taken again to account for probe variability.[2] A consistent saturation differential is considered significant. Thus an upper body oxygen (O_2) saturation of 98% and lower body saturation of 92% implies right-to-left shunting through the PDA. Patients with

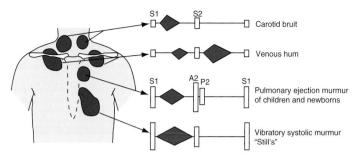

Figure **7-9** Anatomical locations of physiologic murmurs. (Adapted from Park M: P*ediatric cardiology for practitioners,* ed 4, St Louis, 2002, Mosby, p. 32.)

any reduction in arterial O_2 saturation or a significant differential should be referred for further evaluation by a cardiologist.

Chest X-ray

A chest x-ray is helpful in determining overall heart size and shape, enlargement of specific heart chambers, size and position of the great vessels, degree of pulmonary blood flow, and abdominal situs. Heart size is determined by comparing the width of the cardiac silhouette at its widest diameter to the width of the chest at its maximal internal dimension (Figure 7-10). This is referred to as the cardiothoracic (CT) ratio. A CT ratio of greater than 0.65 is considered cardiomegaly. It is important to use a good inspiratory film, as one taken on expiration may make the heart appear larger than it is. Thymic tissue in newborns also may distort the normal cardiac silhouette giving the false impression of cardiomegaly.[2]

The position of the cardiac apex provides information about ventricular enlargement. Normally, the apex points down and to the left. An upward turned apex is indicative of right ventricular enlargement, whereas an apex that is pushed more downward and leftward than normal is caused by left ventricular enlargement. The main pulmonary artery (MPA) is normally seen as a small knob at the left upper sternal border (Figure 7-10). The prominence or absence of this shadow provides clues about the size, position, and presence of the MPA.[2]

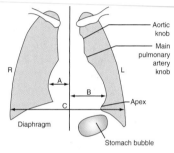

Figure **7-10** Anatomical landmarks for chest radiographs. (Adapted from Park M: *Pediatric cardiology for practitioners,* ed 4, St Louis, 2002, Mosby, p. 52.)

Pulmonary vascular markings provide important information about the degree of pulmonary blood flow and should be noted as normal, increased, or decreased. It is also important to note the heart size and shape, position of the heart apex, and determination of abdominal situs. The location of the cardiac apex is normally on the left and should be on the same side as the stomach bubble and opposite the liver shadow. When these structures are not aligned, that is, the stomach bubble is on the right and the apex is on the left, or vice versa, or the liver is midline, then heterotaxy or situs abnormality is present, which is often associated with serious heart defects.

Electrocardiogram

An electrocardiogram (EKG) provides information about the rhythm, conduction, and

TABLE 7-3 PHYSIOLOGIC OR INNOCENT MURMURS

Murmur	Characteristics/Evaluation	Age of Occurrence
Still's murmur	Localized between LLSB and apex Grade 1-3/6 systolic ejection (outflow murmur), decreasing with inspiration, when upright, or disappearing with Valsalva maneuver Low frequency, vibratory, musical in quality Often confused with VSD murmur	Most commonly heard at 2-7 years old
Peripheral pulmonic stenosis	Also known as *newborn pulmonary flow murmur* Heard at LUSB with radiation to back, axillae Grade 1-2 systolic ejection, crescendo-decrescendo	Often heard in premature infants, infants with low birth weight, and infants up to 4 months of age Need to document resolution by 4-5 months of age to rule out organic cause or valve involvement
Pulmonary ejection	Well localized to LUSB Grade 1-3/6 systolic ejection crescendo-decrescendo Heard loudest when supine and decreases or disappears with Valsalva maneuver Does not radiate Similar to ASD murmur, but S$_2$ is normal.	Common in 8- to 14-year-olds with greatest frequency in adolescents
Venous hum	Heard best just below clavicles at either RUSB or LUSB Grade 1-3/6 low-frequency continuous murmur Loudest when sitting, diminishes or disappears when supine; can be increased by turning patient's head away from the side of the murmur, and can be obliterated by light jugular vein compression; can be mistaken for PDA	Common in 3- to 6-year-olds
Supraclavicular carotid bruit	Heard above the right or left clavicle with radiation to the neck Grade 1-3/6 holosystolic, crescendo-decrescendo Decreases or diminishes with shoulder hyperextension Can be confused with murmur of aortic stenosis	Common at any age

Data from Brook MM, Moore P, Van Hare G. In Rudolph AM, Kamei R, Overby K, editors: *Rudolph's fundamentals of pediatrics*, New York, 2002, McGraw-Hill.
LLSB, Left lower sternal border; *VSD,* ventricular septal defect; *LUSB,* left upper sternal border; *ASD,* atrial septal defect; *RUSB,* right upper sternal border; *PDA,* patent ductus arteriosus.

forces of contraction in the heart and is particularly useful in the diagnosis of arrhythmias and ventricular hypertrophy. However, EKG patterns vary within diagnostic groups, and it is entirely possible for an EKG to be normal in infants with serious heart disease such as in transposition of the great arteries (TGA). **Therefore, except for arrhythmias, EKGs are used most often to confirm a diagnosis of structural CHD as opposed to establishing one.**[2]

Exercise Testing

Exercise testing or stress testing is a diagnostic tool used to evaluate chest pain in adolescents—heart block, arrhythmias or potential for arrhythmias, change in outflow gradient, and the effectiveness of medication in treating hypertension. It is also helpful for determining the safety of sports participation in patients with exercise-induced arrhythmias. During testing, adolescents are monitored for sensations of faintness, complaints of chest pain, ischemic changes or arrhythmias on EKG, and blood pressure and heart rate response. Given the potential threat of a serious arrhythmia or hemodynamic response, testing should always be performed under the supervision of a cardiologist who knows the indications and contraindications for testing and what parameters warrant terminating the test.

Echocardiogram

In many cases, cardiac ultrasound, or *echocardiogram*, has replaced cardiac catheterization as the definitive diagnostic tool for the evaluation of infants with symptomatic or suspected heart disease. An echocardiogram can be done safely and noninvasively at the bedside and provides accurate information for all age-groups including premature infants. The addition of Doppler ultrasound techniques now makes it possible to evaluate valve function and flow patterns throughout the heart and proximal vessels. This is particularly useful in quantifying degrees of shunting and obstruction. Advances in technical resolution have made

fetal cardiac echocardiography an accepted prenatal evaluation tool for parents with a family history of CHD or other risk factors. Echocardiograms are expensive, however, and they should only be ordered by a cardiologist after a thorough evaluation has been done to determine whether one is warranted. All referrals to a cardiologist should be as complete as possible and include data about the history, physical examination, chest x-ray, EKG, and oxygen saturation that have raised suspicion of CHD.

Invasive Procedures

Cardiac Catheterization

Cardiac catheterization remains the only way to directly measure pressures in the heart and precisely calculate shunt flows, pressure gradients, and cardiac output. Angiography is the best way to evaluate peripheral pulmonary vasculature. The vast majority of cardiac catheterizations are for interventional procedures such as device closures, and outnumber purely diagnostic cases. Types of interventional procedures include the following: balloon valvuloplasty for aortic and pulmonic stenosis, device closure for secundum ASD, and coil closure of a PDA. In addition, abnormalities of the conduction system also can be diagnosed and treated in the cardiac catheterization lab.

CARDIAC SYMPTOMS

Arrhythmias and Palpitations

It is not unusual for children to complain of skipped beats, a fast heart rate, or extra heartbeats. Most complaints are benign in origin, but a history of chest pain, light-headedness, or syncope can be indicative of a serious arrhythmia. Family history should be directed toward any structural heart disease or history of sudden death, and the patient history should include any association of symptoms with exercise, food intake (especially caffeine), medications (especially cough preparations), or specific positioning. Physical findings, outside of the arrhythmia, are usually not found. Evaluation begins with an EKG. Documentation of the rhythm on an EKG is essential for determining diagnosis and treatment; however, obtaining this documentation can be challenging, especially if the symptoms are infrequent. For a complete evaluation, referral to a pediatric cardiologist or electrophysiologist is essential, and if the symptoms persist or worsen, additional testing with continuous Holter monitoring or event recording is recommended.[2]

Syncope

Syncope is a common complaint in older children and adolescents. It is usually characterized by a loss of consciousness, falling, and then a quick recovery once the child or adolescent is lying down. The episodes are usually preceded by dizziness, light-headedness, pallor, weakness, blurred vision, or cold sweats. A tonic-clonic seizure also may occur, especially if there is a delay in regaining consciousness. The majority of syncopal events are benign, but a careful evaluation is always warranted, because it may be the first symptom of serious cardiac, neurologic, or metabolic disease. The most common neurologic cause is a seizure disorder, and possible metabolic causes include hypoglycemia, electrolyte imbalance, or profound anemia. In toddlers, the causes

may include breath-holding, and in adolescents, hyperventilation.[2]

Cardiac etiologies include vagal neural reflexive syncope, which is the most common; arrhythmias; prolonged Q-T syndrome; and *hypertrophic cardiomyopathy* (HCM), a primary abnormality of the myocardium causing an asymmetrical, hypertrophied, nondilated LV. The only evidence on physical examination may be the increased intensity of a cardiac murmur from supine to standing.[2]

Information gathering should include careful details of the event and a family history of similar events or sudden death. An EKG should be obtained, and referral to a cardiologist is warranted if laboratory tests are normal (no metabolic disturbance) and there are no neurologic findings on physical examination.[2]

Chest Pain

Most children who complain of chest pain do not have cardiac disease.[5] It is important to elicit the duration of the pain and whether it is related to breathing, or activity, or whether it is accompanied by palpitations (racing heart) or syncope (feeling faint). Chest pain of cardiac origin is usually triggered by exercise and, with the exception of pericarditis, it is not affected by respirations.[1] Complaints of chest pain occur often in school-age children and can be caused by a variety of problems

TABLE 7-4   CHARACTERISTICS OF ACUTE AND CHRONIC CHEST PAIN

Acute Onset Chest Pain	Chronic or Recurrent Chest Pain
Less common	More common
Pain is intense	Pain is mild, vague, often over entire chest; not well localized, not associated with exercise/pleasurable activities
Care is immediately sought	Care sought after several episodes
Caused by serious medical illness	Etiology difficult to determine, often nonorganic

Data from Brook MM, Moore P, Van Hare G. In Rudolph AM, Kamei R, Overby K, editors: *Rudolph's fundamentals of pediatrics*, New York, 2002, McGraw-Hill; Park M: *Pediatric cardiology for practitioners*, St Louis, 2002, Mosby.

TABLE 7-5 **CARDIAC ASSESSMENT SUMMARY AND ABNORMAL FINDINGS**

Assessment	Abnormal Findings
NEWBORN AND INFANT	
History	Persistent lethargy, irritability
	Decreased feeding tolerance or sweating with feeds
	Failure to thrive
	Frequent respiratory infections
	Frequent "staring" episodes
Vital signs	Tachycardia, bradycardia
	Tachypnea
	Hypertension
	Low oxygen saturation, oxygen saturation differential between upper and lower extremities
	Persistent low-grade fever
Inspection	Cyanosis, pallor, or hypoperfusion
	Respiratory distress
	Persistent sweating with feeding
	Grunting
	Dysmorphic features
Palpation	Hepatomegaly
	Decreased or asymmetric pulses, bounding pulses
	Increased RV or LV impulses
	Heaves, thrills
Auscultation	Single S_2, widely split S_2, any S_4, gallop
	Clicks or extra heart sounds
	Grade 2-3 holosystolic murmur
	Grade 3 and higher systolic ejection murmur
	Any diastolic murmur, any continuous murmur
	Rales
Chest x-ray	Enlarged heart
	Pulmonary edema
Electrocardiogram	Abnormal rate, rhythm, axis, voltages, ST segment or T wave changes
	Prolonged QT interval, AV block
TODDLER AND PRESCHOOLER	
History	Tires easily, prolonged irritability/cyanosis
	Frequent respiratory infections
	Syncope

Continued

TABLE 7-5 CARDIAC ASSESSMENT SUMMARY AND ABNORMAL FINDINGS—CONT'D

Assessment	Abnormal Findings
Vital signs	Tachycardia, bradycardia
	Tachypnea
	Persistent low-grade fever
	Blood pressure differential between upper and lower extremities
Inspection	Rash with persistent low-grade fever
Palpation	Hepatomegaly
	Decreased or asymmetric pulses, bounding pulses
Auscultation	Widely split S_2, S_4 gallop
	Any new murmur
	Rales
Chest x-ray	Enlarged heart
	Pulmonary edema
Electrocardiogram	Abnormal rate, rhythm, voltages
	ST segment or T wave changes
	Prolonged QT interval
	Pre-excitation (delta wave)

SCHOOL-AGE CHILD AND ADOLESCENT

History	Syncope, dizziness
	Chest pain, palpitations
	Easily fatigued, unable to keep up with peers
Vital signs	Tachycardia, bradycardia
	Hypertension, blood pressure difference between upper and lower extremities
	Persistent low-grade fever
	Extreme height or weight for age
Palpation	Decreased/absent lower extremity pulses
Auscultation	New murmur
	Midsystolic click
Chest x-ray	Enlarged heart
Electrocardiogram	Abnormal rate, rhythm, voltages
	ST segment or T wave changes
	Prolonged QT interval

RV, Right ventricle; *LV,* left ventricle.

including viral illness, stress (both physical and emotional), trauma, or a cardiac condition. Chest pain also can be due to periodic inflammation of the chest wall, *costochondritis*, and is sharp, short, and well localized and can be reproduced with pressure on palpation. The pain may be associated with muscular movement and exercise or a history of recent viral illness.

Chest pain can present as either acute in onset or recurrent (Table 7-4). The severity, location, and radiation of the pain should be documented as well as its relationship to movement, exercise, or other activities. The physical exam should note the child or adolescent's color, perfusion, pulses, respiratory effort, and degree of acute pain. Auscultation includes the evaluation of breath sounds and their symmetry, as well as the identification of abnormal heart sounds, murmurs, or muffled heart sounds. If an acute chest pain of cardiac origin is suspected, an EKG should be

obtained along with a referral to a pediatric cardiologist.

 Key Points

Assessment of the heart and vascular system in infants, children, and adolescents should be performed in a systematic manner, and no one finding is generally taken in isolation (Table 7-5).

 CHARTING

1-Month-Old Infant With Murmur

Cardiac: Increased RV (right ventricular) impulse, normal S_1, split S_2, 2-3/6 low frequency SEM (systolic ejection murmur) heard best at lower left sternal border. No diastolic murmur, extra heart sounds, thrill, or clicks.

REFERENCES

1. Artman M, Mahony L, Teitel D: *Neonatal cardiology,* New York, 2002, McGraw-Hill.
2. Brook MM, Moore P, Van Hare G. In Rudolph AM, Kamei R, Overby K, editors: *Rudolph's fundamentals of pediatrics,* New York, 2002, McGraw-Hill.
3. Momma K, Hagiwara H, Konishi T: Constriction of the fetal ductus arteriosus by non-steroidal anti-inflammatory drugs: study of additional 34 drugs, *Prostaglandins* 28(4):527-536, 1984.
4. Alano MA, Ngougmna E, Ostrea EM Jr, Konduri GG: Analysis of non-steroidal anti-inflammatory drugs in meconium and its relation to persistent pulmonary hypertension of the newborn, *Pediatrics* 107(3):519-523, 2001.
5. Park M: *Pediatric cardiology for practitioners,* ed 4, St Louis, 2002, Mosby.

CHAPTER 8

CHEST AND RESPIRATORY SYSTEM

Concettina Tolomeo

DEVELOPMENT

Lung development begins in utero at approximately 4 weeks' gestation. The lungs form from a sac on the ventral wall of the alimentary canal. As branching of the lung bud occurs, the trachea, bronchi, and bronchioles are formed by 16 to 17 weeks' gestation. The primitive alveoli begin to form by 17 weeks' gestation and by 24 to 28 weeks are capable of gas exchange. Alveolar cells begin secretion of surfactant by 24 to 26 weeks' gestation. *Surfactant* acts to prevent the alveolar sacs from collapsing during the expiratory phase of respiration. Maturation and expansion of alveoli occur between 30 and 36 weeks' gestation and continue to replicate into early childhood with the most growth occurring during the first 4 years of life.[1,2]

Breathing movements occur in utero. The movements are irregular, range from 30 to 70 breaths per minute, and become more rapid as gestation advances.[3] Gas exchange occurs via the placenta, and movement of fluid in and out of the potential air spaces conditions the respiratory muscles and stimulates lung development.

At birth, the lungs fill with air for the first time and take on the role of ventilation and oxygenation. The fluid in the lung moves into the tissues surrounding the alveoli and is absorbed into the lymphatic system. At this point, gas exchange occurs via diffusion across the alveolar-pulmonary capillary membranes.[1,2]

PHYSIOLOGICAL VARIATIONS

Table 8-1 presents variations in growth and development that impact the function of the respiratory system in the infant and young child.

ANATOMY AND PHYSIOLOGY

Thorax

The thorax is the bony cage that surrounds the heart and lungs. It is composed of the *manubrium,* the *sternum,* the *xiphoid process,* and the ribs (Figure 8-1). The *sternum* is a flat, narrow bone composed of highly vascular tissues enclosed by dense bone. The *manubrium*

TABLE 8-1 PHYSIOLOGICAL VARIATIONS OF THE CHEST AND LUNGS

Age	Developmental Stage
Preterm infant	Respiratory muscles are weak, poorly adapted for extrauterine life; periodic breathing occurs that is similar to fetal breathing; preterm infants become easily hypoxic and apnea occurs
Newborn	Diaphragm is flatter, more compliant; paradoxical breathing occurs in neonate with inward movement of chest during inspiration; predominantly nose breathers until 4 weeks of age; chest circumference very close in size to head circumference at birth
Infant	Smaller airways with increased resistance to airflow; rapid respiratory rate; minimal nasal mucus causes mild to moderate upper airway obstruction
Toddler and preschooler	Rapid growth and maturation of alveoli improve ventilation; respiratory rate decreases dramatically from newborn period
School-age child	Alveoli continue to increase in number; lung development is complete by 5-6 years of age
Adolescent	Alveolar size matures to adult capacity

is roughly triangular and attaches to the first and second ribs. It provides a place of attachment for the *sternocleidomastoid* and *pectoralis major* muscles. The *xiphoid process* is the small, thin cartilaginous end of the sternum, which varies greatly in shape and prominence in infants and children because of the influence of heredity, intrauterine environment, and nutrition. *Pectus carinatum*, pigeon breast,

is the abnormal protrusion of the xiphoid process and sternum, and *pectus excavatum,* funnel chest, is the abnormal depression of the sternum[1,2,4] (Figure 8-2). The chest cavity is divided, with the middle portion known as the *mediastinum.*

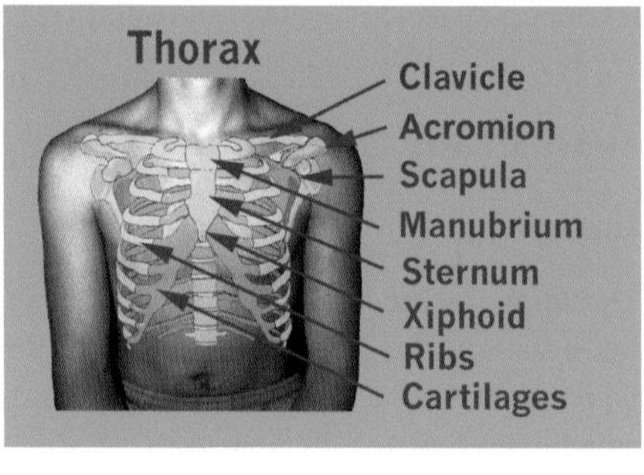

There are 12 pairs of ribs in all, and the first 7 pairs of ribs attach anteriorly via their corresponding costal cartilages to the sternum. Ribs 8, 9, and 10 are attached to the costal cartilage on the rib above them, and ribs 11 and 12 do not attach anteriorly. All 12 pairs of ribs attach posteriorly to the thoracic vertebrae. There are 11 intercostal muscles anteriorly and posteriorly and 8 thoracic muscles, all of which help to increase the volume of the rib cage with inspiration and decrease the thoracic volume with expiration (Figure 8-3).

Thorax
- Clavicle
- Acromion
- Scapula
- Manubrium
- Sternum
- Xiphoid
- Ribs
- Cartilages

Figure **8-1** Anatomy of the rib cage and thorax. (From Lemmi FO, Lemmi CA: *Physical assessment findings multi-user CD-ROM,* Philadelphia, 2000, Saunders.)

⚿ Key Points

Hypotonia in preterm and term infants impacts the chest wall muscles and compromises normal ventilation.

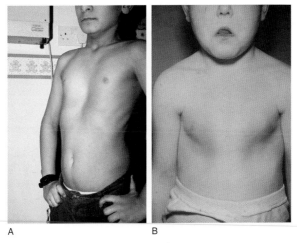

A   B

Figure **8-2 A,** Pectus excavatum. **B,** Pectus carinatum. (**A,** From Chaudhry B, Harvey D: *Mosby's color atlas and text of pediatrics and child health,* St Louis, 2001, Mosby. **B,** From Lissauer T, Clayden G: *Illustrated textbook of paediatrics,* ed 2, St Louis, 2001, Mosby.)

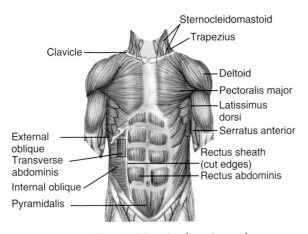

Figure **8-3** Anterior thoracic muscles.

The following landmarks are often used in describing the location of physical findings of the chest: the midsternal line (MSL), which runs down the middle of the sternum; the midclavicular line (MCL), located on the right and left sides of the chest, runs parallel to the MSL and through the middle of the clavicles bilaterally. Laterally, there are three lines on each side, the anterior axillary line (AAL), the midaxillary line (MAL), and the posterior axillary line (PAL). The AAL begin at the anterior axillary folds, the MAL begin at the middle of the axilla, and the PAL begins at the posterior axillary folds. Posteriorly is the vertebral line that runs down the middle of the spine and the scapular line, which runs down the inferior angle of each scapula (Figure 8-4).

Lower Respiratory Tract

The respiratory system is divided into two parts, the *upper respiratory tract* and the *lower*

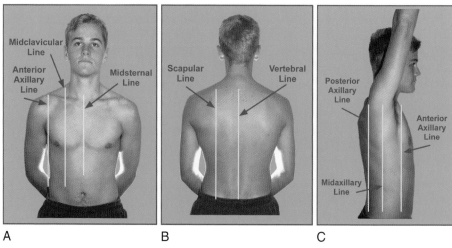

A   B   C

Figure **8-4** Anatomical landmarks of the chest. **A,** Anterior chest. **B,** Posterior chest. **C,** Lateral chest. (From Lemmi FO, Lemmi CA: *Physical assessment findings multi-user CD-ROM,* Philadelphia, 2000, Saunders.)

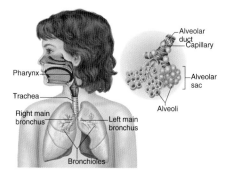

Figure **8-5** Lower respiratory tract.

respiratory tract. The upper respiratory tract consists of the nasal cavity, pharynx, and larynx and is reviewed in Chapter 13. The *lower respiratory tract* consists of the lungs, trachea, bronchi, bronchioles, alveolar ducts and sacs, and alveoli (Figure 8-5). The *trachea* is a tube that lies anterior to the esophagus. The distal end of the trachea splits into the right and left mainstem *bronchi.* This bifurcation occurs at the level of T3 during infancy and childhood. By the time the child is an adult, this bifurcation occurs at T4 or T5. The right mainstem bronchus is shorter and more vertical than the left and, therefore,

more susceptible to aspiration of foreign bodies in the young child.[2] Beyond the bifurcation, the bronchi continue to branch into *bronchioles.* There are three branches on the right and two on the left; each branch supplies one of the lung lobes. These branches further divide into segmental smaller bronchi called *respiratory bronchioles* to supply each segment of the lungs. Ultimately, the respiratory tract terminates with the alveolar ducts, alveolar sacs, and alveoli where gas exchange takes place.[1,2,4] The bronchial arteries branch from the aorta and supply blood to the lung parenchyma. The blood supply is returned primarily by the pulmonary veins.

Lungs

The lungs are positioned in the lateral aspects of the thorax, separated by the heart and the mediastinal structures. The right lung has three lobes (upper, middle, and lower), and the left lung has two lobes (upper and lower). The *apex* is the top portion of the upper lobes, which extend above the clavicles. On the right side, the minor or horizontal fissure, located at the fourth rib, divides the right upper lobe (RUL) from the right middle lobe (RML).

On the left side, there is a tongue-shaped projection that extends from the left upper lobe (LUL), called the *lingula*. Laterally, the right lower lobe (RLL) and the left lower lobe (LLL) occupy most of the lower lateral chest area. Only a small portion of the RML extends to the midaxillary line, and it does not go beyond that point. Posteriorly, the vertebral column helps in identifying the underlying lung lobes. T3 and T4 mark the inferior portion of the upper lobes and the superior portion of the lower lobes. The *base* is the bottom portion of the lower lobes and is marked by T10 or T12 depending on the phase of respiration.[2,4] The principal function of the lungs is to maintain an acid-base balance by supplying oxygen to organs and tissue and eliminating carbon dioxide.

SYSTEM-SPECIFIC HISTORY

Complete and accurate information gathering is essential when assessing an infant, child, or adolescent with respiratory symptoms. Questions should be open-ended and age-specific to allow the parent or caregiver an opportunity to give a full explanation of past and present concerns. Always obtain information directly from the older child or adolescent during the visit (Tables 8-2 and 8-3).

PHYSICAL ASSESSMENT

Equipment

The size of the stethoscope being used is extremely important when evaluating respiratory sounds. Stethoscopes with a smaller bell and diaphragm always should be used on infants and toddlers. Isolating cardiac and respiratory sounds is difficult in small children with too large a diaphragm, and using a diaphragm that is too small on adolescents or on children who are overweight or obese causes practitioners to miss findings of cardiac and respiratory sounds on auscultation.

Positioning

Young children, especially toddlers, may be more relaxed on their parent's lap during the examination of the chest. Children also should be allowed to help as much as possible during the exam. Have them hold the stethoscope in place once you position it in the appropriate location. Other techniques include letting children role play by allowing them to listen to their parent, a doll, or stuffed animal. Taking a few extra minutes to incorporate the child's developmental level into your exam will result in more thorough and reliable findings.

School-age children are very curious and respond well to games. Therefore, explain what you will be doing during the exam. In addition, pictures of lungs in the exam room can be helpful with older children when you are explaining what you are looking for and listening to.

Chest

Pediatric practitioners begin the physical examination by assessing the chest. The "quieter" parts of the exam, the cardiac and respiratory exam, require astute listening skills and less active participation of the child so are best performed first—an effective approach to assessing children among pediatric experts. The practitioner must take a systematic approach to examining the chest and use all the components of physical assessment. This includes inspection, palpation, percussion, and auscultation. Examination of the chest should always include both the anterior and the posterior chest.

A thorough assessment of the chest and lungs is not complete without examination of the upper airway and the extremities. Nasal passages should be examined for the presence of rhinitis, any nasal secretions, polyps, or nasal obstruction. When looking at the oropharynx, note the presence of postnasal drip and tonsillar size. An abnormal finding in any of these areas can be a cause of respiratory symptoms. Finally, you need to examine the extremities for signs of digital clubbing.

TABLE 8-2   INFORMATION GATHERING FOR CHEST AND LUNG ASSESSMENT AT KEY DEVELOPMENTAL STAGES

Age	Questions to ask
Preterm infant	How many weeks' gestation? Any episodes of apnea, tachypnea? Need for oxygen? Admitted to newborn intensive care unit? Length of stay? Need for ventilation? For how long? Infant discharged to home on a ventilator/on oxygen? Infant discharged home on any medications? Any maternal substance abuse?
Newborn	Birth weight? How many weeks' gestation? Any birth complications? Meconium aspiration? Breathing problems at birth? Any episodes of apnea, tachypnea?
Infant	History of respiratory infections as infant (respiratory syncytial virus [RSV], Rhinovirus, etc)? Frequent upper respiratory infections (URIs)? History of wheezing? Hospitalizations? History of intubations? History of eczema/skin allergy? In daycare? Immunization status? Frequent vomiting after feeds/"choking" episodes? Arches back after feeding?
Toddler	Does child's speech have nasal or congested resonance? Multiple URIs or symptoms of respiratory allergies? In daycare? History of apnea/breath-holding spells? Does child suck a finger/pacifier? Still use bottle for milk/juice? Frequently puts objects in mouth/nose?
Preschooler	History of nasal congestion, chronic rhinorrhea, tonsillitis? Exposure to group A streptococcal infection? Does child snore at night? Injuries to mouth/nose? Concerns about child's speech? In preschool? Exposure to ill contacts? Foreign travel/recent immigrant?
School-age child	History of nasal congestion, chronic rhinorrhea, sinusitis, tonsillitis? Does child snore at night? Exposure to group A streptococcal infection? History of asthma? Exposure to ill contacts? Foreign travel or recent immigrant?
Adolescent	History of chronic URIs, allergic rhinitis/asthma, recurrent tonsillitis? History of oral sex? Tobacco use? How many cigarettes per day? Marijuana use? Any oral piercings?
Environmental risks	Year home was built? Location (inner city, suburb, rural)? Number of people in home? Anyone smoke in home? Pets in home? Type of heating system? Wood burning stove? Humidifier? Mold? Carpets? Drapes? Mice or roaches? Presence of chemicals/fumes?

TABLE 8-3　PRESENTING RESPIRATORY SYMPTOMS

Symptom	Questions to Ask
Cough	Onset of cough symptoms? Coughing for how long? Is cough worsening or changing character? Was onset sudden or gradual? Is cough wet, dry, hacking, barking, whooping? *Pattern:* Occasional, regular, paroxysmal, or coughing spasms? Worse during day or at night? Worse with feeding, sleeping, running? Shortness of breath, chest pain, tightness with cough? Choking episodes? History of aspiration (small toy, food, etc.)? Rhinorrhea or nasal congestion? *In older child/adolescent:* Is cough productive with sputum or nonproductive?
Wheeze	Onset of wheezing? Onset sudden or gradually worsening? *Pattern:* Occasional, regular, increase with exercise? History of aspiration (small toy, food, etc.)? *Other symptoms:* Cough? Shortness of breath? Chest pain/tightness?
Shortness of breath	Is it difficult to get air in, out, both? History of aspiration (small toy, food, etc.)? Chest excursion asymmetrical? Accompanying symptoms of cough, wheezing? History of breath-holding spells, seizures?
Chest pain	Is it difficult to get air in, out, or both? Chest pain occurs with movement or rest? Type of pain (sharp, dull)? Ask verbal child to point to area of pain. History of trauma or recent sports injury or weight lifting? Accompanying symptoms of cough, wheezing, shortness of breath?

Clubbing is the bulbous-shaped enlargement of the soft tissue of the distal phalanges (Figure 8-6). Clubbing can be hereditary or can be the result of cardiac disease, respiratory disease, or severe malnutrition.

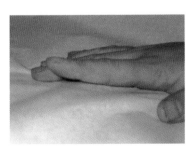

Figure **8-6** Digital clubbing.

Inspection

Ideally, start the exam by visually inspecting the infant or child undressed from the waist up. This allows you to make general observations about the child's respiratory rate, breathing pattern, respiratory effort, inspiratory to expiratory ratio (I:E ratio), skin color, presence of noisy breathing, chest symmetry, and chest shape. Optimally, the observation of the respirations should be made when the infant or child is calm and relaxed in the parent's lap.

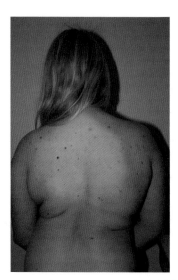

Figure **8-7** Scoliosis in a 12-year-old child. (From Lemmi FO, Lemmi CA: *Physical assessment findings multi-user CD-ROM, Philadelphia,* 2000, Saunders.)

This is usually best accomplished while you are taking a history and before you approach the child for physical examination. In an irritable, ill, or fearful child, observation of respiratory pattern and rate may be the most helpful part of the examination if the child exhibits resistance to auscultation.

Assess the shape of the chest and note any abnormalities. The normal anterior-posterior (AP) to transverse ratio is 1:2. In the infant, the chest is round with a diameter roughly equal to the head circumference until 2 years of age and has a 1:1 AP/transverse ratio, giving a barrel chest appearance.[2,4] As the child grows, the chest takes on the shape of the adult chest, and by the age of 6 has a ratio of 1:1.36.[1] A barrel chest shape also can be seen when chronic air trapping is present, such as in advanced stages of cystic fibrosis. Other deformities of the chest that can have an impact on the child's respiratory status and decrease expansion of the lungs include *pectus*

carinatum, pectus excavatum, or scoliosis (Figure 8-7).

Assessment of Respirations

Resting respiratory rates vary with the age of the child: the younger the child, the higher the respiratory rate (Table 8-4). The child's rhythm of breathing should be regular. Many factors can increase or decrease the respiratory rate, such as fever, exercise, and medications.

Pediatric Pearls

The child's respiratory rate should not be evaluated in isolation of other respiratory parameters and should be correlated with the other physical findings.

Periodic breathing is characterized by rapid breathing followed by periods of *apnea,* cessation of breathing. This is normal in the first few hours of life in healthy full-term newborns. Periodic breathing is more likely to persist in preterm infants, but the episodes of apnea should improve as infants approach term age.[2,4,5]

TABLE 8-4   EXPECTED RANGE OF RESPIRATORY RATES FOR AGE

Age	Rate
Preterm	40-70
Newborn to 3 months	35-55
3 to 12 months	30-45
Toddlers	24-40
Preschoolers	20-30
School-age children	14-22
Adolescents	12-20

Data from Behrman RE, Kleigman RM, Jenson HB: *Nelson textbook of pediatrics,* ed 17, Philadelphia, 2004, Saunders.

If the apnea is prolonged (>15 seconds) or it is accompanied by central cyanosis, it is abnormal and requires immediate further evaluation. *Paradoxical breathing*, or seesaw breathing, is often seen in newborns and infants because they use abdominal muscles more than intercostal muscles.[1,2] *Cheyne-Stokes breathing* is characterized by cycles of increasing and decreasing tidal volume separated by apnea. It occurs in children with congestive heart failure and increased intracranial pressure.

Noisy breathing includes stridor, grunting, and snoring. *Stridor* is a high-pitched, loud, inspiratory sound produced by upper airway obstruction. Causes of upper airway obstruction include edema status post intubation, subglottic stenosis, laryngotracheobronchitis, and foreign body aspiration. *Grunting* is a low-pitched expiratory sound caused by a partial closure of the glottis. Snoring is a rough, snorting sound that can be present on inspiration or expiration. It may be present during sleep in healthy children who have an upper respiratory infection, in children experiencing respiratory distress, or with chest pain. Snoring is often heard in the presence of nasal polyps, adenoidal and tonsillar hypertrophy, or congenital anomalies that involve the upper airway or facies.[1,2,4]

Inspect for nasal flaring and use of accessory muscles in the infant and toddler. Mild nasal flaring can be seen in newborns because they are preferential nose breathers in the first month of life. However, increased nasal flaring should be investigated because it is a sign of labored breathing. Other signs of increased effort and respiratory distress include retractions, bulging of the intercostal muscles, and head bobbing. Although mild retractions may be seen in some healthy young children, increased retractions can be a sign of airway obstruction. The chest wall of newborns and infants is more compliant than that of older children, making them more prone to retractions. Bulging of the intercostal spaces also may be seen with airway obstruction as a consequence of increased expiratory effort. *Head bobbing*, the forward movement of the infant's head, is a sign of respiratory distress due to the contraction of the scalene and sternocleidomastoid muscles.[2,4,5]

An abnormal inspiratory to expiratory (I:E) ratio is an additional sign of respiratory distress. A normal I:E ratio in the infant is 1:2 seconds except in the newborn, when it is variable. Obstructive diseases such as cystic fibrosis or an acute asthma exacerbation can increase the expiratory time. Restrictive diseases can give a ratio of 1:1, and acute upper airway obstruction can produce a ratio of 2:2 to 4:2.

Assess for *cyanosis*, a bluish color to the skin or mucous membranes. *Acrocyanosis*, cyanosis of the hands and feet, is normal in the newborn and can persist for days if the infant is in a cool environment. *Central cyanosis*, which occurs in the conjunctiva, lips, mucous membranes, and tongue, is an abnormal finding at any age and warrants immediate further evaluation. In the anemic child, it may be difficult to detect cyanosis early on because the arterial oxygen saturation at which cyanosis becomes apparent varies with the total hemoglobin level.[2,4,5]

Auscultation

Auscultation is best performed at the beginning of the examination when the infant and child are more cooperative and attentive. Auscultation is performed with the diaphragm of the stethoscope placed firmly on the chest. The child's chest should be bare because clothing can change the quality of the breath sounds. You want to auscultate moving from side to side across the chest so that you can compare one side to the other. Be sure to listen at each location for one full breath (Figure 8-8). Breath sounds are also identified by their intensity, pitch, and duration. In children breath sounds tend to be louder because of the thinness of the chest wall. There has been much confusion about the terminology

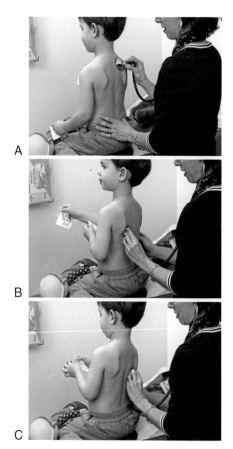

A

B

C

Figure **8-8 A,** Auscultation of upper right lobe. **B,** Auscultation of lower left lobe. **C,** Auscultation of lower right lobe.

used to describe breath sounds. Table 8-5 presents the most accurate description of normal breath sounds in the respiratory cycle.

Transmitted voice sounds or an infant's cry also can be assessed with a stethoscope. Voice sounds are typically muffled on auscultation. If you hear the voice sound or cry loud and clear, it is termed *bronchophony*. Again, this technique can be used to examine an infant or uncooperative child even while he or she is crying. If the verbal child speaks the sound "ee" and it sounds like "ay," it is called *egophony*. If the child whispers a word and it is

heard loudly, it is called whispered *pectoriloquy*.[1,2,4] *If any of these signs are positive*, it is evidence of a consolidation.

Abnormal Lung Sounds

In addition to normal lung sounds, you may hear adventitious or abnormal breath sounds (Table 8-6). Adventitious lung sounds are sounds that are superimposed on normal breath sounds.

Palpation

Palpation is performed to identify anatomical landmarks, respiratory symmetry, and areas of tenderness or abnormalities. Begin by counting the ribs, locate the sternal angle, the *angle of Louis*, where the manubrium meets the sternum, and move your fingers laterally to feel the second rib and corresponding costal cartilage. Directly below this rib is the second intercostal space, the important landmark for cardiac examination. From there, count downward to the other ribs and their respective intercostal spaces.[2,4]

To assess chest excursion, place your hands along the lateral rib cage and squeeze the thumbs toward each other so that you gather a small amount of skin in between your thumbs. As the child inhales, note the symmetry of the chest excursion. Again, this should be done both anteriorly and posteriorly. Asymmetry is an abnormal finding. In the newborn period, asymmetrical chest excursion may be a sign of a diaphragmatic hernia. Other possible abnormalities associated with asymmetrical chest excursion during the newborn period or later include pneumothorax, mass, foreign body, or abnormal chest wall shape. An important part of the exam that should not be ignored in the newborn is palpation of the trachea to assess for a mediastinal shift. A shift in the trachea occurs when there is a difference in volume or pressure between the two sides of the chest, as is seen in a pneumothorax or pleural effusion.[5]

To complete the palpation portion of the exam, assess for tactile fremitus. To do this,

TABLE 8-5 NORMAL BREATH SOUNDS

Sound	Description	Duration of Inspiration and Expiration	Sound Diagram
Vesicular	Soft sound heard over entire surface of lungs; inspiration louder, longer, higher-pitched than expiration	Inspiration > expiration 2.5:1	
Bronchovesicular	Loud, high-pitched sounds heard over intrascapular area; inspiration and expiration are equal	Inspiration = expiration 1:1	
Bronchial (tubular)	Very loud over trachea near suprasternal notch; inspiration is shorter than expiration	Inspiration < expiration 1:2	

Adapted from Lemmi FO, Lemmi CA: *Physical assessment findings multi-user CD-ROM,* Philadelphia, 2000, Saunders.

TABLE 8-6 ABNORMAL BREATH SOUNDS

Sound	Description
Crackles or rales	Discontinuous sounds, heard primarily on inspiration, do not clear with cough; associated with pneumonia, bronchopulmonary dysplasia, cystic fibrosis • Fine crackles—Higher in pitch, generally indicative of fluid in smaller airways in infants, children • Coarse crackles—Lower in pitch, usually signify fluid in larger airways
Wheezes	Continuous, high-pitched musical sounds heard primarily on expiration; associated with partial obstruction of one or more bronchi caused by narrowing of airways due to an inflammatory response, as with asthma and aspiration of a foreign body
Rhonchi	Continuous low-pitched sounds; clears with coughing; caused by secretions/mucus in larger airways as in bronchitis and lower respiratory tract infections.

Data from Bickley LS: *Bates' guide to physical examination and history taking,* Philadelphia, 1999, Lippincott; Engel JK: *Pocket guide to pediatric assessment,* ed 4, St Louis, 2002, Mosby; Pasterkamp H, Kraman S, Wodicka GR: Respiratory sounds: advances beyond the stethoscope, *Am J Respir Care Med* 156(3 Pt 1):974-987, 1997; Seidel HM, Ball JW, Dains JE, Benedict GW: *Mosby's guide to physical examination,* ed 5, St Louis, 2003, Mosby.

use your palm, the ulnar surface of your hand, or your fingers depending on the size of the chest wall, and ask the verbal child to say "1-2-3." In an infant or uncooperative child this technique can be performed while the child is crying. Perform this exam on the left side and the right side, both anteriorly and posteriorly. Increased or decreased fremitus can be the result of consolidation or pneumothorax.[1,2,4]

Percussion

Percussion is used to determine the sounds of the underlying organs and tissues. It helps to distinguish whether the tissue is air filled, fluid filled, or solid. There are five sounds that are produced with percussion: *resonance, hyperresonance, dull, flat,* and *tympany.* The sounds are distinguished by their intensity, pitch, and duration. In infants and toddlers, the sound produced is more resonant because the chest wall is thinner than in older children and adolescents (Table 8-7). To perform percussion, hyperextend the middle finger of your nondominant hand and press the distal interphalangeal joint firmly on the chest. With the middle finger of your dominant hand, strike down on the hyperextended interphalangeal joint. The movement must be sharp and quick and the only portion of the nondominant finger that should be touching the chest should be the hyperextended joint. Strike each area two or three times and then move to the opposite side for comparison (Figure 8-9). Lastly, it

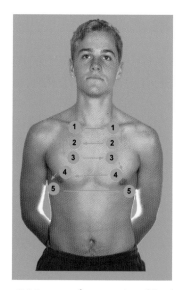

Figure **8-9** Sequence for percussion of the thorax. (From Lemmi FO, Lemmi CA: *Physical assessment findings multi-user CD-ROM,* Philadelphia, 2000, Saunders.)

may be necessary to repeat auscultation to confirm findings that were revealed during palpation and percussion. Percussion is sometimes deferred in infants and children.

ABNORMAL CONDITIONS

Table 8-8 presents the most common abnormal conditions seen in infants, children, and adolescents by the pediatric healthcare practitioner.

TABLE 8-7 PERCUSSION SOUNDS

Tone	Intensity	Pitch	Quality
Tympanic	Loud	High	Drumlike
Resonant	Loud	Low	Hollow
Dull	Moderate	Medium to high	Dull thud
Flat	Soft	High	Very dull

TABLE 8-8   ABNORMAL CONDITIONS OF THE CHEST AND LUNGS

Condition	Description
Acute bronchiolitis	Inflammatory obstruction of small airways caused by edema, mucus plugging; occurs during first 2 years of life with peak incidence at 6 months of age *Etiology:* viral etiology common with >50% caused by respiratory syncytial virus (RSV)
Acute epiglottitis	Obstructive inflammatory process of airway that is supraglottic; abrupt onset of high fever, sore throat, drooling, dysphagia, dyspnea, increasing airway obstruction; occurs between 2 and 7 years of age *Etiology:* Bacterial with marked decrease in incidence because of widespread use of *Haemophilus influenzae* vaccine
Asthma or reactive airway disease	Inflammatory process initiated by irritability/hyperreactivity of airway to variety of stimuli, obstruction/bronchoconstriction; inflammation plays key role in factors leading to cough, wheezing, tachypnea, dyspnea with prolonged expiration
Croup or laryngotracheobronchitis	Acute upper airway obstruction; inflammation, edema of airway leads to hoarse, barking cough, intermittent stridor; respiratory distress occurs in some cases, which is worse at night; most common between 3 months and 5 years of age *Etiology:* ~75% parainfluenza virus
Cystic fibrosis	An inherited autosomal recessive trait causing multisystem disorder in children; characterized by obstruction, infection of airways caused by dysfunction of epithelial surface leading to thick, retained secretions *Overall incidence:* 1:4 births, most common occurrence in whites
Foreign body aspiration	Lodging of object in larynx, trachea, bronchi with degree of obstruction dependent on size/location of object in respiratory tract; hot dogs, bread are most common causes of fatal aspiration; possibility of foreign body must be considered in infants, young children with acute respiratory distress regardless of history
Gastroesophageal reflux	A passive transfer/reflux of gastric contents across lower esophageal sphincter, which may lead to tissue damage causing gastroesophageal reflux disease (GERD); GERD may be associated with respiratory conditions such as bronchospasm, pneumonia

Continued

TABLE 8-8 ABNORMAL CONDITIONS OF THE CHEST AND LUNGS—CONT'D

Condition	Description
Laryngomalacia or tracheomalacia	A congenital deformity of larynx or trachea often termed "floppy airway;" manifests as harsh noise/stridor on inspiration caused by airway collapse; onset in early neonatal period; diagnosed by laryngoscopy
Pneumonia	Inflammation of parenchyma of lungs; may be primary condition or manifestation of another illness *Etiology:* Most commonly caused by viral microorganisms— RSV, parainfluenza, adenovirus; bacterial pneumonia is less common, but *Mycoplasma pneumoniae* accounts for ~70% of all pneumonias in 9- to 15-year-olds; noninfectious causes such as foreign body should be considered
Respiratory distress syndrome	A condition related to developmental delay of maturation of lungs; deficient production of *surfactant,* a phospholipid secreted by alveolar epithelium, in preterm infant produces severe respiratory compromise; inadequate pulmonary perfusion and ventilation develop resulting in long-term respiratory complications

Data from Behrman RE, Kleigman RM, Jenson HB: *Nelson textbook of pediatrics,* ed 17, Philadelphia, 2004, Saunders; Wong DL, Hockenberry-Eaton M, Wilson D, Winkelstein ML, Schwartz P: *Essentials of pediatric nursing,* ed 6, St Louis, 2001, Mosby.

CHARTING

2-Week-Old Infant

Chest: Respiratory rate 45, rate regular, respirations quiet. No nasal flaring, retractions or intercostal bulging. I:E 1:2, AP diameter 1:1. Chest excursion symmetrical. Trachea midline. Vesicular lung sounds across lung fields.

CHARTING

5-Year-Old With Asthma Exacerbation

Chest: Respiratory rate 30, audible wheeze present. Mild nasal flaring. Mild intercostal retractions. Symmetrical chest excursion. Lung sounds diminished bilaterally with expiratory wheezes scattered throughout lung fields. No rales noted.

REFERENCES

1. Engel J: *Pocket guide to pediatric assessment,* St Louis, 2002, Mosby.
2. Seidel HM, Ball JW, Dains JE, Benedict GW: *Mosby's guide to physical examination,* ed 5, St Louis, 2003, Mosby.
3. Porth CM: *Pathophysiology: concepts of altered health status,* Philadelphia, 1998, Lippincott.
4. Bickley LS: *Bate's guide to physical examination and history taking,* Philadelphia, 1999, Lippincott.
5. Hilman BC: Clinical assessment of pulmonary diseases in infants and children. In Hilman BC: *Pediatric respiratory disease: diagnosis and treatment,* Philadelphia, 1993, Saunders.

CHAPTER 9

HEAD AND NECK

Karen G. Duderstadt

DEVELOPMENT

The rapid growth of the head begins during the fifth week of embryonic life, as the brain simultaneously undergoes a similar period of rapid growth. By the eighth week, the embryo is human-like in form, but the head size is disproportional to the body. During this early fetal development, the head is the fastest growing part of the body and at 8 weeks' gestation constitutes 50% of the body length. The head growth then slows during the period from the ninth to the twelfth weeks in the developing fetus while spine growth accelerates. During the thirteenth week, ossification of the cranium takes place in one of the primary ossification centers of the skeletal system, which is located in the skull; the other is located in the long bones. The hair patterns on the scalp also develop during the thirteenth week of fetal development, and the scalp hair present in the term infant is established by the twentieth week.[1] During the last half of pregnancy, the head size becomes proportional to the body. The fetus continues to grow and gains 85% of its birth weight during this final period of growth.

The normal growth of the skull depends on placental function, hereditary factors, growth potential within the uterus, and optimum nutrition during pregnancy and early childhood.

If growth retardation occurs in the fetus as a result of either intrinsic or extrinsic factors, it impacts skull growth and affects potential development of the brain. Depending on the time of the insult during fetal development, the infant can suffer long-term consequences of delayed growth and development.

ANATOMY AND PHYSIOLOGY

The cranium provides a protective housing for the brain and parts of the central nervous system. There are eight skull plates, or bones, in the cranium joined together by sutures (Figure 9-1). These skull plates are movable and separate at birth. The *fontanels* are the membranous spaces between the frontal and parietal bones and the parietal and occipital bones. The *anterior fontanel* lies along the *coronal* and *frontal* sutures (Figure 9-2). The *posterior fontanel* lies at the juncture of the *sagittal* and *lambdoidal* sutures. There are small fontanels located bilaterally in the lower skull. The *sphenoid fontanel* is located at the lower juncture of the frontal and parietal bones superior to the ear, and the *mastoid fontanel* is posterior to the ear at the juncture of the occipital and posterior parietal bones. The cranial sutures accommodate brain growth. Ossification of the skull begins in infancy

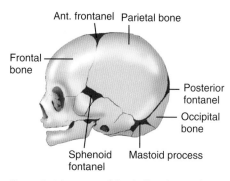

Figure **9-1** Anatomy of the skull in the newborn.

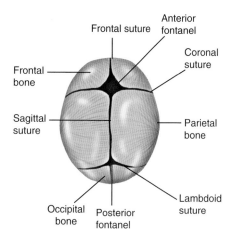

Figure **9-2** Fontanels and sutures.

and continues throughout childhood and into adulthood. The cranium is supported by the first cervical vertebra, the *atlas*. The *atlas* is a solid vertebra and rests on the second vertebra, the *axis*. These bones form the rotational bones of the skull.

The facial bones are pliable at birth, except for the maxilla and the mandible, which are then very small and underdeveloped. The facial skeleton consists of the larger bones of the frontal area, zygomatic processes, *maxilla,* and *mandible* (Figure 9-3). The two *nasal plates* and the *lacrimal, ethmoid,* and *sphenoid* bones comprise the smaller bones in the head.

The muscular structure of the head and neck is an intricate part of the underlying fascia of the cranium and neck structures. The connections between the muscular fascia and the facial orifices control facial expressions such as smiling, raising the eyebrows, and wrinkling the forehead. The superficial and deep muscles of the neck support the pivotal rotation of the head. The large lateral cervical muscles are the sternocleidomastoid and the trapezius. The *sternocleidomastoid* muscle is the largest muscle in the neck, running from the mastoid area at the base of the ear to the clavicle and sternum, and is primarily responsible for turning the head from side to side. It can be particularly susceptible to the effects of viral infections and gastrointestinal conditions in the pediatric patient. The *trapezius*

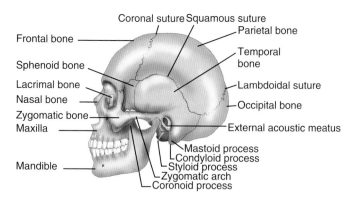

Figure **9-3** Facial skeleton.

muscle lies at the back of the neck and has a triangular shape. The origin of the trapezius muscle is in the back at the twelfth thoracic vertebra extending to the lateral border of the clavicle and attaches at the posterior edge of the occipital bone. It supports the head movement from side to side and the shoulder movement.

The structures in the neck, the trachea, thyroid gland, and parathyroid glands, are protected by the deep vertebral muscles, which support the side movements of the head. The *trachea* is the cartilaginous tube that extends from the larynx to the bronchi in the upper chest beneath the sternum. In infants and children, it is more mobile and more deeply recessed in the vertebral muscles than in adults. The *thyroid gland* lies in the midneck region surrounding the fifth or sixth tracheal ring. There are two lobes joined by an anterior *isthmus* connecting the lobes. The gland is extremely vascular and secretes *thyroxine* directly into the bloodstream, which promotes normal growth. The *parathyroid glands* are located on the lateral lobes of the thyroid gland on the dorsal side. Like the thyroid gland, they do not contain ducts and secrete the *para-thyroid* hormone, which regulates calcium metabolism.

The *carotid arteries* provide circulation to the head and neck region. The *external carotid* supplies the head, face and neck, and the *internal carotid* supplies the cranium. Blood is drained carried through the *subclavian* and *jugular* veins.

PHYSIOLOGICAL VARIATIONS

Newborn

Some variations of the skull are to be monitored during the first few months of life and throughout the first year. The *anterior fontanel* ranges in size from an average of 2 cm to 4 to 5 cm in the term infant. It may be small or fingertip size at birth because of the compression of the skull during the vaginal birth and then enlarge in the

neonatal period. Slow progression of closure of the fontanels occurs during the first year of life. Head growth in the first year is determined by the normal increase of the occipital-frontal head circumference, not the size of the fontanel. The *posterior fontanel* may or may not be palpable at birth. It enlarges by a range of 0.5 to 1 cm and closes by 6 weeks to 2 months of age. *Caput succedaneum,* edema or swelling over the sagittal suture, is often noted at birth. *Cephalhematoma* is a soft, fluctuating effusion of blood trapped beneath the pericranium that is confined to one cranial bone and does not cross the sagittal suture at the crown. It often persists until 2 weeks of age. *Microcephaly,* a small head for gestational age, is considered 1 to 2 SD *below* the norm, and *macrocephaly,* a large head, is 1 to 2 SD *above* the norm for age and size.

Infant

Rapid growth in the infant brings rapid changes in the head and neck. Suture lines can be overlapping or protuberant and often are palpable until 6 months of age from molding at birth. A term infant should hold the head in midline position by 2 months of age and achieve head control by 4 months of age. Head lag is normal in the term infant when pulled to a sitting position until 3 to 4 months of age. Persistent head lag after 6 months of age indicates developmental delay. The *anterior fontanel* may begin closure by 9 months, with only a fingertip concavity present at the crown of the scalp. The neck is shortened in the infant and musculature is underdeveloped. The *thyroid gland* is most often not palpable in the first year of life (Table 9-1).

SYSTEM-SPECIFIC HISTORY

The normal growth of the skull is critical to the early development of the infant and young child. It is important for the practitioner to focus on this early period and obtain history of falls or any head trauma in the growing child (Table 9-2).

TABLE 9-1 PHYSIOLOGICAL VARIATIONS OF THE HEAD AND NECK DURING DEVELOPMENT

Age	Physiological Variations
Preterm infant	Symmetrical or asymmetrical head shape with a flattened temporal/parietal region giving head an elongated shape *Craniotabes*, abnormal softness of cranium, related to incomplete bone and ossification of widened sutures, is often present
Newborn	Symmetrical or asymmetrical head shape with head circumference > chest circumference; ridges over suture lines are common in neonate because of pressure on skull during vaginal birth *Craniotabes* may be present until 6 months of age
Infant	Symmetrical brain growth is reflected in *occipital-frontal circumference* (OFC) of skull; abnormal growth patterns of skull are indicated by a misshapen skull or growth rate of head
Toddler	Closure of *anterior fontanel* is expected from 12-18 months of age in healthy term infant; after 18 months, chest circumference exceeds head circumference by 5-7 cm; brain reaches 80% of adult size by 2 years of age
Preschooler	Cranium continues to ossify; sutures are proximate and immobile; neck lengthens at 3-4 years of age and neck to body proportion is closer to adult size; musculature of neck is strong with full range of motion; nasal sinus cavities widen and deepen with skull growth
School-age child	Size and distribution of sinuses approximates those of an adult; thyroid gland is more readily palpable and approximates adult size

PHYSICAL ASSESSMENT

Examination of the head and neck region is best reserved for the latter part of the physical exam in the infant and young child. Palpation around the head and neck region often makes young children very uncomfortable. Careful visual inspection of the head should begin with the practitioner's initial contact with the patient. It is important to view the overall head size and shape. In the infant and young child, begin at the crown of the head and evaluate the scalp, the fontanels, and the bony structures of the skull. The examination proceeds with a thorough inspection of the scalp area, viewing the condition of the scalp around the base of the hair follicles, particularly with long and/or thick hair.

Fontanels

The fontanels should be palpated for size, level of tenseness, or pulsations (Figure 9-4). The length and width of the fontanel should be noted in the medical record for accuracy and to monitor head growth. Overlapping sutures may occur in the first 6 months of life and are not considered abnormal in the presence of a normal occipital-frontal head circumference (see Chapter 2). Suture lines are not normally palpable after 6 months of age in the term infant. Infants should be evaluated for *cranio-synostosis,* premature closure of the sutures, if the skull shows asymmetrical growth. Occasionally, an infant in the first few months of life develops a visible or palpable ridge at the crown of the head known as a *metopic ridge.*

TABLE 9-2   INFORMATION GATHERING FOR HEAD AND NECK ASSESSMENT AT KEY DEVELOPMENTAL STAGES

Age	Questions to Ask
Preterm infant	History of intraventricular insult? History of maternal substance or alcohol abuse or infections?
Newborn	Vaginal or cesarean birth? Prolonged labor with prolonged third stage? Precipitous? Forceps delivery? Shoulder presentation? Respiratory distress at birth? Head tilt? Neonatal screen results? History of maternal hyperthyroidism, thyroid disease, gestational diabetes?
Infant	Neonatal screen results? History of maternal infection? Neonatal infections? Meningitis? Quality of muscle tone and strength, head control? Achieving developmental milestones?
Toddler	Achieving developmental milestones? History of falls, clumsiness? Stable gait? Persistent lymph gland swelling? Head tilt, neck pain/stiffness?
Preschooler	History of head trauma or falls, neck pain/stiffness? Use of bike helmet?
School-age child	History of headache? Onset and duration? History of head injury? Neck pain/stiffness? Use of bike or skateboarding helmet? Other protective sports equipment?
Adolescent	History of head injury? Recurrent headaches? Blurred vision? Neck pain/stiffness? Weight loss or gain? Neck/lymph gland swelling? Use of bike or skateboarding helmet, other protective sports equipment?
Environmental risks	Contact with chemical cleaning agents, hazardous chemicals or smoke, radiation, hazardous waste?

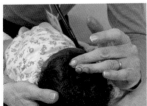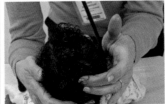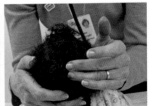

Figure **9-4** Palpation of the fontanels.

This is a normal variant when the head shape appears normal and the head circumference grows at a normal rate. Infants with a wide margin along the frontal or sagittal suture may have a communicating *anterior* and *posterior* fontanel. This is often referred to as a *metopic suture*, or pertaining to the forehead. Separation of the sagital suture is one of the most common findings in Down syndrome, along with a flattened occiput and a small rounded head.[2] Infants should be monitored closely for increasing head size or other indications of abnormal growth and development in the first year.

The level of the fontanel is indicative of the health and hydration status of the infant. Normally, there is a slight pulsation in the *anterior fontanel,* and it tenses or bulges slightly when the infant is crying but flattens when the infant calms. In the ill infant, the tense, bulging *anterior fontanel* can be a sign of increasing intracranial pressure due to infection or head trauma and is a medical emergency. Tumors in the brain and meninges also can cause increased intracranial pressure indicated by a bulging fontanel. Infants can have a sunken fontanel, unaccompanied by other symptoms, which may indicate mild dehydration due to the metabolic demands of growth or fluid loss due to perspiration. If accompanied by gastrointestinal symptoms, infection, or loss of normal turgor of skin and mucous membranes, a sunken fontanel indicates an urgent need for further medical evaluation (see Chapter 6). Infants and young children with increased intracranial pressure will have a resonant or cracked-pot sound, *Macewen sign,* when tapping or percussing on the scalp with the forefinger.

CULTURAL CONSIDERATIONS

Native-American infants have an additional horizontal suture line over the occipital bone. African-American infants have a slightly larger anterior fontanel than do Caucasian infants.

Skull

Craniotabes

Craniotabes, or abnormal softness of the cranium noted on palpation of the skull in the term infant, may be a normal variant in the first 6 months because of incomplete ossification of bone or widened sutures. However, if accompanied by abnormal facies or if persistent, craniotabes should be investigated. Craniotabes may be associated with hydrocephalus or rickets. If swelling or masses are detected, the size, mobility, and location on the cranium should be noted. The cranial swelling related to minor birth trauma of the scalp and periosteal space resolves in the first 6 weeks of life. All other swelling or masses require urgent medical investigation.

Transillumination

Transillumination, although rarely used today because of the availability of computed tomography (CT) imaging, is still useful in detecting excess fluid or densities on the scalp. A flashlight or penlight is placed firmly against the scalp in a darkened room. The light creates a halo effect on the scalp, which is concentric and consistent as the light is moved over the scalp. The dimension decreases slightly over the occiput because of the density of the bone. Irregularities are detected by a change in the size and consistency of the halo pattern.

A flattened occipital region or a unilateral flattening of the parietal region occurs in young infants because of positional placement. In early infancy, often infants prefer lying on one side to mimic the fetal position. There has been an increase in the number of cases of flattening of the occiput, or *posterior plagiocephaly,* causing an increase in the referrals to neurosurgery centers.[3] This increase has been related to the change in the infant's sleep position. The American Academy of Pediatrics Task Force on Infant Positioning and SIDS (1992) recommended putting infants to sleep on their backs to reduce the risk of sudden infant death syndrome (SIDS).[4]

The resulting positional deformities in the skull that can occur in the young infant require careful monitoring in the first 3 months of life. Usually positional misshaping of the occiput will normalize by 3 months of age but any persistence in a misshapen head or abnormal head growth should be carefully evaluated and referred.

Key Points

Persistent positioning of the infant on the back may result in flattening of the pliable bones in the cranium.

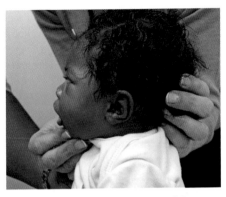

Figure **9-5** The normal alignment of the ear.

Facies

Examination of the facial area begins with initial observation of the infant, child, or adolescent for symmetry of facial features and facial movements. Observing the smile, laugh, facial creases, and facial wrinkles reveals normal function as well as innervation of the facial structures. Observing the symmetry of the facial features in the newborn and infant during crying will assist the practitioner in facial and neurological assessment of the young infant. Often, birth injury to the facial nerves can be detected when observing the infant while crying. Unusual facies with disproportional features, frontal bossing of the forehead, and small or low-set ears are indicative of a genetic insult and need prompt medical investigation (Figure 9-5).

Head

Inspection of the head includes observation by the practitioner for head movement and head control. Head lag when pulling the infant to the sitting position is normal until 3 to 4 months of age in the term infant. Head lag should be evaluated in all infants in the first 6 months of life as an indicator of muscle tone. Persistent head lag between 3 and 6 months of age in the term infant is suspect and should be considered abnormal. Head alignment in the infant and young child should be evaluated in the resting position after 3 to 4 months of age with the infant or young child being supported in a sitting position with head at midline. Persistent head tilt may indicate *hypotonia, congenital torticollis,* muscular or gastrointestinal abnormalities, or vision and hearing deficits. Range of motion and movement of the head should be examined to determine tone and flexibility. In examining the infant younger than 3 months, the practitioner should move the head passively on the examining surface to the left and right to determine mobility and range of motion. Children between 3 and 6 months of age can begin to follow a light or small toy to determine the full range of motion of the head and the function of the musculature. Any limited range of motion, head bobbing or jerking, tremors, or involuntary muscle contractions or spasms should be investigated.

Infants and young children with unexplained fever, irritability, or a bulging fontanel indicating increased intracranial pressure, may indicate pain or neck stiffness during examination of the neck region. *Meningismus* or *meningitis,* inflammation of the brain and spinal cord, can manifest in the neck. Flexion of the head forward or ventrally with the infant or young child lying on a flat surface or examining table causes pain, irritability, and resistance to movement and range of motion. Often flexion of the lower extremities will occur spontaneously with flexion of the head forward in an effort to guard or protect the body. The infant or young child with *meningitis* will resist extension of the knees and lower extremities. A positive *Kernig* or *Brudzinski* sign for *meningeal irritation occurs when the examiner notes* pain and resistance to extension of the knees when the infant or young child is lying with knees flexed in the supine position. *Opisthotonos*, hyperextension of the neck and spine, indicates severe meningeal irritation.

Neck

The neck should be inspected for symmetry, shape, and mobility. To examine the neck in the very young child, it is best to have the newborn or infant on a firm surface for inspection. While supporting the neck and shoulders cradled with the thumb and forefingers, use the opposite hand to extend the head back slightly to expose the shortened neck region. This position allows the examiner to inspect not only for symmetry and strength of the musculature of the neck but also for the alignment of the trachea and the condition of the skin in the infant and young child, who is vulnerable to fungal and bacterial infection in the anterior neck region. Palpation of the *sternocleidomastoid muscle* in the infant and young child examines for masses, strength, and tone. Palpation should include the clavicular area at the base of the sternocleidomastoid muscle. Palpable masses in the clavicular area in the newborn could include a fracture of the *clavicles* sustained during the birth process. Any sign of pain or irritability, or resistance to range of motion in the infant, child, or adolescent indicates an abnormality. Resistance to lateral motion of the neck may indicate lymph gland swelling, infection, or trauma to the sternocleidomastoid muscle. If webbing of the neck is noted, it may indicate *Turner syndrome* (Table 9-3).

Pulsations in the jugular vein in the neck can be seen when the child is in the supine position on the examining table. The pulsations should be of normal rate and amplitude without bruits, or blowing sounds, heard on auscultation over the vessel. The jugular venous pulsation is normally a gentle undulation visible in good lighting.

Thyroid Gland

Examination of the *thyroid gland* is more easily accomplished from the front of the neck in the young child to minimize any fear that may occur during the exam. Standing or sitting in front of the child, the practitioner tilts the head forward slightly while maintaining a sitting position with the back straight. The child may be guided gently in this activity with the practitioner's hand on the back of the head. Using the opposite hand, palpate with the thumb and forefingers in the anterior region of the midneck surrounding the trachea. Extend the forefingers and thumb, and apply slight pressure for deep palpation along both sides of the trachea. Fingernails must be groomed short for effective examination of the thyroid in children. The choking sensation from deep palpation often makes children fearful and then they are not able to cooperate with swallowing during the exam to assist the practitioner in locating and sizing the gland. The thyroid gland is difficult to palpate in infants and is often omitted from the exam, unless masses or nodular lesions are noted in the neck. Screening for thyroid disease in newborns is required in all states. Thyroid disease in infants and young children presents with systemic symptoms (including hypotonia, lethargy, distended abdomen, and enlarged tongue), as compared to adults, in whom develop thyroid nodules or glandular enlargement are often the initial point of diagnosis.

In the older school-age child and adolescent, the thyroid gland can be examined from behind with the head tilted slightly forward (Figure 9-6). The practitioner uses the forefingers of both hands to palpate deeply between the trachea and sternocleidomastoid muscle.

TABLE 9-3 ABNORMAL CONDITIONS OF THE HEAD, FACE, AND NECK

Condition	Description
Bell palsy	Acute unilateral paralysis of cranial facial nerve VII related to postinfectious viral neuritis
Congenital hypothyroidism	Thyroid dysgenesis characterized by prolonged gestation, large for gestational age (LGA), delayed first stool and constipation, poor feeding; infant may have dysmorphic facial features, enlarged tongue, sparse hair/eyebrows with low-set hairline
Congenital syphilis	Bacterial infection transmitted placentally characterized by frontal bossing, depressed nasal bridge, chronic rhinitis, facial lesions circumorally
Congenital torticollis	Contracture of sternocleidomastoid muscle causing tilting of head to one side; occurs secondary to birth trauma, cervical spine or spinal cord congenital deformities
Craniostenosis	Narrowness of skull caused by premature closure of sutures
Craniosynostosis	Premature closure of the cranial sutures
Down syndrome	Microcephaly or small rounded head, thick epicanthal folds, almond-shaped eyes or oblique palpebral fissures; flattened nasal bridge, large protuberant tongue; ears are low-set, small, and protuberant
Facies of fetal alcohol syndrome	Fetal alcohol exposure characterized by dysmorphic features: microcephaly, short palpebral fissures, wide and flattened philtrum/thin lips; associated with developmental delay
Hydrocephalus	Ventricle enlargement in dura caused by increased production and blockage of or impaired absorption of cerebral spinal fluid; increased head circumference
Hypothyroidism	Acquired thyroid condition usually caused by lymphocytic thyroiditis
Micrognathia	Underdeveloped mandible
Plagiocephaly	Asymmetrical head shape or flattening from persistent positioning of infant on one side during first 6 months of life
Potter syndrome	Renal agenesis characterized by low-set ears, broad nose, underdeveloped chin line, blank appearance
Torticollis	Contraction of sternocleidomastoid muscle causing tilting of head toward involved side; can be sequela of upper respiratory infection
Turner syndrome	Genetic disorder, a female phenotype; characterized by short stature, webbed neck, pectus excavatum, primary amenorrhea, no development of secondary sexual characteristics

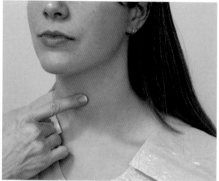

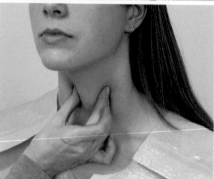

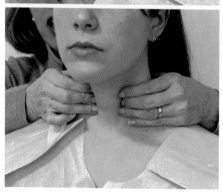

Figure **9-6** Examination of the thyroid gland.

Locating the *cricoid cartilage,* the prominent ring of the tracheal cartilage, with the forefinger provides a landmark the examiner can use as a guide in determining the position of the thyroid gland in the older child or adolescent. Tilting the head to one side, or rotating the neck very gently in a circular motion may help to evaluate the size, quality, and firmness of the gland. A soft, mushy gland, masses, or nodules are abnormal and require prompt medical investigation.

ABNORMAL CONDITIONS

Table 9-3 presents the most common abnormal conditions seen in infants and children by the pediatric healthcare practitioner.

 CHARTING

Healthy Newborn

Head and neck: Normocephalic, anterior and posterior fontanel patent and soft, overriding sagittal suture, neck supple.

REFERENCES

1. Porth CM: *Pathophysiology: concepts of altered health states,* ed 7, Philadelphia, 2005, Lippincott Williams & Wilkins.
2. Engel JK: *Pocket guide to pediatric assessment,* ed 4, St Louis, 2002, Mosby.
3. Huang MH, Mouradian WE, Cohen SR, Gruss JS: The differential diagnosis of abnormal head shapes: separating craniosynostosis from positional deformities and normal variants, *Cleft Palate Craniofac J* 35(3):204-211, 1998.
4. American Academy of Pediatrics AAP Task Force on Infant Positioning and SIDS: Positioning and SIDS, *Pediatrics* 89(6 Pt 1):1120-1126, 1992.

CHAPTER 10

LYMPHATIC SYSTEM

Karen G. Duderstadt

DEVELOPMENT

The lymphatic system is established in the mesoderm layer during the third week of embryonic development. The mesoderm gives rise to the bone marrow and excretory organs, and the ectoderm gives rise to the epithelial linings of the glandular cells of the large organs that make up the lymphatic system.[1] Developmental changes of the lymphatic system occur from birth throughout childhood and into early adolescence (Table 10-1).

PHYSIOLOGICAL VARIATIONS

The lymphatic system is one of the most sensitive indicators of infection and toxins in the pediatric age span. The lymph glands that occur throughout the body, both superficially and embedded deep in the tissues, form the drainage and filtering system. The lymphatic tissue plays a role in the immune system as a first responder to fight infection through phagocytosis, the destruction of harmful cells, and the production of lymphocytes and antibodies. Lymphatic tissue increases throughout infancy and early childhood and peaks in the later years of middle childhood. During adolescence, the volume of lymphatic tissue begins to decrease and assumes an adult level, which is 2% to 3% of total body weight.[2]

ANATOMY AND PHYSIOLOGY

Lymphatic System

The *lymphatic system,* composed of capillaries, collecting vessels, lymph nodes, and lymphatic glands or organs, forms an extensive network throughout the body. *Lymph* is a clear, colorless fluid filtered and collected from the organs and tissues through the *lymphatic capillaries.* The *collecting vessels* carry the lymph from the lymphatic capillaries to the bloodstream. The lymph nodes throughout the body are filters for the collection vessels. The *lymph* is deposited into the bloodstream through the jugular and subclavian veins in the neck. The lymphatic system also absorbs fat and fat-soluble substances from the intestinal wall. The lymph and fat are transported from the lymph glands to the larger ducts and through the venous return to the heart.

A *lymph node* is an accumulation of lymphatic tissue lying along a lymphatic vessel and consists of an outer cortical layer and an inner medullary layer. The terms *gland* and *node* are often used interchangeably in relation to the lymphatic system. Both terms can be applied to the lymphatic system. Figure 10-1 illustrates the lymph glands in the head and neck area and gives a view of the lymphatic chain in the body.

TABLE 10-1 PHYSIOLOGICAL VARIATIONS OF THE LYMPHATIC SYSTEM

Age-Group	Variations
Preterm	Minimal amount of palpable lymphatic tissue present in preterm infant
Newborn	The lymphatic system is underdeveloped in term newborn; although amount of lymphatic tissue is small, *lymphadenopathy* can be detected as result of perinatal infections particularly in occipital region; *thymus gland* is prominent in newborn, often shadowing cardiac silhouette on radiographs
Infant	Amount of lymphoid tissue increases throughout first year and cervical lymph nodes become more pronounced with respiratory infections by first birthday
Toddler	Mild infections of any type result in swollen lymph glands and often splenomegaly
Preschooler	Period of increased upper respiratory infection with mild to moderate swelling in cervical and occipital nodes common
School-age child	Tonsillar and adenoid tissue approximately same as adult size by 6 years of age and reach peak size by 12 years of age, which is twice adult size
Adolescent	Tonsillar size reduces to adult norm

Pediatric Pearls

Occipital nodes are located high above the hairline in the infant and are often missed by the examiner palpating too low at the nape of the neck. Occipital adenopathy may be an indicator in the newborn of maternal infection during pregnancy or of an acute viral infection in the infant. They may be visible on inspection and are often noted by the parent of a young infant.

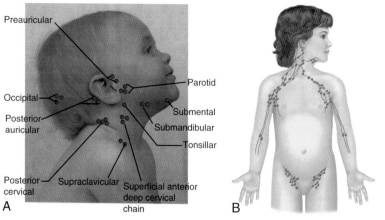

Figure **10-1 A,** Lymph glands in the head and neck area. **B,** Lymph glands in the body.

TABLE 10-2 INFORMATION GATHERING FOR LYMPHATIC SYSTEM ASSESSMENT AT KEY DEVELOPMENTAL STAGES

Age-Group	Questions to Ask
Preterm infant and newborn	History of maternal substance/alcohol abuse? Maternal infections? HIV+ mother? Prenatal results of TORCH screen? Neonatal meningitis or sepsis? Immunization history in NICU?
Infant	Neonatal screen results? History of maternal/neonatal infection? History of fever/respiratory infection?
Toddler	Lymphadenopathy? History of fever/respiratory infection, exposures? International travel? Persistent lymph gland swelling? Head tilt? Neck pain/stiffness? Anemia?
School-age child	Lymphadenopathy? History of fever/respiratory infection? Exposures? Fatigue? Loss of appetite? History of anemia? International travel? Family history of infections, tuberculosis?
Adolescent	Lymphadenopathy? History of fever/respiratory infection? Neck pain/stiffness? Fatigue? Weight loss or gain? Neck swelling?
Environmental risks	Contact with chemical cleaning agents, hazardous chemicals, smoke, radiation, hazardous waste? Recent professional carpet cleaning?

TORCH, Toxoplasmosis, other (congenital syphilis and viruses), rubella, cytomegalovirus, and herpes simplex virus; *NICU,* neonatal intensive care unit.

⌐ Key Points

A *gland* is an organ that produces a product or secretion, and a *node* is a swelling or protuberance.

The tonsils, adenoids, thymus, and spleen are all organs of the lymphatic system, as is the *bone marrow.* The buds of *tonsillar tissue* are present in the oropharynx at birth, but are underdeveloped. As the immune system develops and reacts to respiratory triggers—viral, bacterial, and fungal infections and environmental toxins—the *tonsils* are the first line of defense.

The *thymus gland* is embedded beneath the sternum, the bony prominence at the apex of the chest wall. In the infant and young child, the thymus is important to the development of the immune system in regard to the

production of T-lymphocytes, which have a role in cell-mediated immunity.[3] The thymus gland is prominent in the mediastinum of the newborn and infant in the first year of life and is usually undetectable in the adult[4] (Figure 10-2).

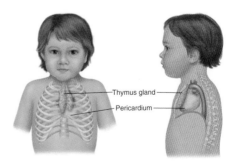

Figure **10-2** Thymus gland in infant.

The *spleen* lies in the upper left quadrant of the abdomen protected by the rib cage. It is composed of lymphoid tissue and reticuloendothelial cells and is a densely vascular organ. The spleen acts as a part of the immune system and is the response organ in regard to blood-borne infections. In the infant and young child, the spleen stores erythrocytes and filters the blood through the large presence of phagocytes.

SYSTEM-SPECIFIC HISTORY

Obtaining a complete history of exposure to infections is key to an accurate assessment of lymphadenopathy in the pediatric population. Table 10-2 reviews the pertinent areas of information gathering for each age-group and developmental stage.

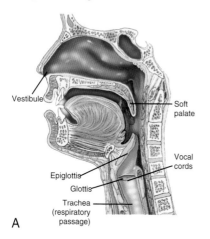

Vestibule

Soft palate

Vocal cords

Epiglottis

Glottis

Trachea (respiratory passage)

A

PHYSICAL ASSESSMENT

Inspection and Palpation

Because the lymph glands are distributed throughout the body, it is important to include the *inspection* and *palpation* of the lymph glands regionally during the physical examination. The examination includes palpating lymph glands accessible in four areas: the head and neck, arms, axillae, and inguinal areas of the body. Most effective for palpation are the pads of the examiner's second, third, and fourth fingers. It is important to distinguish between massage and palpation. Massaging an area superficially may not detect nodes, but superficial then deep palpation with the forefingers can better determine the size and mobility of a lymph gland. Lymph nodes are generally mobile, nontender, and do not feel warm to the touch.

Lymph nodes normally range in size from 3 mm in the head to 1 cm in the neck and inguinal area. In children, lymph glands are often palpable and the practitioner will feel small, firm, mobile lymph glands along the *cervical* chain on physical examination. These are occasionally referred to as "shotty" nodes because of the pellet-like distribution. Lymph nodes that are immobile, tender, and warm to the touch indicate infection or an abscess. The healthcare provider must be an astute observer

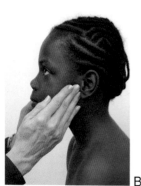
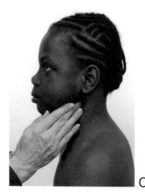
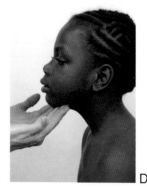

B   C   D

Figure **10-3 A,** Parotid and submandibular gland. **B-D,** Palpation of the cervical chain in a school-age child.

TABLE 10-3   REGIONAL AND SYSTEMIC CAUSES OF LYMPHADENOPATHY

Region	Related Causes
Occipital	Scalp infections such as seborrheic dermatitis, tinea capitis, pediculosis/head lice; viral syndromes such as varicella, measles, rubella, roseola; viral respiratory infections (i.e., rhinovirus, RSV, post immunization)
Preauricular, parotid, postauricular, and superficial cervical	Infection of pinna (ear), otitis externa, middle ear infection; parotitis
Cervical glands— tonsillar, sublingual, submandibular, deep cervical	Tonsillitis, pharyngitis, stomatitis; tooth decay, dental abscess; ear infection; oral mucosa/mucous membrane infections, tongue; cervical adenitis from systemic infections; neoplasm or cancer; postimmunization response
Axillary	Breast infections, thoracic wall inflammation, infections of shoulder and arm, systemic infection, or neoplasm in lymphatic system
Supraclavicular and subclavian	Neoplasm or cancer—metastatic cancers from respiratory, gastrointestinal, or lymphatic system
Epitrochlear and popliteal	Forearm and finger infections, infection secondary to fractures, skin infections, neoplasm, or cyst in lower extremity
Inguinal	Diaper rash, gluteal and perineal infections; skin infections in lower abdominal area; foot and leg infections, systemic viral infections
Generalized lymphadenopathy	Systemic disease occurring in lymphatic, circulatory, respiratory, gastrointestinal, or genitourinary system; infections such as tuberculosis, HIV

RSV, Respiratory syncytial virus.

when examining the lymphatic system because each region of the body has clusters or chains of lymph glands that can signal infection in adjacent areas (Table 10-3).

Head and Neck

Assessment of the lymph glands begins with the inspection of the clusters of lymph glands in the head and neck area. The *cervical nodes* constitute the largest collection of lymph glands in the body. In children, the cervical glands are often palpable because of the frequency of respiratory infections. The *posterior*

auricular and *preauricular nodes* often are not palpable during routine respiratory infections but palpable only with specific infection related to the external and internal ear, the *pinna,* and surrounding skin. The *occipital nodes* in the infant and young child lie on either side of the occiput just above the base of the skull. In the young infant, the occipital nodes are located well above the hairline adjacent to the occipital bony prominence.

The *parotid* glands are located anterior to the ear and surround the oral cavity. *Parotitis,* or an inflammation of the salivary glands, can

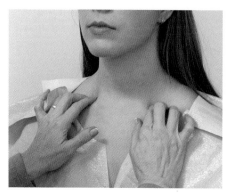

Figure **10-4** Palpation of the supraclavicular nodes.

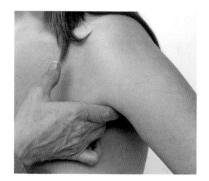

Figure **10-5** Palpation of the subscapular nodes of the axillary chain.

be caused by mumps, a ribonucleic acid (RNA) polymerase virus, or other viruses or bacteria. Incidence is less than 500 reported cases per year. The *mandibular, submandibular,* and *submental* glands are located along the anterior and posterior jaw line and under the anterior jaw. They are palpable when infection occurs in the tongue, the mucous membranes of the mouth, the sublingual area extending to the base of the tongue, or the gum or when decay or abscess occurs in the teeth (Figure 10-3).

The *superficial cervical nodes* are palpable at the juncture of the *mandible* and *sternocleidomastoid muscle* at the neck. This examination requires both superficial and deep palpation depending on the age and developmental stage of the child or adolescent. These glands are almost always palpable during throat and respiratory infections. A lack of findings may indicate incorrect positioning of the fingertips during the assessment of the neck (Figure 10-4). The *deep cervical nodes* are rarely palpable and are only identifiable with deep palpation in the older child. Visible swelling in the lymph glands on inspection is generally of grave concern in the child or adolescent; is a medically urgent condition, and indicates the need for further laboratory investigation of systemic infection.

Torso

The *axillary, brachial,* and *subscapular* nodes lie anteriorly along the brachial artery and in the axillae along the lateral edge of the pectoralis major muscle. They are generally noted in children only on deep palpation unless enlarged. Examination of the subscapular nodes of the axillary chain is illustrated in Figure 10-5. The *epitrochlear* nodes lie along the medial aspect of the arm above the elbow and are palpable over the *humerus.* The *epitrochlear* and *popliteal* nodes are the only peripheral lymph nodes in the lymphatic system and act as collection ducts for the limbs.

Groin

The *inguinal nodes* can be palpated along the juncture of the thigh and abdomen and along the inguinal ligament and the saphenous vein. The horizontal chain of inguinal nodes runs along the inferior groin and the vertical chain can be palpated on deep palpation along the upper inner thigh. If lymph glands are enlarged in the inguinal area, they are often visible when the young child lies supine on the examining table. Figure 10-6 shows a toddler in the supine position for examination of the inguinal nodes. Inguinal lymphadenopathy often occurs with systemic viral infection in the pediatric patient. Table 10-4 reviews commonly used sizing of the lymph nodes on physical exam.

Lymphadenopathy

Lymphadenopathy, disease within the lymph glands, is an indicator of either local or

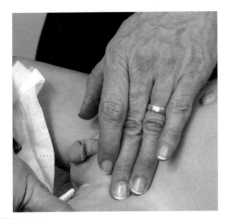

Figure **10-6** Palpation of inguinal nodes in a toddler.

TABLE 10-4 SIZING OF LYMPH GLANDS ON EXAMINATION

Size	Description
1+	Shotty, firm, nontender, <1 cm to > 1-1.5 cm, requires deep palpation
2+	Mobile, detectable on superficial-to-deep palpation, >2-2.5 cm
3+	Palpable superficially, visible on inspection, >3-3.5 cm
4+	Lymph glands are walnut size or larger, nonmobile, tender; skin can be reddened and warm to the touch; >4-4.5 cm; visible on inspection

generalized infection in the pediatric patient. The extensive lymphatic system throughout the body provides the healthcare provider with a map in times of illness. Swelling in regional lymph glands, such as in the neck, indicates a localized source of infection, whereas generalized swelling of the lymph glands indicates a systemic source of infection. The head and neck region is the area of the body with the highest concentration of lymph glands. Even mild infections in children cause swelling in the lymph glands, and general lymphadenopathy is more likely to occur in children than in adults.

The patterns of drainage leading to the lymph glands are indicative of infections that occur in different areas throughout the body. Accurate assessment and diagnosis may depend on the practitioner's knowledge of the lymphatic drainage. Table 10-3 reviews some of the causes of regional and systemic lymph node swelling in infants, children, and adolescents.

ABNORMAL CONDITIONS

Table 10-5 reviews common pediatric infectious conditions presenting with lymphadenopathy.

 CHARTING

Physical Examination Findings on an Adolescent with Lymphadenopathy

Neck: 3+ tonsillar lymph nodes, mobile, warm, tender to touch, neck supple with full ROM (range of motion), no meningismus noted.

REFERENCES

1. Porth CM: *Pathophysiology: concepts of altered health states,* ed 7, Philadelphia, 2005, Lippincott Williams & Wilkins.
2. Engel JK: *Pocket guide to pediatric assessment,* ed 4, St Louis, 2002, Mosby.
3. Seidel HM, Ball JW, Dains JE, Benedict GW: *Mosby's guide to physical examination,* ed 3, St Louis, 2003, Mosby.
4. Muscari ME: *Advanced pediatric clinical assessment: skills and procedures,* Philadelphia, 2001, Lippincott Williams & Wilkins.
5. Hill NL, Sullivan L: Management guidelines for pediatric nurse practitioners, Philadelphia, 1999, FA Davis.

TABLE 10-5   ABNORMAL CONDITIONS OF THE LYMPHATICS

Condition	Description
Cat-scratch fever	Bacterial infection caused by scratch from contact with kitten or cat; initial lesion on face/arm area; fever, lymphadenopathy present after incubation period of 10-14 days or longer
Cervical lymphadenitis	Marked swelling most commonly in anterior cervical node although other lymph glands can be involved; characterized by tenderness, > 4+ swelling *Etiology:* Primarily streptococcal, 20% staphylococcal, 10% of viral origin[5]
Hodgkin lymphoma	Malignant neoplasm of lymph system characterized by painless, enlarged lymph nodes, generally asymmetrical, nontender, firm along cervical/supraclavicular chain; onset common in adolescent or young adult; swelling in left clavicular node in adolescent males is ominous sign of disease
HIV seropositive, AIDS	HIV+ adolescent onset of severe fatigue, weight loss, fever, persistent lymphadenopathy with history of recurrent persistent infections including pneumonias
Leukemia	Most common malignancy of childhood characterized by fever, fatigue, lymphadenopathy, splenomegaly, pallor, loss of appetite; may present with purpura or petechiae
Lymphangitis	Acute onset of inflammation of lymphatic vessels usually extending from finger, forearm, or upper arm infection characterized by erythematous line extending from infection area along collecting vessels
Mononucleosis	Systemic viral etiology characterized by splenomegaly with accompanying tenderness, cervical adenopathy 3+ to 4+; may be tender/firm; tonsillar hypertrophy
Roseola infantum	Viral exanthem of infancy characterized by high fever for 3-4 days and swelling of occipital and postauricular nodes; with defervescence, mildly erythematous morbilliform rash appears over trunk
Streptococcal pharyngitis	Acute onset of bacterial pharyngitis with swollen anterior cervical nodes, accompanying fever, malaise, scarlatinaform rash over trunk, abdominal pain

HIV, Human immunodeficiency virus; *AIDS,* acquired immunodeficiency syndrome.

CHAPTER 11

EYES

Karen G. Duderstadt

The first connection a parent makes with the personhood of the newborn infant is through the eyes. Early on a parent often asks about the color of the infant's eyes and the visual health of the infant. Can my baby see? Will my baby's eyes be dark? When the infant is born, the eyes are anatomically complete, but the sense of vision develops over the first weeks and months. Vision depends on appropriate visual stimulus to the internal structures of the eye and is determined by an individual's heredity, as well as physical health and environmental factors. Any condition that limits or occludes this process of visual development affects the long-term visual health of the infant. A complete and thorough eye examination by the healthcare provider can determine whether conditions are present in the eye that would impact visual development. If congenital conditions are present and not detected, the full potential of vision can be lost.

DEVELOPMENT

The *retina* is a direct extension of the central nervous system that forms as a sensory tissue during embryological development. Vision develops at the very center of the retina in the macula. The *macula* is a circular area surrounding the *fovea*. At birth, the macula is not fully formed but does hold the genetic potential for 20/20 vision. The retina is rod predominant at birth; the cones are located near the outermost layer of the retina. As the retina is exposed to light, the cones migrate toward the center to become the anatomical macula on the *fundus,* the posterior surface of the retina. The *optic nerve* is also developing at that time. There are as many as 8 million cells in the optic nerve and 5 million cells in the optic neuron at birth that compete for synaptic sites on the nerve. Cells that are not oxygenated do not develop. *Hypoxia* in the preterm infant often affects the retina, and consequently a *retinopathy* develops, causing cells to be replaced by fibrous tissue and blood vessels, which results in poor vision or blindness if left untreated.

Term infants from 36 to 40 weeks of gestation perceive shape, color, motion, and patterns at birth. The term infant is *hyperopic,* or farsighted, at birth, which means images are focused behind and not on the retina, so the visual image is blurred. The *ciliary muscles* are responsible for changing the lens shape to make it possible to focus on an image (Figure 11-1). For the infant to see near objects, the ciliary muscles of the eye must work hard to accommodate, or shape, the lens; in time these efforts of the ciliary muscles result in thickening of

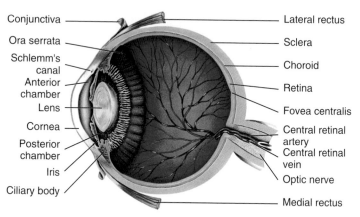

Figure 11-1 The globe, looking down on the right eye. (From Palay DA, Krachmer JH: *Primary care ophthalmology,* ed 2, St Louis, 2005, Mosby.)

the lens, which makes accommodation of the image onto the retina possible. As the eye grows, the hyperopia decreases and the lens hardens.

Research has shown the human face at a distance of 8 to 12 inches holds the most visual interest for a newborn. Central fixation is present shortly after birth in the term infant, but detailed visual acuity is not present until 3 to 4 months of age in the healthy eye and not until 3 to 4 months corrected age for preterm infants. Term infant's eyes often wander in the first 6 weeks when trying to achieve visual fixation in the *central field* of vision. After 6 weeks of early visual stimulus, an infant is expected to focus and visually follow an object or the parent's movements. Any inability to visually focus after an infant is 6 weeks of age is considered suspect and at 3 months of age is considered abnormal (Table 11-1).

PHYSIOLOGICAL VARIATIONS

The eye in the infant undergoes a dynamic developmental process that begins at birth and continues through the first 2 years of life. The majority of the growth of the sensory organ of the eye occurs in the first 2 years;

then growth continues slowly until maturity at 12 to 13 years of age. The visual system remains malleable during the first 8 to 10 years of age. After this age, conditions that affect early visual development cannot be completely corrected (Table 11-2).

ANATOMY

External Eye

The *conjunctiva* is formed by mucous membrane lining the anterior surface of the sclera and eyelids and acts along with the tear film as a protective covering for the cornea. The conjunctiva has two surfaces: the palpebral and bulbar. The *palpebral* portion lines the eyelids, is vascular, and is covered by papillae. The *bulbar* portion covers the sclera, is clear, and contains no papillae and very few blood vessels. The eyelashes add further protection to the surface of the eye. The *sclera,* the outermost layer of the exterior wall of the eye, is the firm collagenous layer that protects the intraocular structures (Figure 11-2).

The *cornea* is the most anterior aspect of the eye and acts as a refractory surface for the eye. The *anterior chamber* is directly posterior

TABLE 11-1 VISUAL DEVELOPMENT

Age	Developmental Stage of Vision
Birth	Awareness of light and dark
Neonatal	Rudiments of fixation on near object
2 weeks	Intermittent fixation
4 weeks	Follows moving objects
6 weeks	Fixates and follows moving objects
8 weeks	Convergence beginning to stabilize
4 months	Inspects hands and small held objects; vision 20/300
6 months	Retrieves small objects; hand-eye coordination appears
9 months	Binocular vision clearly established; beginning of depth perception
12 months	Vision 20/180; looks at pictures with interest; fusion is established
18 months	Convergence established; visual localization peripherally poor
2 years	Accommodation well developed; vision 20/40 in normal eyes

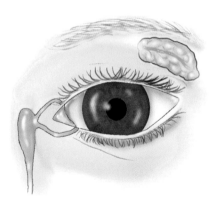

Figure **11-2** External eye and lacrimal apparatus.

to the cornea. It is filled with aqueous humor, and when inflamed or injured collects white blood cells. Because the young child's eye occupies a greater portion of the orbit than does the adult's eye, it is more vulnerable to injury. The *limbus* is the junction of the cornea and the sclera. The *iris* is the pigmented structure containing the sphincter and dilator muscles, connective tissue, and pigmented epithelium. An absence of color in the iris may indicate *albinism*. The center of the iris forms the aperture, or pupil, controlled by the *ciliary body* and *iris muscles*. The *pupil* constricts or dilates depending on the amount of light entering the eye. The iris lies behind the anterior chamber and in front of the *crystalline lens* and is protected by a thin clear capsule. This capsule is attached by small filaments to the ciliary body. The ciliary body produces aqueous humor and controls accommodation. The *posterior chamber* is the vitreous body, which contains a clear gel, and is attached to the inner eye at the *optic nerve* head and the anterior margin of the *retina*. The *choroid* is the interior layer of the eye between the sclera and the retina and is continuous with the iris and ciliary body. It is highly vascular and

TABLE 11-2 PHYSIOLOGICAL VARIATIONS OF THE EYE

Age-Group	Variations
Preterm infant	• 24 weeks: Partially fused eyelids • 24-28 weeks: Eyelids open spontaneously • 28-30 weeks: Eyes have membranous embryonic vascular network over iris to protect lens, producing dull *red light reflex* • 36-40 weeks: Membrane over iris normally resolves; persistent membrane may result in anterior cataracts
Newborn	• Macula not fully developed, eyes tend to drift in initial newborn period • Benign scleral hemorrhage often present after birth • Definite ability to follow object not developed until 4 weeks • Lacrimation present at 6 weeks of age
Infant	• 3-4 months: Fully fixates and follows object • Sucking often stimulates infant to open eyes and focus attention on surroundings • 3-5 months: Color discrimination present • 6 months: Eye color generally established • Infants may have visible sclera above and below cornea • Intermittent convergent strabismus common until 6 months
Toddler	• 2 years of age: Binocular vision and depth perception are developed in healthy eye • Visual acuity should be 20/40 to 20/50
Preschooler	• Visual acuity should be 20/30 • Accommodation and convergence are smooth and well established
School-age child	• Refractive error is common beginning at 9 years of age • Visual concerns about near vision in school-age child often are related to learning differences
Adolescent	• Hormonal changes during early and middle adolescence often cause change in visual acuity

nourishes the receptor cells of the retinal epithelium.

The *lacrimal gland* is located in the lateral aspect of the frontal bone in the orbital cavity (Figure 11-2). It is a peanut-size gland similar to the salivary glands. In each eyelid, a *lacrimal duct* opens onto the eyelid margin, and the *nasolacrimal duct* opens into the *lacrimal sac,* which is buried in the frontal process of the maxillary bone. The *lacrimal puncta* are noted at the edge of the upper and lower eyelids at the medial or inner canthus. Tear production

is present by 6 to 12 weeks of age. The sebaceous glands, known as the *meibomian glands,* are located near the hair follicles of the eyelashes in the upper and lower lids. In individuals with allergic reactions, these glands exude a yellowish sebaceous material onto the base of the eyelids. Finally, six *ocular muscles,* inserted into the scleral surface, control the movement of the eye (Figure 11-3). The *oblique* muscles arise from the anterior and posterior orbit. The superior oblique tendon passes through the *trochlea,* the small,

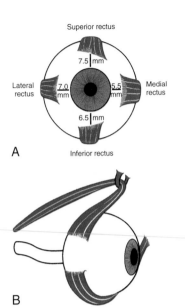

A

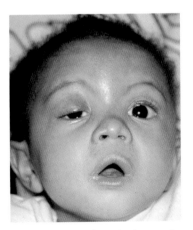

B

Figure **11-3 A,** Four extraocular recti muscles. **B,** Oblique extraocular muscles. (From Palay DA, Krachmer JH: *Primary care ophthalmology,* ed 2, St Louis, 2005, Mosby.)

Figure **11-4** Congenital ptosis. (From Palay DA, Krachmer JH: *Primary care ophthalmology,* ed 2, St Louis, 2005, Mosby.)

cartilaginous pulley on the frontal bone. The upper eyelid is elevated by the *levator muscle,* which inserts into the tarsal plate in the upper eyelid, and is innervated by the third cranial nerve. *Ptosis,* an eyelid that droops or has an absent or faint lid crease, may be a normal variant or the result of a brachial plexus injury during a difficult delivery. *Ptosis* that extends partially over the pupil and causes the infant to tilt the head in an effort to see constitutes an impact on the visual field and requires prompt referral to a pediatric ophthalmologist (Figure 11-4).

Internal Eye

The eye visible on gross inspection is only one third of the entire organ that must be examined in an infant or child. The *retina* contains photoreceptors, which are stimulated by light focused from the anterior lens, and translates impulses received by the brain, which are then perceived as visual images. The retinal vessels and optic nerve fibers enter and exit through the *optic cup* and divide into two branches on the surface of the optic disc. The *optic disc* is pink to orange-red or pale with a yellow cup at its center (Figure 11-5). The *macula* lies medially to the optic nerve on the *fundus,* the posterior surface of the retina. The *fovea* is a central depression in the macula without vessels and is darker in pigmentation than the retina. This is the area where vision is most perfect.

The *arteries* on the fundus appear thinner and more orange-red than the *veins,* which are larger and darker (Figure 11-5). The normal arterial-to-venous ratio (A:V) is approximately 2:3 in the healthy individual. Vascular changes present in the retina reflect abnormal conditions in the systemic vasculature.

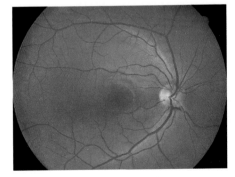

Figure **11-5** Normal fundus. (From Palay DA, Krachmer JH: *Primary care ophthalmology,* ed 2, St Louis, 2005, Mosby.)

Papilledema, bilateral optic disc edema, is associated with increased intracranial pressure. *Retinal hemorrhage* is associated with acute trauma.

CULTURAL VARIATIONS

Thick epicanthal folds are seen more commonly in infants and young children of Asian and Latino descent. They partially or completely cover the inner canthus and diminish by school age. Tiny pigmented areas sometimes found on the scleral surface are within the range of normal variations in darkly pigmented children. These usually become evident in the preschool or school-age child and persist into adulthood. The intensity of the "red" light reflex varies in darkly pigmented individuals, and the *fundus* appears pale or more "light brown" than red. The optic disc is often a pale yellow.

SYSTEM-SPECIFIC HISTORY

Detecting vision problems early is critical to the healthy development of the visual system in infants and young children. Table 11-3 reviews the pertinent areas of information gathering for each age-group.

PHYSICAL ASSESSMENT

Inspection of the External Eye

Note any asymmetry in the eyelids or brows, the size of the orbit, and whether the eyelashes are normally distributed. The palpebral fissure or opening appears horizontal on a plane between the medial and lateral canthus in pediatric patients of Caucasian descent and slants upward laterally in children of Asian descent or children with Down syndrome. The upper eyelids should appear symmetrical and when closed should completely cover the cornea and sclera. Incomplete closure of the eyelid may indicate *hyperthyroidism.*

Inspection of the Upper Lid

Inspection of the inside of the upper eyelid is necessary in the case of conjunctival irritation, infection, foreign body, trauma, or possible injury or abrasion of the cornea. To evert the upper eyelid for examination in the cooperative child, give the child a bright object and ask the child to look down at the object. Grasp the upper eyelashes at the base and *gently* pull out and up while pushing in and down with a cotton applicator on the upper *tarsal plate* (Figure 11-6). Gently remove the applicator stick and hold the eyelid while inspecting the *adnexa.* The palpebral conjunctiva should have a pink and glossy appearance and the adnexa should be clear. To return the lid to a normal position, have the child look up as the lid is released. This procedure is well tolerated by school-age children and cooperative preschool children. In a toddler, administration of a topical anesthetic, such as proparacaine, may be necessary or referral to an ophthalmologist may be made if warranted to ensure a thorough assessment. Newborn infants will occasionally have an inverted eyelid, which is within the normal range of variations.

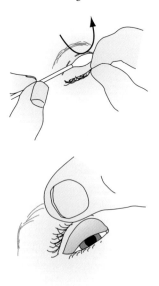

Figure **11-6** Examination of the upper eyelid.

TABLE 11-3 INFORMATION GATHERING FOR EYE ASSESSMENT AT KEY DEVELOPMENTAL STAGES

Age-Group	Questions to Ask
Preterm	History of oxygen exposure in early neonatal period? Prolonged phototherapy? History of intraventricular insult? History of maternal substance or alcohol abuse? Maternal rubella immunization status?
Newborn	Significant neonatal or maternal infections? Does infant focus on face of parent when alert? Any eye discharge or swelling? Family history of congenital cataracts or glaucoma? History of maternal substance or alcohol abuse?
Infant	When did infant begin visually following parent? Does infant blink/react to bright light? Any *rapid* involuntary movement of eyes? Persistent discharge or tearing on one or both sides? Any parental concern about visual development? Significant jaundice in neonatal period? History of maternal infection? Neonatal meningitis? Has infant been vigorously shaken?
Toddler	Does child sit close to TV? Able to see birds/plane in sky? Any clumsiness/ bumping into objects? Holds books close to face? Abnormal head positioning? Appropriate response to visual cues? Has toddler been vigorously shaken?
Preschooler	Frequent eye rubbing? Repeated blinking? Eye pain? Does child sit close to TV? Holds books close to face? Difficulty with color recognition? Family history of color vision deficit?
School-age child	History of visual problems? Family history of myopia, strabismus? Is the child squinting? Does child have corrective lenses or refuse to wear them? Date of most recent eye exam? Where is child seated in classroom? Any difficulty reading? Does child learn at grade level? Protective eyewear for sports?
Adolescent	History of eye trauma? Any difficulty with eyestrain when studying? Wears corrective lenses or refuses to wear them? Contact lens wearer? History of corneal abrasion? Date of most recent eye exam? Protective eyewear for sports? History of concussion or head trauma? Driver's license? Restricted license?
Environmental risks	Exposure to eye irritants? Contact with chemical cleaning agents, hazardous chemicals, or smoke?

Accommodation

To test for *accommodation* and *pupillary reaction*, shine a bright light momentarily into the eye. As the light approaches the iris, the pupil should begin to dilate. Bringing the light of the large aperture of the ophthalmoscope near the pupil from a distance, the pupils constrict as the light nears. Compare the pupil and iris in both eyes for color, size, shape, movement, and clarity. A *coloboma,* an irregular

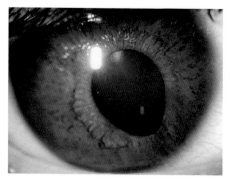

Figure **11-7** Iris coloboma. (From Palay DA, Krachmer JH: *Primary care ophthalmology,* ed 2, St Louis, 2005, Mosby.)

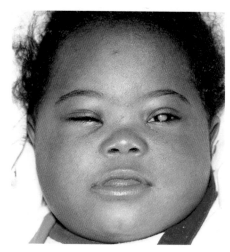

Figure **11-8** Leukokoria. (From Palay DA, Krachmer JH: *Primary care ophthalmology,* ed 2, St Louis, 2005, Mosby.)

or teardrop-shaped iris, indicates a deficit in the visual field and requires immediate referral (Figure 11-7). To inspect for opacities, illuminate the cornea by shinning the light of the ophthalmoscope obliquely about 15 degrees from the lateral canthus.

Red Light Reflex

The *red light reflex* determines the clarity of the posterior chamber of the eye, the receptivity to light, and the sensitivity of the *retina* to visual stimulus. Any serious defect of the cornea, aqueous chamber, lens, and vitreous chamber can be detected in the infant and young child by assessing the quality of the red light reflex.

Position the ophthalmoscope obliquely at a 15- to 25-degree angle laterally to the eye about 12 inches from the infant or child. Use the ophthalmoscope on the "0" setting to view the fundus. In dimmed light, bring the red light reflex into view. Inspect for symmetry and brightness, or brilliance, of the red light reflex. Any asymmetry or darkness in the uniformity of the red light reflex indicates the need for immediate referral to an ophthalmologist. *Leukokoria,* a whitish opacity of the pupil visible in dim light or in room light, is highly abnormal and appears as an absent red light reflex or a partially darkened reflex if

the opacity does not cover the entire pupil (Figure 11-8). This finding is usually *unilateral. Congenital cataracts* and *retinoblastoma* are associated with an absent or incomplete red light reflex and may have a presenting sign of leukokoria. A lens that is congenitally dislocated or abruptly dislocated because of trauma also appears as a darkened or asymmetrical red light reflex. An alert infant should blink at a bright light directed at the eye and follow a light or an object horizontally for 90 degrees.

Pediatric Pearls

To visualize the red light reflex, hold the infant upright, cradling the head, and gently rock the infant. As the head is lowered to the exam table, the eyes usually will open.

Alignment

The initial screening test to assess alignment of the extraocular muscles in the infant and young child is the *corneal light reflex,* or *Hirschberg test.* The reflection of the light from the cornea at a distance of about 12 inches

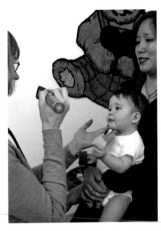

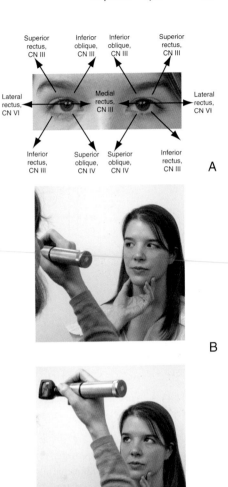

Superior rectus, CN III   Inferior oblique, CN III   Inferior oblique, CN III   Superior rectus, CN III

Lateral rectus, CN VI   Medial rectus, CN III   Lateral rectus, CN VI

Inferior rectus, CN III   Superior oblique, CN IV   Superior oblique, CN IV   Inferior rectus, CN III

A

Figure **11-9** Position for testing corneal light reflex.

determines the clarity of the lens as well as the alignment and the position of the *pupil* in the visual field (Figure 11-9). In the older school-age child and adolescent, evaluation of the extraocular muscles in the six cardinal fields of gaze should be included in the complete physical examination (Figure 11-10, *A*). The older child or adolescent can follow a penlight or the examiner's finger through the visual field to evaluate the six extraocular muscles and the oculomotor (III), trochlear (IV), and abducens (VI) cranial nerves (Figure 11-10, *B-D*).

B

C

Cover Test

The *cover-uncover test* further evaluates ocular alignment and can be performed as early as 4 months of age in an alert infant. The young infant should be assessed on the examination table. The infant or toddler should be seated in the parent's lap. Begin by having the infant or child fixate on the light of the otoscope, the light of the large aperture on the ophthalmoscope, or a bright object. If the infant is alert but distracted, it is helpful to dim the lights and use a toy. Use the opposite hand or an occluder brought in laterally over the eye while the infant or child is fixating on the light or bright object. Observe the uncovered eye for fixation on the object. Note any

D

Figure **11-10 A,** Six cardinal fields of gaze with associated cranial nerves. **B,** Testing lateral rectus, CN VI; **C,** testing superior rectus, CN III; **D,** testing superior oblique, CN IV.

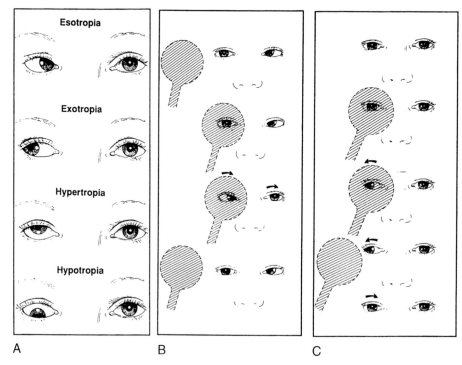

Figure 11-11 A, Types of strabismus. B, Cover test for tropia. C, Cover test for phoria. (From Magramm I: Amblyopia: etiology, detection, and treatment, *Pediatr Rev* 13[1]:7-14, 1992.)

deviations, movement of the covered or uncovered eye that may indicate abnormal alignment (Figure 11-11). An inward deviation of the eye is referred to as *esotropia*; an outward deviation is referred to as *exotropia*. Remove the hand or occluder and observe immediately for any refixation movement in the eye that was covered. If *phoria* is present, the covered eye will deviate, which indicates focusing problems.

Abnormalities in ocular alignment noted on examination can be congenital or acquired and may involve conditions affecting the muscle or nerve. *Congenital esotropia* occurs in the first 6 months and *accommodative esotropia* occurs between 12 months and 7 years of age.[3] *Cover-uncover testing* should be performed with the child fixating on a distant toy or poster as visual acuity develops and should continue to be part of the exam throughout childhood until 10 years of age in order to detect strabismus.

Strabismus

Strabismus is nonbinocular vision or nonalignment of the eyes causing the visual image to fall on the retina at a distance from the fovea. This keeps the eyes from working simultaneously and disrupts visual fusion. The resultant double vision and loss of depth perception from the blurred image are symptoms of which the very young child is usually unaware. If strabismus goes undiagnosed, amblyopia develops. *Amblyopia* is a monocular loss of vision due to insufficient visual stimulation during the critical period of visual development. The *cover test* and the *corneal light reflex* are both required in a complete ophthalmological examination in order to detect strabismus (Figure 11-12). A common finding in the young infant is *pseudoesotropia*, a crossed appearance of the eyes caused by the large epicanthal folds covering the sclera (Figure 11-13).

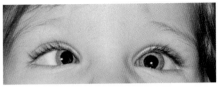

A

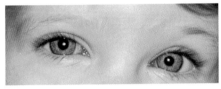

B

Figure **11-12 A,** Esotropia. **B,** Shortly after corrective muscle surgery. (From Palay DA, Krachmer JH: *Primary care ophthalmology*, ed 2, St Louis, 2005, Mosby.)

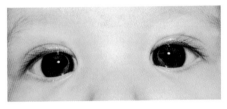

Figure **11-13** Pseudoesotropia. (From Palay DA, Krachmer JH: *Primary care ophthalmology*, ed 2, St Louis, 2005, Mosby.)

Nystagmus

Nystagmus is spontaneous, involuntary movement of one or both eyes and is an indication of poor visual acuity. In the preterm infant, *persistent* or *horizontal nystagmus* can be indicative of retinopathy of prematurity, intracranial hemorrhage, or tumor. In the term infant, *congenital nystagmus* can be associated with Down syndrome, atrophy of the optic nerve, congenital cataracts, abnormalities of the ocular muscles or nerves, vestibular disturbances, and decreased visual acuity. In the older child or adolescent, drug overdose or chemical toxicity is a possible cause.[1] Children with

amblyopia exhibit nystagmus because of loss of vision in the affected eye. If nystagmus is noted, a thorough neurological examination is warranted as well as an evaluation by a pediatric ophthalmologist.

Inspection of the Internal Eye

In the preterm infant, examination of the internal eye should be done by a pediatric ophthalmologist. In the full-term infant, eliciting a red light reflex during the initial newborn examination is the screening test used to determine the health of the internal eye. The ophthalmoscopic exam permits the healthcare provider to clearly visualize the internal structures of the eye in a child who is able to sit for examination and focus steadily on a distant point. This generally occurs in the prekindergarten or early school years.

Using the lens selector disc, focus the ophthalmoscope on the palm before examining the child to determine the clarity of the image and accommodate for any visual deficit in the examiner. The lens indicator may read "0" or +/– to produce the clearest image depending on the visual acuity of the examiner. Resting the left hand on the child's forehead just above the eyebrow, begin with the ophthalmoscope positioned laterally about 2 inches from the eye to decrease *miosis*, constriction of the pupils (Figure 11-14). The rubber pad on the face of the ophthalmoscope should be resting on the

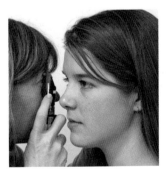

Figure **11-14** Positioning ophthalmoscope for exam.

eyebrow of the examiner. Use a distant focal point to attract the child's attention and help him or her fixate. As the examiner moves medially toward the central field of vision, the vessels of the *fundus* should come into view. Once a vessel in the *retina* is in focus, follow along the vessel; where it "branches" will point toward the *optic nerve*. The *optic disc* should come into view in the medial aspect of the fundus. The macula is examined last to minimize miosis.

Forcibly opening the eyes, except in the initial newborn period, results in a frustrated child and an incomplete examination. If examination is immediately necessary but cooperation is not achieved through verbal preparation, proper positioning, and distraction of the child, then referral to a specialist is warranted.

EVALUATION OF VISUAL ACUITY

Visual Acuity Testing

Visual acuity testing begins at 2 to 3 years of age with the Allen near card (Figure 11-15 and Table 11-4). Children should be allowed to practice with a parent or caretaker to familiarize themselves with the figures. Then testing should proceed starting at a near distance, testing each eye separately using an occluder held by the parent. The examiner should then show the Allen cards while walking backward and continue testing one eye and then both eyes until the distance is 15 feet to 20 feet for the 3- to 5-year-old child. Allen cards test to

20/30 or 15/30 depending on the distance from the child and the figure size of the cards.[2]

The Snellen *Tumbling E test* begins in the prekindergarten age-group and is used until the child knows standard letters with accuracy or for children and adolescents with low literacy. The examiner asks the child which way the "legs of the table" are pointing. Using this directional approach may be difficult for children with learning disabilities or attention or behavior problems. The Snellen distance acuity chart can be used when the child achieves literacy. Children of school age may become *myopic* (nearsighted) as the eye matures. This condition is most often noted in girls between 9 and 11 years of age and slightly later in boys. *Myopia* increases throughout adolescence and into early adulthood.

Testing the eyes separately to detect a difference in refractive error is extremely important in young children. Occluding the eye properly is the key to accurate testing of visual acuity. *Anisometropia*, a difference in refraction between the eyes, can lead to *amblyopia*. It is difficult to detect in the young child because the eye initially remains in alignment. Referral is indicated if accurate visual testing yields a >20 difference in refraction between the eyes, for example 20/40 in left eye and 20/70 in right eye.

Color Vision Testing

Visual testing for color sensitivity should occur at 4 years of age or before school entry. Children should be tested between 4 and 8

  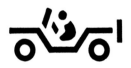

Figure **11-15** Allen card figures. (From Palay DA, Krachmer JH: *Primary care ophthalmology,* ed 2, St Louis, 2005, Mosby.)

TABLE 11-4 VISUAL ACUITY TESTING

Age-Group	Examination at All Well Visits	Referral Criteria
Preterm	Red light reflex Penlight exam of cornea Evaluate for nystagmus	Require pediatric ophthalmologic evaluation Criteria for high-risk preterm infants: <1500 g, <33 weeks, oxygen required >48 hours; referral required for preterm infants
Newborn	Red light reflex Penlight exam of cornea Evaluate for nystagmus	Asymmetrical, absent, or white reflexes Cloudiness of cornea Presence of *rapid* involuntary ocular movement
Infant	Red light reflex Penlight exam of cornea Evaluate for nystagmus Corneal light reflex Cover test Fixation to light/follow 90 degrees	Asymmetrical, absent, or white reflexes Objects to occlusion for *cover test* Strabismus: Any ocular misalignment or deviation of eye from central axis
Toddler	Red light reflex Corneal light reflex Cover test Visual acuity: Allen cards	Acuity of 20/50 in one or both eyes with accurate testing Difference of >20 between right and left eye Strabismus
Preschooler	Red light reflex Corneal light reflex Cover test Visual acuity: Allen cards, Blackbird test, Tumbling E Funduscopic exam	Acuity of 20/40 in one or both eyes Difference of >20 between right and left eye Strabismus
School-age child	Red light reflex Corneal light reflex Cover test Extraocular muscle testing Visual acuity: Tumbling E, Snellen Funduscopic exam	Acuity of 20/40 in one or both eyes Difference of >20 between right and left eye Strabismus Abnorml fundus
Adolescent	Visual acuity: Snellen Tumbling E for low literacy Extraocular muscle testing Funduscopic exam	Refractive error Abnormal fundus

years of age for any history of difficulty with color recognition. Difficulty or confusion when identifying colors may be related to cognitive learning differences and should alert parents and teachers. The incidence of *color vision deficit*, previously referred to as *color blindness*, is 8% in Caucasian males and 4% in African-American males. The incidence in females is from 0.4% to 1%. Testing should be completed with the *Hardy-Rand-Rittler (HRR) test*. The *HRR test* uses a series of symbols rather than numbers, which allows reliable testing to be done on young children. The *Ishihara test*, which uses a series of figures and letters composed of spots of certain colors can be used on the older child. Letters or figures of a certain color are not seen by the child with a *color vision deficit*.

ABNORMAL CONDITIONS

Table 11-5 presents the most common abnormal conditions seen in infants, children, and adolescents by the pediatric healthcare practitioner

 CHARTING

Healthy Preschooler

Eye: Vision with Allen figure cards 20/40 bilaterally. Extraocular movements intact, sclera and conjunctiva clear, corneal reflex intact bilaterally, irides brown, pupils accommodate. Ophthalmoscopic examination reveals a symmetrical red light reflex.

 CHARTING

Well Adolescent

Eye: Sclera and conjunctiva clear, extraocular movements (EOMs) normal (nl), irides brown, PERRLA (*P*upils, *E*qual, *R*ound, *R*eact to *L*ight, and *A*ccommodate), ophthalmoscopic examination—without opacities, optic disc visualized, pale yellow, disc margins clear (cl). Vessels nl, arteries/veins (A/V) ratio 2:3.

TABLE 11-5 ABNORMAL CONDITIONS OF THE EYES

Condition	Description
Sundowning	Downward deviation of the eyes associated with hydrocephalus, intracranial hemorrhage, other pathological brain conditions, or early sign of cerebral palsy; a sign of increased intracranial pressure when symptoms of lethargy, poor feeding, vomiting, bulging fontanel, or rapidly increasing head circumference are noted
Conjunctivitis	Acute inflammation of palpebral and bulbar conjunctiva; etiology includes viral, bacterial, corneal abrasion, allergy, or environment irritation
Pterygium	Overgrowth of conjunctival tissue extending from the lateral canthus to cornea; begins in childhood with overexposure to sun and constant dust/environmental irritants
Scleral icterus	Yellowish coloration of sclera extending to the cornea; most often first indication of systemic jaundice and liver dysfunction in neonate

TABLE 11-5 ABNORMAL CONDITIONS OF THE EYES—CONT'D

Condition	Description
Lacrimal duct obstruction	Abnormal tearing pattern; upward pressure on lacrimal sac often yields mucoid discharge; massage of nasolacrimal duct with downward pressure on lacrimal sac may open duct to normal drainage by 6 months of age
Dacryocystitis	Inflammation of nasolacrimal sac; swelling and redness occur around lacrimal sac in area of inner canthus
Retinoblastoma	Solid intraocular tumor; presents as abnormal red light reflex in newborn or as white pupillary reflex in infant; can be associated with proptosis, protruding eye bulb
Congenital glaucoma	Triad of symptoms in 30% of infants: photophobia (sensitivity to bright light), epiphora (excessive tearing), and blepharospasm (eyelid squeezing); conjunctival injection, ocular enlargement, and visual impairment may occur in some infants

REFERENCES

1. Leitman MW: *Manual for eye examination and diagnosis,* ed 5, Malden, Mass, 2001, Blackwell Science.
2. Palay DA, Krachmer JH: *Primary care ophthalmology,* ed 2, St Louis, 2005, Mosby.
3. Magramm I: Amblyopia: etiology, detection, and treatment, *Pediatr Rev* 13(1):7-14, 1992.

CHAPTER *12*

EARS

Patricia Jackson Allen

The ear is a complex organ system that functions as the sensory organ for hearing and vestibular equilibrium. Visual inspection of the ear is only the first step in determining the normal function of this complex organ. The role of the pediatric provider is to maintain optimum function of the ear and detect any abnormalities early to preserve hearing in the infant, child, and adolescent, and support the normal development of verbal communication.

DEVELOPMENT

External Ear

The ear is located in the temporal bone of the skull and is composed of the inner, middle, and external ear (Figure 12-1). The structures of the ear evolve in the mesoderm, and development of the external ear begins during the sixth week of gestation when the six *hillocks of His* develop from the first and second branchial arches. The individual portions of the *auricle*, or flap of the ear, begin to fuse and assume the classic adult shape by the twelfth week of gestation, and fusion is complete by the twentieth week (Figure 12-2). The normal auricle should be no greater than 10 degrees off vertical plane or slope, and the superior portion should be in line with the outer canthus of the eye (for illustration of ear alignment, see Chapter 9). Abnormality of the auricle does not necessarily indicate other abnormalities of the ear but may provide a clue to other alterations in development occurring during the same gestational period. External, middle, and inner ear deformities are rare, and mixed deformities are usually seen only in children with conditions such as craniofacial deformities and trisomy 13, 18, and 21.[1]

Inner Ear

Although the external ear formation coincides in time with the gestational formation of the internal ear structures, they develop separately. The auditory placode and the acousticofacial ganglion are present the fourth week of gestation. Over the next month, the first of the three turns in the cochlea develops. Arrest in development during this phase results in a common bony abnormality of the inner ear associated with congenital sensorineural hearing loss known as *Mondini's deformity*. The final 2.5 turns of the cochlea occur by the ninth week of gestation. The *organ of Corti* develops from the epithelium of the cochlea and is responsible for transmission of sound impulses to the eighth (acoustic) cranial nerve. Improper development of the membranous labyrinth of the organ of Corti results in a

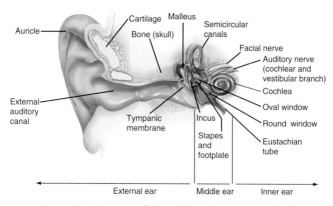

Figure **12-1** Anatomy of the middle and inner ear in skull.

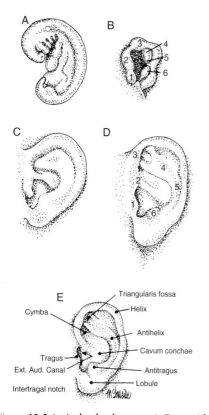

Figure **12-2** Auricular development. **A,** Fetus with branchial arch development. **B,** Six hillocks develop from arches. **C,** Newborn auricle. **D,** Hillocks fully developed. **E,** Anatomy of young adult ear. (From Bluestone CD, Stool, SE, Alper CM et al: *Pediatric otolaryngology,* ed 4, Philadelphia, 2002, Saunders.)

Scheibe deformity, the most common congenital abnormality of the cochlear duct, resulting in sensorineural hearing loss (see hearing loss section later in this chapter). The semicircular canals first appear in the sixth week of gestation with differentiation of canal structures being complete by the sixteenth week. The sensory cells needed for equilibrium actually attain adult size by the twenty-third week of gestation.

Middle Ear

Simultaneous with the early development of the inner ear is the formation of the first pharyngeal pouch in the oropharynx. The proximal portion of the pharyngeal pouch develops into the eustachian tube, and the distal portion becomes the tympanic cavity and supporting structures. The eustachian tube is 17 to 18 mm long at birth and lies 10 degrees off the horizontal plane. The development of the tympanic cavity with ossicles is not complete until the eighth month of gestation. The *manubrium, malleus,* and *stapes* and their supporting ligaments are formed by the *Meckel's* and *Reichert's cartilage.* Failure of ligaments to form properly results in a conductive hearing loss (see hearing loss section later in this chapter).[3] A conductive hearing loss is also seen in children with *osteogenesis imperfecta,* which causes *otosclerosis,* an abnormal destruction and redeposition of the bony structures of the labyrinth.

TABLE 12-1 PHYSIOLOGICAL VARIATIONS OF THE EAR

Age-Group	Physiological Variations
Preterm	Vulnerable to hearing loss, particularly before 33 weeks, from noise exposure, hypoxia, ototoxic drugs, hyperbilirubinemia, persistent pulmonary hypertension[3]
Newborn	At birth, tympanic membrane is almost adult size but lies in a more horizontal plane compared to the adult ear, which alters visual assessment Intrauterine positioning may result in disfiguring of the pinna, which will usually resolve after birth with proper positioning because of the elastic quality of the ear cartilage Whitish material including vernix caseosa covers external auditory canal
Infant	Fluid easily trapped in the middle ear causing eustachian tube dysfunction, particularly common in infants with Down syndrome, preterm infants, and any infant with craniofacial abnormalities
Toddler	External auditory canal ossifies by 2 years of age, straightening the canal and improving visualization of tympanic membrane
Preschooler	The pinna is approximately 80% of the adult size in the 4- to 5-year-old
School-age child	In a 9-year-old, the pinna and external auditory canal have attained adult size The canal measures 2.5 cm and has become somewhat "S" shaped

PHYSIOLOGICAL VARIATIONS

Table 12-1 presents variations in the pediatric age-group from the preterm infant to the school-age child.

ANATOMY AND PHYSIOLOGY

External Ear (Pinna)

The ear is divided into sections: the outer portion is called the *helix*, just medial and parallel to the helix is the *antihelix*, and the *concha* is the cavity leading to the opening of the external canal (Figure 12-3). A firm protuberance on the anterior portion of the ear just at the entrance to the auditory canal is the *tragus* and across from the tragus on the border of the antihelix is the *antitragus*. The soft fold of skin beneath the tragus is the ear lobe. Although the shape of the auricle varies slightly

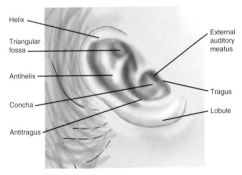

Figure 12-3 Anatomy of the external ear.

from person to person, the ears should be comparable in size, shape, and position and not significantly varied from the norm.

The external auditory canal connects the outer ear to the middle ear and funnels sound

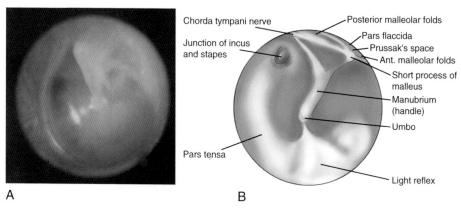

A   B

Figure **12-4 A,** Normal left tympanic membrane. **B,** Normal right tympanic membrane. (**A** from Lemmi FO, Lemmi CA: *Physical assessment findings multi-user CD-ROM,* St Louis, 2000, Saunders.)

waves to the tympanic membrane. The auricular muscles are innervated by the seventh (facial) cranial nerve. The medial portion of the canal is innervated by the fifth (trigeminal) cranial nerve and the posterior canal by the tenth (vagus) cranial nerve. The exterior third of the ear canal contains hair follicles, ceruminous glands (a modified apocrine sweat gland), and sebaceous glands. The ceruminous glands secrete a milky substance that when exposed to the secretions of the sebaceous glands and air form cerumen. *Cerumen* is a skin lubricant, a barrier to foreign objects entering the interior canal, and has protective antibacterial properties to reduce the incidence of skin infection in the external canal. Natural lateral movement of skin in the external canal facilitates drainage of cerumen and other debris from the external ear canal.

Middle Ear

The tympanic membrane is a thin layer of oval-shaped skin attached to the wall of the external canal and is approximately 9 to 10 mm in diameter (Figure 12-4, *A*). It is surrounded by a fibrous band called the *annulus.* The medial surface of the tympanic membrane is attached to the manubrium and lateral process of the malleus. The tympanic membrane has a resonance frequency of 800 to 1600 Hz, approximating the normal speech frequency

of 500 to 2000 Hz found in humans. The tympanic membrane is divided into sections: (1) the *pars flaccida* is superior to the lateral process of the malleus, (2) the *pars tensa* comprises the majority of the tympanic membrane inferior to the lateral process of the malleus, and (3) *Prussak's space,* which lies medial to the pars flaccida (Figure 12-4, *B*). *Prussak's space* is the most common location of retraction pockets and congenital or acquired *cholesteatoma* (Figure 12-5), an asymptomatic white mass in the middle ear that is thought to arise from the continued growth of the epidermoid layer over the tympanic membrane.[3] Tympanosclerosis, thickening and scarring of the tympanic membrane, is

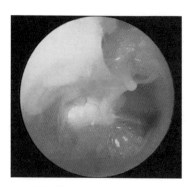

Figure **12-5** Cholesteatoma. (From Zitelli BJ, Davis HW: *Atlas of pediatric physical diagnosis,* ed 4, St Louis, 2002, Mosby.)

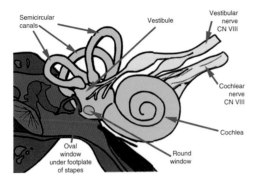

Figure **12-6** Anatomy of the inner ear. (From Lemmi FO, Lemmi CA: *Physical assessment findings multi-user CD-ROM*, St Louis, 2000, Saunders.)

commonly seen after chronic infections of the middle ear.

The three ossicles of the inner ear, the malleus, incus, and stapes, the smallest bones in the body, transmit the movement of the tympanic membrane to the oval window and subsequently to the eighth (acoustic) cranial nerve (Figure 12-6). The head of the *malleus* articulates with the body of the *incus* at the incudomalleolar joint. The long crus or leg-like structure of the incus, articulates with the head of the *stapes* at the incudostapedial joint. These joint areas are the most vascular regions of the ossicles, and therefore are the most susceptible to trauma or infection. The footplate of the stapes sits upon the oval window of the inner ear at the fibrous stapediovestibular joint. Because of the mechanical function of the three ossicles and the transmission of sound waves from the larger surface area of the tympanic membrane to the smaller surface area of the oval window, there is a net increase of 22 times the sound energy radiating from the tympanic membrane to the oval window.

The *eustachian tube* is the drainage and ventilatory structure for the middle ear. In the adult, the eustachian tube averages 35 mm in length, but in the infant it is half that length (Figure 12-7). The musculature of the eustachian tube, which controls function, is innervated by the motor division of the fifth *(trigeminal)* cranial nerve. Muscle maturation, elongation of the eustachian tube, and a more

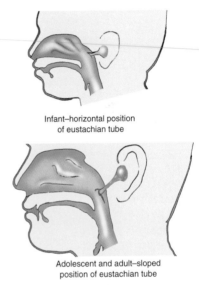

Infant–horizontal position of eustachian tube

Adolescent and adult–sloped position of eustachian tube

Figure **12-7** Position of eustachian tube in infant and in adult.

vertical position all contribute to the decreased incidence of otitis media and middle ear effusions in adolescents and young adults. In infants and children with cleft palate, the dilator muscle functions poorly, resulting in eustachian tube dysfunction.

Inner Ear

The inner ear is the sensory end organ and is directly responsible for hearing and balance (see Figure 12-6). The inner ear contains the *vestibule, semicircular canals*, and *cochlea* and is bathed in fluid that facilitates the transmission of sound waves to the auditory nerve and

TABLE 12-2 INFORMATION GATHERING FOR EAR ASSESSMENT AT KEY DEVELOPMENTAL STAGES

Age-Group	Questions to Ask
Preterm	History of maternal infection, TORCH infections? Maternal drug use or maternal diabetes? Antibiotic treatment with aminoglycosides, other ototoxic antibiotic use, salicylates?
Newborn	Newborn hearing screening results? ABO incompatibility? Elevated bilirubin level >20 mg/100 ml serum? Premature infant? History of anoxia, pulmonary hypertension, ECMO therapy, or meningitis? Any craniofacial abnormalities noted?
Infant	Does infant react to sound with startle response or change in activity? Turn head or body toward sound? Does the infant make cooing or babbling noises? Does infant have frequent colds? History of recurrent ear infections or ruptured tympanic membrane?
Toddler	Do you have any concerns about child's ability to hear? How many words does child use? How clear is child's pronunciation? How many languages are spoken at home or by care providers? Does child play with his ears? Has he ever put small objects in his ears or nose? History of ear infection? Was it treated with antibiotics? Does child have frequent colds or respiratory allergies?
Preschooler	Do you have any concerns about child's ability to hear or speak? If in daycare or preschool, do care providers have any concerns about child's hearing or speech? Does child combine words into meaningful sentences? Has child ever had a hearing test done? Were the results normal? How many languages are spoken at home or by care providers? Does child play with his ears? Has he ever put small objects in his ears or nose? Has child had a documented ear infection? Was it treated with antibiotics? Does child have frequent colds or respiratory allergies?
School-age child	Do you or child's teachers have any concerns about child's hearing or speech? Does child have difficulty following directions in school? Has child been exposed to unusually loud noises? Does child use headphones to listen to music? Is the volume loud? Has child ever complained of ringing in ears, dizziness? Does child have frequent colds or respiratory allergies? Has child ever had any drainage from ears? Ear pain? Does child spend a lot of time in water?

TABLE 12-2 **INFORMATION GATHERING FOR EAR ASSESSMENT AT KEY DEVELOPMENTAL STAGES—CONT'D**

Age-Group	Questions to Ask
	Previous injury/trauma to head, ears, or mouth?
	History of meningitis? Mumps?
	History of cancer therapy?
Adolescent	History of frequent colds, nasal allergies, or ear infections?
	Does adolescent use headphones to listen to music? Is the volume loud?
	Has adolescent been exposed to unusually loud music or noises (e.g., rock concerts)?
	Has adolescent ever complained of ringing in ears, dizziness?
	Does adolescent spend a lot of time in water?
	Any recreational or work activities potentially affecting ear (i.e., swimming, scuba diving, flying, boxing)?
Environmental risks	Crowded living conditions?
	Exposure to secondhand smoke?
	Exposure to loud noises?

TORCH, Toxoplasmosis, other (congenital syphilis and viruses), rubella, cytomegalovirus, herpes simplex virus; *ECMO,* extracorporeal membrane oxygenation.

sensations of balance in the *semicircular canals.* The sound waves pass over approximately 30,000 innervated hair cells in the cochlea that are the primary receptors, transducers, and conveyers of sound energy to the brain.

SYSTEM-SPECIFIC HISTORY

Table 12-2 presents the important information to be gathered for each age-group and developmental stage. Table 12-3 presents a symptom-focused history for those children or adolescents presenting with health problems.

PHYSICAL ASSESSMENT

Equipment

Equipment for examining the ear includes an otoscope with halogen light and speculum; pneumatic bulb attachment, and gloves if any apparent skin infection or ear drainage is present.

Positioning

Proper positioning of the infant and young child will ensure the least discomfort during the examination, prevent accidental injury to the canal or membrane by the examination, and ensure the healthcare provider has sufficient opportunity to visualize the canal and tympanic membrane. Letting the young child become familiar with the otoscope often decreases the anxiety of the ear exam (Figure 12-8, *A*). The infant is best positioned lying on the examination table until he or she is able to sit securely in the parent's lap (Figure 12-8, *B*). The curve of the pediatric ear canal can be lessened by pulling the auricle inferiorly and posteriorly in the young child, as compared to superiorly and posteriorly in the adult. Another examination technique that is very useful in the pediatric patient is for the examiner to position the hand above the ear, supporting the ear with the forefingers, and pulling the tragus forward or anteriorly with the thumb or forefinger (Figure 12-8, *C*). The

TABLE 12-3 SYMPTOM-FOCUSED HISTORY FOR EAR ASSESSMENT

Symptom	Questions to Ask
Ear pain	Onset, duration, and intensity of pain? Associated symptoms (i.e., fever, rhinorrhea, cough, ear drainage, hearing loss, vertigo, ringing in ears, swelling or redness around ear, mouth sores, dental pain, sore throat, difficulty sucking or swallowing, vomiting, neck swelling, tenderness)? Concurrent illness (i.e., upper respiratory infection, mouth infection, skin infection)? Home management of pain (i.e., medications/home remedies): type, how much, how often, effective? Changes in activities of daily living (i.e., loss of sleep, change in appetite, ability to attend daycare, school, or work)? Changes in activity level, talking, or movement of temporomandibular joint? Change in interaction with others (i.e., playful, withdrawn)? What makes the pain feel better, worse? Others at home, daycare, school, or work with similar symptoms? What do you think might be the cause of the pain?
Ear drainage	Onset, duration, and intensity of discharge? Associated symptoms (i.e., fever, rhinorrhea, cough, ear pain, hearing loss, vertigo, ringing in ears, swelling or redness around ear, vomiting)? Concurrent illness (i.e., upper respiratory infection, mouth infection, skin infection)? Changes in activities of daily living (i.e., loss of sleep, change in appetite, ability to attend daycare, school, or work)? Changes in activity level, interaction with others (e.g., playful, withdrawn)? Home management of pain (i.e., medications/home remedies): type, how much, how often, effective?

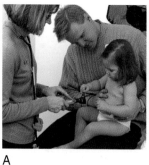 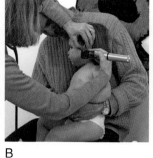 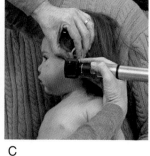

A   B   C

Figure 12-8 A, Preparing the young child for the ear exam. B, Positioning of the toddler for ear exam. C, Positioning of tragus forward with hand above the ear.

TABLE 12-3   SYMPTOM-FOCUSED HISTORY FOR EAR ASSESSMENT—CONT'D

Symptom	Questions to Ask
	Injury caused by pressure or trauma (i.e., laceration or barotraumas)?
	Others at home, daycare, school, or work with similar symptoms?
	How do you care for/clean your child's ears?
	What do you think might be the cause of the ear drainage?
Hearing difficulty relevant in school-age child and adolescent	Gradual or sudden onset?
	Bilateral or unilateral?
	Associated with other symptoms (i.e., ear pain, sense of fullness, drainage, systemic symptoms of illness)?
	Concurrent illness (i.e., otitis media, otitis media with effusion, respiratory allergies)?
	Trauma or exposure to loud noises?
	Changes in activities of daily living (i.e., difficulty hearing in school, at home, watching television, talking on phone)?
	Home management of hearing difficulty (i.e., sitting closer to television or in front of classroom, increasing visual cues for communicating)?
	What conditions make hearing better or worse?
	What do you think might be the cause of the hearing difficulty?
Dizziness or vertigo relevant in school-age child and adolescent	Gradual or sudden onset?
	Associated with other symptoms (i.e., nausea, vomiting, tinnitus, ear pain, ear drainage, hearing loss, systemic symptoms of illness)?
	Concurrent illness (i.e., viral illness, gastroenteritis, respiratory allergies/illness)?
	Use of medications or recreational drugs?
	Changes in activities of daily living (i.e., ability to attend school and work)?
	Home management of dizziness? Others in home with similar symptoms?
	What makes dizziness better or worse?
	What do you think might be the cause of the dizziness?

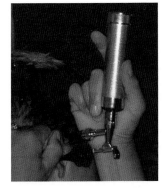

Figure 12-9 Holding the otoscope handle in the upright position. (From Lemmi FO, Lemmi CA: *Physical assessment findings multi-user CD-ROM*, St Louis, 2000, Saunders.)

handle of the otoscope also can be held upright when examining children to help stabilize the head and prevent accidental movement of the otoscope during the examination (Figure 12-9).

Pediatric Pearls

The technique of pulling the tragus forward straightens the auditory canal for ease in examination and causes less discomfort than pulling on the pinna.

External Ear

Inspection

Before examining the ear, inspect the head and neck for any asymmetry or indication of craniofacial defect or infection. The superior portion of the auricle should be equal in height to the outer canthus of the eye and vertical with no more than a 10-degree tilt. An ear that is set lower than an imaginary horizontal line drawn from the outer canthus of the eye or tilted greater than 10 degrees may indicate chromosomal abnormality or renal disorders.

Inspect the auricles for size, shape, and color. The size and shape of the ears should be similar and may have familial characteristics. In the newborn, the cartilage should have instant recoil, but in the premature infant, the cartilage may not be so elastic and may appear flattened and have less prominent incurvings of the helix or concha. The color of the auricle should be similar to the facial skin.

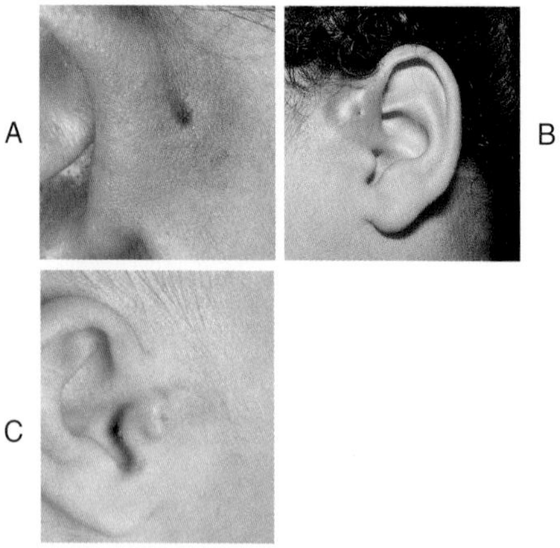

Common normal variations of the auricle include auricular sinus and preauricular skin tags (Figure 12-10). Occasionally an infection can occur in the preauricular pit resulting in inflammation and redness. Any ear piercings should be examined for signs of infection or trauma.

Palpation

Palpate the auricle for any masses or areas of tenderness. Scar tissue may be palpable around piercings and is generally nontender. Sebaceous cysts may occur around the auricle or in the external canal and are often mildly inflamed and tender. If movement of the auricle results in pain, the examiner should suspect an otitis media, otitis externa, or other inflammation of the auditory canal. A foul-smelling cheesy discharge is commonly found with otitis externa and often is caused by the bacterium *Pseudomonas.*

External Canal

Inspection

Inspect the external auditory canal for patency, discharge, odor, and foreign bodies. The largest speculum that will fit comfortably into the external canal should be used to increase the field of vision. The smallest ear speculum is often used for the infant. During the initial newborn examination, patency or atresia of the external auditory canal must be determined. If the canal is not patent or is abnormally narrow or curved, additional abnormalities of the auditory system should be suspected and referral to a specialist for further evaluation should be made immediately. Because of the normally curved "S" shape of the canal, visualization is improved with minimal discomfort if the tragus is pulled forward to visualize the auditory canal and the tympanic membrane. Another frequently used technique for the infant and young child is to pull the ear gently back and down for visualizing the auditory canal. For the older child and adolescent, pull the ear up and back for examination of the ear.

A

B

C

Figure **12-10 A,** Preauricular sinus. **B,** Abscessed preauricular sinus. **C,** Preauricular skin tags. (**A** and **B** from Zitelli BJ, Davis HW: *Atlas of pediatric physical diagnosis,* ed 4, St Louis, 2002, Mosby; **A** courtesy Michael Hawke, MD; **C** from Field et al: *Paediatrics: An illustrated color text,* Edinburgh, 1997, Churchill Livingstone.)

⊙━ Key Points

Foreign objects in the ear, such as small parts from toys, insects, food particles, cotton, or tissue will obstruct the canal, interfere with hearing, and may result in an infection in the canal.

Internal Ear

Inspection

Inspect the tympanic membrane for contour (normally concave), intactness (no perforations, tympanostomy or myringotomy tubes), color (normally gray or silver), translucency (normally translucent without scarring or opacity), and presence of visible landmarks (umbo, handle of malleus, and light reflex) (see Figure 12-5). Mobility of the tympanic membrane, an important indication of middle ear pressure, can be assessed with a pneumatic attachment to the otoscope (Figure 12-11) or by use of a tympanometer. If the middle ear pressure is equalized, the tympanic membrane will flutter in response to air pressure in the outer canal. This can be visualized through the otoscope as movement of the light reflex or recorded on the tympanometer as a rise and fall of pressure over the normal pressure setting of zero (Figure 12-12). Decreased or limited movement indicates either *increased*

negative pressure in the middle ear, with the tympanic membrane being retracted and taut and the bony landmarks accentuated, which is associated with eustachian tube dysfunction and *serous otitis media*, or *decreased movement* due to fluid buildup behind the membrane secondary to infection and *otitis media*, which causes the membrane to become inflamed, convex in shape, and taut and also causes a loss of visible bony landmarks (Figure 12-13).[1] A ruptured tympanic membrane will result in discharge in the canal.

Pediatric Pearls

It is important to emphasize that the color of the tympanic membrane is less important in diagnosing middle ear problems than the movement and shape of the tympanic membrane. A red or pink tympanic membrane may occur as a result of irritation, crying, or fever and may not be an indication of an acute otitis media.

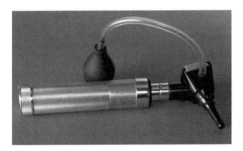

Figure **12-11** Insufflator or pneumatic attachment to otoscope. (From Lemmi FO, Lemmi CA: *Physical assessment findings multi-user CD-ROM*, St Louis, 2000, Saunders.)

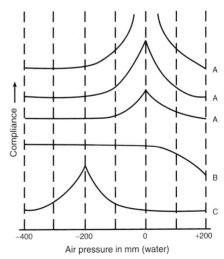

Figure **12-12** Tympanometry readings. (From Martin R: *Introduction to audiology*, Boston, 1991, Allyn & Bacon, © by Pearson Education. Reprinted by permission of the publisher.)

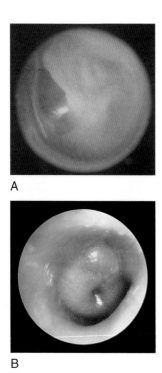

A

B

Figure **12-13 A,** Retracted tympanic membrane (TM). **B,** TM with otitis media. (From Lemmi FO, Lemmi CA: *Physical assessment findings multi-user CD-ROM,* St Louis, 2000, Saunders.)

EAR CERUMEN

Parents and caretakers should always be told that cerumen is a normal and a protective ear secretion and that some infants and children just normally have more wax than other children. They should be encouraged to clean the child's ears only with warm soapy water and should not use cotton-tipped applicators for fear of injuring the ear canal or tympanic membrane. Removal of cerumen or debris may be necessary to visualize the tympanic membrane. If the child can cooperate, a plastic or metal cerumen spoon can be used for removal. An infant or young child must be secured on the examination table before attempting cerumen removal. If the child cannot hold still for removal of cerumen when necessary, then irrigating the ear canal with warm water will

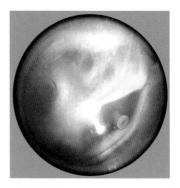

Figure **12-14** Tympanostomy or ventilation tubes in serous otitis media. (From Lemmi FO, Lemmi CA: *Physical assessment findings multi-user CD-ROM,* St Louis, 2000, Saunders.)

usually loosen and flush out built up wax. Irrigation should never be attempted if a ruptured tympanic membrane is suspected. Tympanostomy or myringotomy tubes inserted into the tympanic membrane for eustachian tube dysfunction are also a contraindication for irrigation of the external auditory canal (Figure 12-14). If the child is asymptomatic, cerumen buildup can be reduced and the canals cleared by daily use of eardrops made of mineral oil and hydrogen peroxide or commercially prepared eardrops for dissolving earwax.

Cultural Variation

Cerumen has two predominant types. Dry cerumen, which is gray and flaky, is found in 84% of Asians and Native Americans. Wet, honey-colored to dark brown cerumen is found in 97% of whites and 99% of blacks.[2]

HEARING ASSESSMENT

Testing for hearing is a critical component of the assessment of the ear. An infant or child's ability to hear cannot be determined by physical examination or radiological evaluation. Given the incidence of permanent hearing loss detectable in newborns of 4 per 1000 and of treatable conductive hearing loss of 2 per 1000 in

TABLE 12-4   PHYSIOLOGICAL MEASURES OF HEARING

Screening Test	Response
Auditory brainstem response	Measures electrical activity via scalp electrodes in the auditory nerve to midbrain level in response to sound delivered by air conduction or bone conduction
Otoacoustic emissions	Records sounds in the ear canal that are generated by the cochlea; absence of otoacoustic emission sounds may indicate a nonpatent ear canal, nonaerated middle ear, or lack of normal outer hair cell function needed for auditory nerve function

newborns, the Joint Committee on Infant Hearing (2000) recommends that auditory brainstem response screening tests or acoustic reflex testing be performed on all newborns before 3 months of age and preferably before discharge from the hospital (Table 12-4).[3] Newborn hearing screening determines the newborn's gross ability to hear and identifies those infants needing further evaluation. The practitioner should not assume that if the newborn screening is normal the growing infant or child's hearing is normal and no further hearing screening is necessary. Ten percent of childhood hearing loss is acquired after birth.

The American Academy of Audiology recommends that all children and adolescents be screened annually via conventional pure tone audiometry starting at age 3 years.[3] Any child under age 3 whose parents have concern regarding the child's hearing or who has a history indicating high risk for hearing loss should be referred to an audiologist or otolaryngologist for testing. If significant concerns are present at any age, generated either from history or initial screening, then referral is indicated. Most primary care practices have access to conventional pure tone audiometry, but a variety of other screening tests are available for infants and young children (Table 12-5).

Behavioral audiometry determines the weakest intensity at which a child shows behavioral awareness of the presence of sound. Sound

fields include 250 to 6000 Hz, but screening often is done between 500 and 4000 Hz at 25 decibels. Physiological measures of hearing determine the infant's physiological response to stimulation of the auditory system (Table 12-4). Speech audiometry determines the child's response to speech stimuli and tests the clarity of sound received and perceived (Table 12-6).

WEBER AND RINNE HEARING SCREENING TESTS

In older children and adolescents the *Weber* and *Rinne* tests can be performed in the practitioner's office as additional screening tests to determine deficits in either conductive hearing or sensorineural hearing, although they are seldom used outside of the laboratory or specialty setting (Figure 12-15). The *Weber* test is performed by placing a vibrating tuning fork (512 Hz) midline on the skull, making sure the examiner's hand does not touch the prongs of the tuning fork or the child's head. The child/adolescent is then asked if he or she hears the sound of the tuning fork better on one side or the other, or equally well on both sides. If the child/adolescent indicates the sound is heard better on one side, this is called *lateralization* and indicates a conductive hearing deficit in the ear perceived as hearing the tuning fork better.

TABLE 12-5 BEHAVIORAL AUDIOMETRY IN INFANTS AND YOUNG CHILDREN

Test	Age	Method
Conventional audiometry	4 to 5 years	Child is instructed to listen quietly for the test tone and to raise a hand or give a verbal response when it is heard
Bone-conduction testing	5 years	Calibration standards have not been established on infants and children; responses to bone-conducted stimuli may be inferred by head-turn response or as in conventional testing; young children may object to wearing oscillator
Hear test	Infants	Infant reaction to different frequency sounds is observed; elicited with standardized toys (i.e., bell, squeak toy) that make noises at different frequencies
Conditional play audiometry	2 to 5 years	Child performs a repetitive play task (i.e., places block in dish or peg in pegboard) in response to transmitted tone
Visual reinforcement audiometry	Developmental age 6 months to 2 years	Loudspeakers, earphones, or bone-conduction oscillator is used to observe child's ability to hear and localize sound (by turning head or body); visual reward (i.e., lighted toy) provided for accurate responses
Behavioral observation audiometry	Developmental age birth to 5 months	Similar to visual reinforcement audiometry but used for infants or children unable to move head or eyes reliably; any repeatable response to sound may indicate hearing

TABLE 12-6 SPEECH AUDIOMETRY

Screening Test	Response
Speech detection threshold	Speech stimulus used to determine the ability to hear at varying decibels and frequencies via sound field, earphones, or bone conduction
Speech reception threshold	Word stimulus given and child repeats word or points to picture to indicate word heard
Central auditory processing tests	Tests evaluate school-age children with normal pure tone audiograms to determine speech perception with background noise, sounds in contralateral ear, rapid rate of presentation, or filtering

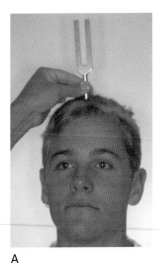

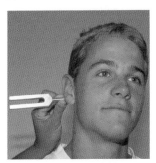

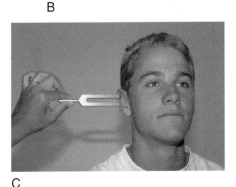

A, Rinne test—bone conduction.

C

Figure **12-15 A,** Rinne test—bone conduction.
B, Rinne test—air conduction. **C,** Weber test.
(From Lemmi FO, Lemmi CA: *Physical assessment
findings multi-user CD-ROM,* St Louis, 2000,
Saunders.)

The *Rinne test* compares air conduction to bone conduction. A vibrating tuning fork is placed on the child's mastoid bone to determine hearing via bone conduction. When the sound is no longer heard, the tuning fork should be moved to a position 1 to 2 cm from the external auditory canal. Sound is then being processed via air conduction in that area. Air conduction should be twice as long as bone conduction. If bone conduction of sound is heard longer than air conduction, then a conductive hearing loss is present in the affected ear. If the ratio of air conduction to bone conduction is less than 2:1, then a sensorineural hearing loss is present. The Weber and Rinne tests are not done on children until school age.

ABNORMAL CONDITIONS

Hearing Loss
Conductive Hearing Loss
Conductive hearing loss is caused by an abnormality in the transmission of sound waves through the ear canal, the tympanic membrane, middle ear space, or middle ear ossicles. The auditory nerve system is intact, but the sound impulses do not reach the nerve. Transient hearing loss is common during episodes of otitis media with effusion or acute otitis media. Recurrent or chronic bilateral ear effusions during the early years of rapid language, speech, and communication development may impede development. *Cholesteatoma,* with its associated destruction of the middle ear, is another common cause of conductive hearing loss, but this hearing loss will be permanent and progressive unless the cholesteatoma is surgically removed and middle ear reconstructed. Chronic or recurrent ear infections can cause *tympanosclerosis,* visualized as white scarring and thickening of the tympanic membrane, but this alone never results in measurable hearing loss. Acquired ossicular fixation from chronic diseases of the

ear is almost never seen in children although it is a relatively common cause of acquired hearing loss in older adults. Children with osteogenesis imperfecta do develop otosclerosis and must be followed by an ear specialist.

Congenital Conductive Hearing Loss

Congenital conductive hearing loss can occur with any gestational abnormality of the craniofacial structures. Isolated malformations of the external ear or microtia, malformations of the ear canal, congenital stenosis or congenital atresia, or congenital fixation of the stapes in the middle ear, all will result in conductive hearing loss. Down syndrome also can be associated with a congenital conductive hearing loss.

Sensorineural Hearing Loss

Sensorineural hearing loss is caused by abnormalities of the cochlea, auditory nerve, or the auditory pathways, which traverse the brainstem ending in the auditory cortex of the brain. Sensorineural hearing loss is often congenital and of unknown etiology although genetics is thought to play a role. It is less often associated with congenital syndromes than is conductive hearing loss. Syndromes that do include sensorineural hearing loss are Alport's, Jervell and Lange-Nielsen, and Usher's syndromes.

Infections, either gestational or acquired, are common causes of sensorineural hearing loss. Any newborn with a history of TORCHS infection (toxoplasmosis and other diseases: rubella, cytomegalovirus [CMV] infections, herpes simplex, syphilis) must be carefully tested and monitored for sensorineural hearing loss. Infants and children with symptomatic congenital cytomegalovirus infection have a 44% chance of developing progressive hearing loss, and asymptomatic infants have a 7.4% chance of developing progressive hearing loss. The onset of sensorineural hearing loss in infants with CMV infection often occurs after 3 months of age.[4]

Premature infants and graduates of the neonatal intensive care unit have a higher incidence of hearing loss than full-term infants. Newborns with a history of persistent pulmonary hypertension or extracorporeal membrane oxygenation (ECMO) therapy have a 20% to 25% incidence of late-onset or progressive hearing loss. Children of any age who develop meningitis also must be carefully tested for hearing loss due both to the consequences of the infections and the ototoxic side effects of many antibiotics used to treat meningitis. Children treated for malignancies with platinum compounds (cisplatin or carboplatin) or who are receiving cranial radiation may develop delayed sensorineural hearing loss and must be followed carefully with audiometry testing.

The management of hearing deficits has advanced with new surgical techniques, and bone-anchored, bone-conduction hearing aids once piloted in adults are now being used in children. Cochlear implantation and advances in hearing aids have improved the treatment of hearing loss dramatically, providing some sound to most children with even severe hearing loss.

CHARTING

Healthy Newborn Infant

Ear: Auricle well formed, symmetrical, with superior portion on equal plane with outer canthus of eye. Canals patent, pink, with small amount of white flaky residue. Tympanic membrane partially visible, gray, opaque, without visible light reflex or bony landmarks. Startle response with sudden loud noise.

REFERENCES

1. Wetmore RF, Muntz HR, McGill TJ: *Pediatric otolaryngology: principles and practice pathways,* New York, 2000, Thieme.
2. Jarvis C: *Pocket companion for physical examination and health assessment,* ed 4, Philadelphia, 2004, Saunders.
3. Joint Committee on Infant Hearing et al: Year 2000 position statement: principles and guidelines for early hearing detection and intervention programs, *Pediatrics* 106(4):798-817, 2000.
4. Bluestone CD, Stool SE, Alper CM et al: *Pediatric otolaryngology,* ed 4, Philadelphia, 2002, Saunders.

 CHARTING

Comprehensive Ear Exam of an Adolescent

Ear: Auricles well formed, symmetrical, with two healed piercings on outer border of helix and one healed piercing center of lobe. No masses, erythema, or tenderness noted. External canals partially blocked with dark brown cerumen. Tympanic membranes are pearly gray, concave, with bright light reflex and visible bony landmarks. Membranes move with insufflation. Weber—lateralizes equally to both ears; Rinne—air conduction greater than bone conduction. Audiometric—able to hear in both ears 500-6000 frequency (Hz) at 25 decibels (dB).

CHAPTER 13

NOSE, MOUTH, AND THROAT

Patricia Jackson Allen

DEVELOPMENT

The facial structures develop in the embryo during the first few weeks of gestation. The tongue, lips, gums, and tooth enamel all evolve from the ectoderm of the primitive mouth, the *stomodeum*, early in the fourth week. The lips are formed during the fourth to eighth weeks of gestation. The teeth and salivary glands are formed between the sixth and eighth weeks of fetal life. By the sixth fetal month, the ducts are hollow and begin producing saliva. Calcification of the *primary teeth* begins in the fourth month of fetal life and is complete by the first year of age. Any insult to the sensitive process of tooth formation can result in an anomaly in the color, size, or shape of the primary or permanent dentition.

Early development of the nose begins during the fourth week of gestation, with development of muscle, bone, and cartilage being completed by the twelfth week of gestation. The *palate* evolves from fusion of the maxillary prominences during the seventh and eighth weeks of gestation and is completely formed by the twelfth week of gestation during the fusion of the primary and secondary palates.

Failure in fusion results in cleft palate. *Cleft palate* is a relatively common congenital anomaly (1/700 births) (Figure 13-1). The specific etiology is usually unknown, but folic acid deficiency, ingestion of some teratogens such as alcohol, Dilantin, retinoic acid, and family genetics have been implicated. A *subcutaneous cleft* also can occur during this period with incomplete fusion of the palate and often goes undetected until preschool age when persistent abnormal speech patterns are investigated.

PHYSIOLOGICAL VARIATIONS

Table 13-1 presents the variations to be monitored from infancy to school age. Table 13-2 reviews the development of the sinuses from infancy through adolescence.

⚷ Key Points

Calcification of the dentition and tooth eruption occurs earlier in girls and in African Americans and Native Americans than in other racial groups.

155

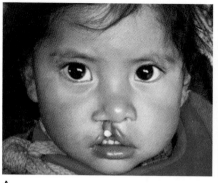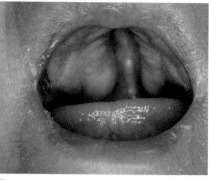

A   B

Figure **13-1 A,** Cleft lip and palate. **B,** Posterior cleft soft palate. (**B** from Chaudhry B, Harvey D: *Mosby's color atlas and text of pediatrics & child health,* St Louis, 2001, Mosby.)

TABLE 13-1 PHYSIOLOGICAL VARIATIONS OF THE NOSE, MOUTH, AND THROAT

Age-Group	Physiological Variations
Newborn	Nose cartilage is soft, malleable; deformities in external appearance from intrauterine or birth positioning usually resolve spontaneously Natal teeth may be present Epstein pearl—small whitish nodules or cysts—at juncture of hard and soft palates visible first month of life; Bohn nodules, or mucous gland cysts, may be present on gum surface in first 2 to 3 months Rooting, gag, sucking reflexes are present
Infant	Anatomically small airway passages Occlusion of nasal pathways can occur with nasal secretions Deciduous teeth appear between 6 and 24 months Rooting, sucking reflexes wane about 4 to 6 months Drooling increases as salivary gland production increases Anterior permanent teeth begin to calcify at 3 to 12 months
Toddler	Tonsils, adenoids enlarge to size 2+ to 3+ Nasal passages enlarge allowing easier airflow Swallowing coordination improves; drooling decreases Permanent molars begin to calcify at 18 months to 3 years
Preschooler	Sinuses not normally assessed in children until school age because of their limited development Tonsils, adenoids remain enlarged to size 2+ to 3+ Maxillary sinuses present but sphenoid, ethmoid, frontal sinuses limited in size, function
School-age child	Tonsils and adenoids usually begin to atrophy returning to size 1+ to 2+ Horizontal creases on anterior nose may develop in children with nasal rhinitis Deciduous teeth begin to shed; permanent teeth erupt causing change in facial structure, appearance Bridge of nose becomes more prominent Third molar, last permanent tooth, is formed and begins calcifying

TABLE 13-2   DEVELOPMENT OF SINUS CAVITIES

Sinus Cavity	Development
Maxillary	Present at birth; first sinuses to develop significantly; can be seen radiologically at 4 to 5 months of age; rapid growth between birth and 4 years of age and 6 to 12 years of age; final growth completed by 22 to 24 years of age
Frontal	Last sinuses to develop beginning between 4 and 8 years of age and do not develop fully until late adolescence
Ethmoid	Present at birth, but not developed, grow rapidly during the first 4 years and are fully developed by 12 years of age; they are first seen radiologically at 1 year of age
Sphenoid	Undeveloped at birth and do not begin to grow rapidly until after 5 years of age; development complete between 12 and 15 years of age

Data from Wetmore RF, Muntz HR, McGill TJ, et al: *Pediatric otolaryngology: principles and practice pathways,* New York, 2000, Thieme.

ANATOMY AND PHYSIOLOGY

External Nose

The nose of the newborn and young infant is generally flattened and malleable (Figure 13-2). Nasal breathing is the normal breathing pattern, and infants and young children are prone to increased airway resistance because they have anatomically small airway passages. In the past, it was thought that newborns are obligatory nasal breathers for the first few months of life. However, research has demonstrated newborns have the ability to switch from nasal to mouth breathing as needed so are "preferential" nasal breathers.[1] Respiratory compromise or distress occurs rapidly in the young infant when the passages become occluded with mucosal congestion or increased secretions. Nasal resistance may result in 50% of the total airway resistance being largely determined by the size of the airway passages. The nose becomes pyramid-like by adolescence and develops a bony structure. It is divided into four sections: the proximal bony portion, often referred to as the *nasal bridge*; the mid cartilaginous vault; the tip, *columella* and *nares*; and the interior *vestibule* (Figure 13-3).

Internal Nose

The internal nose, the *vestibule,* is divided by the bony and cartilaginous *nasal septum.* The septum is rarely perfectly straight and a

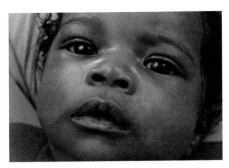

Figure **13-2** Flattened nasal bridge in newborn.

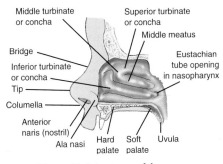

Figure **13-3** Anatomy of the nose.

Middle turbinate or concha — Superior turbinate or concha — Middle meatus — Bridge — Eustachian tube opening in nasopharynx — Inferior turbinate or concha — Tip — Columella — Anterior naris (nostril) — Ala nasi — Hard palate — Soft palate — Uvula

significant deviation of the septum resulting from the birth process or trauma must be assessed to determine whether it causes interference with nasal breathing. The perpendicular plate of the nasal septum ossifies by 3 years of age. The anterior portion of the vestibule is lined with vascular squamous epithelium that has tiny hair follicles and secretes mucus. The posterior portion is lined with fragile respiratory epithelium. The lateral walls of the nose are composed of horizontal bony structures known as the *superior, middle,* and *inferior turbinates,* which mature throughout childhood and resemble those of the adult by 12 years of age (see Figure 13-3). They are covered with vascular mucous membranes. Furrows between the bony structures provide recesses to filter air and form a nasal passage, or *meatus.* The posterior *ethmoid sinuses* drain into the superior meatus, and the *paranasal sinuses* drain into the middle meatus. Until approximately 6 years of age, the inferior meatus is nonfunctioning except for being the drainage outlet for the *nasolacrimal duct.* This is why the nose has increased drainage in children particularly during periods of crying or eye irritation. The space between the posterior portion of the turbinates and the posterior wall of the nasopharynx is called the *choana* and is of little significance in children unless blocked by a congenital abnormality such as *choanal atresia,* a bony or membranous blockage of the naris posterior to the nasal turbinates, resulting in blockage of the airway. It occurs in 1 in 10,000 births.

The *olfactory receptors* in the nose are found only along the superior turbinate and the adjoining septum. Olfactory learning begins in newborns within the first 48 hours after birth. Nasal congestion or mucus plugging limits airflow up to the receptors and can block the sensation of smell. *Cranial nerve I (olfactory)* innervates the nasal area.

Nasopharynx

The *nasopharynx* forms the superior portion of the pharynx. The *eustachian tube* opening is located along the lateral walls of the nasopharynx. Adenoid tissue, or *pharyngeal tonsils,* are found along the superior posterior wall. The inferior border of the nasopharynx is formed by the soft palate. The nasopharynx is surrounded by bone, ensuring patency unless trauma occurs.

Sinuses

The ethmoid sinuses are present at birth, and the maxillary, sphenoid, and frontal sinuses develop during infancy and childhood. They become air-filled cavities as they develop and mature within the skull (Figure 13-4 and Table 13-2).

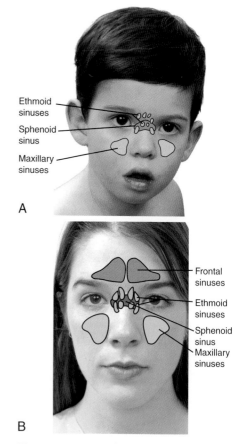

Figure **13-4 A,** Sinus development in childhood. **B,** Sinus development in adolescence.

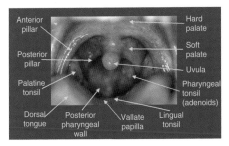

Figure **13-5** Anatomy of the posterior oral cavity. (From Lemmi FO, Lemmi CAE: *Physical assessment findings multi-user CD-ROM,* St Louis, 2000, Saunders.)

TABLE 13-3 TONSILLAR SIZE

Size	Description
1+	Tonsils visible slightly beyond tonsillar pillars
2+	Tonsils visible midway between tonsillar pillars and uvula
3+	Tonsils nearly touching the uvula
4+	Tonsils touching at midline occluding the oropharynx

Mouth and Oropharynx

The *oral cavity* is composed of the lips, cheeks, hard and soft palates, teeth, posterior pharynx, tongue, sensory cells for taste, and the mandible that supports the lower gums and teeth (Figure 13-5). The cheeks form the lateral walls lined with *buccal mucosa.* Cheeks may be particularly prominent in young children because of the buccal fat pad. The cheeks and lips are innervated by *cranial nerves V (trigeminal)* and *VII (facial).* The central nervous system controls the complex mechanisms of the mouth needed for sucking, swallowing, breathing, and vocalization. The *hard palate* is the anterior two thirds of the palate and separates the nasal and oral cavities. The posterior third of the palate is the *soft palate,* which is contiguous with the lateral pharyngeal wall. It provides a slightly mobile barrier between the nasopharynx and oropharynx and is essential for normal articulation.

Tonsils

The *palatine tonsils* form the anterior and posterior tonsillar pillars. Tonsillar size is graded on a scale of 1+ to 4+ (Table 13-3). Additional tonsillar tissues surround the posterior pharynx but are not visible on examination. The *uvula* hangs down from the middle of the soft palate in line with the anterior pillar, or *palatoglossus muscle.* A *bifid uvula,* a cleft with two parts, is an anomaly that results from disruption of the palate development.

Pediatric Pearls

In the infant, the palatine tonsils are not normally visible, but by 2 years of age they are usually easily seen extending medially into the oropharynx. They generally are at their peak size between 2 and 6 years of age and then begin to atrophy or decrease in size along with other lymphatic tissue.

Teeth

The mandibular central incisors are the first to erupt in the majority of infants, followed by lateral incisors, first molars, cuspids, and then the second molars. *Eruption,* movement of the tooth through alveolar bone, normally occurs between 4 and 12 months of age for the first tooth, and takes place when about two thirds of the root is developed. The maxillary incisors usually erupt 1 to 2 months after the mandibular incisors. The eruption of 20 primary teeth should be complete between 24 and 30 months of age (Figure 13-6, *A*). The timing and sequence of tooth eruption depend on genetic, nutritional, environmental, and systemic factors.

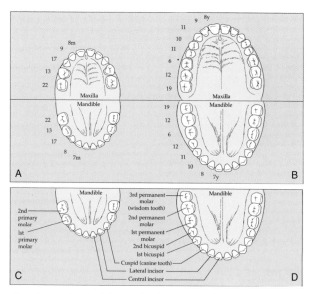

Figure **13-6** Ages of tooth eruption. **A,** Primary dentition of maxilla. **B,** Permanent dentition. **C,** Primary dentition of mandible. **D,** Permanent dentition of mandible. (From Zitelli BJ, Davis HW: *Atlas of pediatric physical diagnosis,* ed 4, St Louis, 2002, Mosby.)

The period of *mixed dentition* occurs between 6 and 13 years of age beginning with the eruption of the first permanent tooth. Exfoliation of the primary dentition often begins with the central incisors and follows the eruption pattern. There are 32 permanent teeth (Figure 13-6, *B*). Low birth weight, infection, and trauma have been associated with delayed eruption of the permanent teeth. Delayed exfoliation of the primary dentition has been associated with Down syndrome, hypothyroidism, osteogenesis imperfecta, and other congenital endocrine disorders.

Tongue

The *tongue* is a mobile muscle, with its anterior two thirds located in the oral cavity and the posterior third located in the oropharynx. The anterior dorsal surface of the tongue is composed of a thick mucous membrane lined with *filiform,* or threadlike, papillae, and the posterior dorsal surface is lined with lymphoid tissue that forms the *lingual tonsil.* The ventral surface of the tongue has a thin mucous

membrane with visible vessels and is anchored to the floor of the mouth by the *lingual frenulum* (Figure 13-7). *Cranial nerves IX (glossopharyngeal)* and *X (vagus)* innervate the tongue for sensation and taste, and *cranial nerve XII (hypoglossal)* innervates the tongue for motor function. The sensation of taste is immature at birth and not fully functional until approximately 2 years of age. Infants also

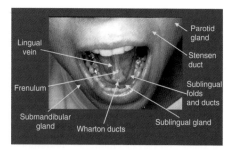

Figure **13-7** Ventral surface of the tongue and salivary glands. (From Lemmi FO, Lemmi CAE: *Physical assessment findings multi-user CD-ROM,* St Louis, 2000, Saunders.)

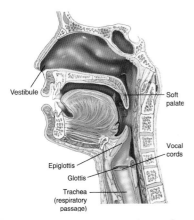

Vestibule

Soft
palate

Vocal
cords

Epiglottis

Glottis

Trachea
(respiratory
passage)

Figure **13-8** Sagittal view of mouth and oropharynx.

have a reflexive tongue-thrusting movement for the first 4 months of life that aids in breast-feeding or bottle-feeding but is counterproductive when trying to feed solids by spoon. At the base of the tongue in the oropharynx lies the *epiglottis,* a glistening pink spoon-shaped appendage that helps direct the passage of food into the esophagus and away from the trachea (Figure 13-8). Normally, it is not visible on examination, but in some children it can be seen protruding upward from the posterior oropharynx almost opposite from the uvula when the tongue is depressed and the child says "ah."

Salivary Glands

The *salivary glands* are paired exocrine glands that secrete enzymes that aid in initial digestion. The *parotid glands* are the largest salivary glands and are the glands that become inflamed with *mumps,* or *parotitis.* The *parotid duct, or Stensen duct,* empties into the oral cavity opposite the upper second molar. The *submandibular gland* is the second largest gland and is located in the floor of the mouth. The *submandibular ducts,* or *Wharton's ducts,* exit into the mouth on either side of the frenulum. The third set of salivary glands is the *sublingual glands,* which release their enzymes

through approximately 12 ducts located on the floor of the mouth. The sublingual glands are not visible on examination. Secretions from the salivary glands increase during the first few months of life, which results in increased drooling by 3 to 4 months of age. As infants mature and become more proficient in swallowing and the lower teeth develop to create a dam, the drooling decreases even though the production of saliva increases. Hundreds of additional salivary glands line the mucous membranes of the mouth and oral pharynx in late adolescence, providing additional serous and mucous secretions.

SYSTEM SPECIFIC HISTORY

Table 13-4 presents important information to gather for different ages and developmental stages when assessing the nose, mouth, and throat.

PHYSICAL ASSESSMENT

Equipment

Equipment needed for examination of the nose, mouth, and throat includes an otoscope with halogen light and speculum; gloves if any nasal drainage or skin lesions are present; tongue depressor.

Positioning

Delay the examination of the mouth and nose in the infant and young child until after the "quiet" parts of the exam and after the ear examination. The young infant is best positioned on the examination table with the arms secured by the sides and head supported to visualize the internal nose and mouth. Securing the arms above the head often increases fear and frustration in the child. Infants and young children are often resistant to the oral and nasal examination, and proper positioning ensures the least discomfort. Take the opportunity to examine the mouth if the infant cries.

TABLE 13-4 INFORMATION GATHERING FOR ASSESSING THE NOSE, MOUTH, AND THROAT AT KEY DEVELOPMENTAL STAGES

Age-Group	Questions to Ask
Preterm and Newborn	History of maternal infection, TORCH infections? Maternal drug use? Perinatal exposure to infection? Any difficulty sucking, feeding? Difficulty breathing through nose? Any natal teeth or lesions in mouth?
Infant	Any nasal discharge? Any difficulty sucking, feeding, introducing solid foods? Any sores, white patches, or bleeding in mouth? Have any teeth erupted? Use of juice in bottle? Is infant on fluoride supplement or is water fluoridated? Plans for weaning from breast or bottle? Does infant habitually put objects in mouth?
Toddler	Does child have difficulty eating solid foods? Use bottle for milk or juice? Frequently puts objects in mouth or nose? Does child's speech have a nasal or congested resonance? Has child had multiple upper respiratory infections or symptoms of respiratory allergies? Does child suck a finger or pacifier? Is child in daycare? Age at first dental visit? Does child brush teeth? History of trauma to mouth or gums?
Preschooler	Are there any concerns about child's speech? Has child had any mouth or nose injuries? History of nasal congestion, chronic rhinorrhea, or tonsillitis? Is child in preschool?
School-age child	Any mouth or nose injuries? History of nasal congestion, chronic rhinorrhea, tonsillitis? Does child snore? Any known exposure to group A streptococcal infection? Or other respiratory infections? Routine dental care? Does child brush and floss?
Adolescent	Any injuries to mouth or nose? History of nasal congestion, chronic rhinorrhea, tonsillitis? Does adolescent snore? Exposure to group A streptococcal infection? History of oral sex? Are there any oral piercings? Routine dental care, brushing, flossing?
Environmental risks	Exposure to smoke? Recreational drug use or exposure to use? Recreational activities with increased risk of injury to mouth or nose.

TORCH, Toxoplasmosis, other diseases, rubella, cytomegalovirus, herpes simplex virus.

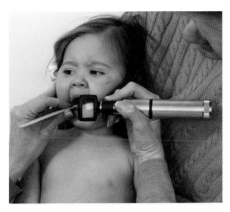

Figure **13-9** Position for the oral examination in the infant and toddler.

Examination of the older infant or young child is easiest while the child is sitting in the caretaker's lap with the head secured at the forehead and hands secured by the sides (Figure 13-9). The feet may need to be secured between the caretaker's legs if the child is uncooperative. An alternative position for conducting the oral exam and inspection of the teeth is to place the child in the "knee-to-knee" position.[2] In this position, the examiner and parent sit face to face with their knees touching to make a comfortable support for the young infant and the examiner can look directly into the child's mouth (Figure 13-10).

External Nose

While the child is comfortable, note any flaring or narrowing of the nares with breathing. If an infant is feeding, watch carefully for indications of nasal obstruction requiring mouth breathing. Note the shape of the nose, any obvious deviation of the bridge or columella, the tip of the nose. An *allergic salute* is a transverse crease across the nose caused by an upward swipe with the hand from chronic nasal drainage. If there is drainage from the nose, note the color, consistency, quantity, and whether it is unilateral or bilateral. Allergic conditions and upper respiratory infections cause bilateral drainage, whereas foreign objects in the nose can cause unilateral, purulent, malodorous discharge. *Epistaxis*, hemorrhage from the nose, occurs from irritation of the nasal mucosa, nasal allergy, or as a result of trauma. Sinus infections, if limited to one sinus, also may cause unilateral drainage. Swelling or discoloration may occur under the eyes with *sinusitis*.

Palpate any areas around the nose that appear discolored or inflamed. If there is a history of facial trauma, palpate the bridge of the nose to determine tenderness or pain. If the child has a recent history of head or face trauma and clear watery nasal discharge, a cerebrospinal fluid leak must be ruled out. Fractures of the protective facial bones increase the risk of meningitis developing. Children with obvious deviation of the nose should be referred to a facial surgeon for evaluation. Patency of each side of the nose can be determined by gently occluding one naris at a time. In the newborn, this technique assists in diagnosis of choanal atresia.

Internal Nose

To inspect the internal nose, use an otoscope with halogen light and nasal speculum. Be careful not to touch the sensitive nasal septum. A large ear speculum can be inserted 2 to 3 mm into the nares in older children and adolescents for inspection of the nasal cavity but is not recommended in infants and young children, to avoid trauma. An otoscope with halogen light used without a speculum is effective for visualizing the nares in infants and young

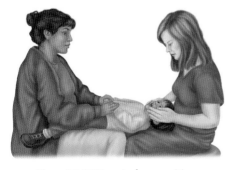

Figure **13-10** Knee-to-knee position.

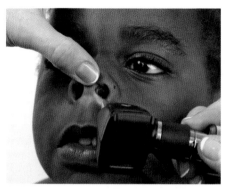

Figure **13-11** View of the nasal vestibule and turbinates.

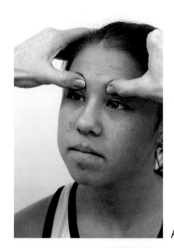

A

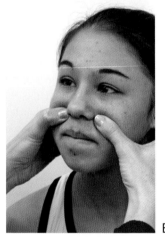

B

Figure **13-12 A,** Palpation of frontal sinuses. **B,** Palpation of the maxillary sinuses.

children who are positioned on the exam table or on the parent's lap.

The vestibule of the nose should be assessed for any blockage by foreign body, polyps, nasal secretions, mucous plugs, or dried blood (Figure 13-11). The mucosal lining should be assessed for consistency of color, abrasions, lesions, and swelling. The color is normally deep pink, and a thin layer of clear mucus gives it a shiny appearance. The septum should be examined for alignment, perforations, abrasions, bleeding, or crusting. It should be relatively straight and midline in the nose. Significant deviations of the septum may interfere with breathing. The turbinates should be assessed for color and swelling. Pale, swollen mucosa and edema of the turbinates is associated with allergic rhinitis and occlusion of air passage; and inflamed, reddened mucosa and turbinates is associated with respiratory infections. Children with chronic respiratory conditions may develop polyps that appear as shiny sacs extending into the vestibule.

If a foreign body is suspected, attempt to have the child blow out the object while occluding the unaffected side. If this is not successful in dislodging the object, a gentle probe with a curette or tweezers can be attempted but often is unsuccessful if the object has become adhered to the wall or septum. Position the child on the exam table for removal of the object or refer to a pediatric otolaryngologist if necessary for removal.

Sinuses

Only the maxillary and frontal sinuses can be assessed by physical examination through inspection and palpation. The facial area over the maxillary and frontal sinuses should be evaluated for swelling and erythema in school-age children and adolescents. Percuss or apply mild pressure with the thumb or forefinger over the maxillary and frontal sinus area.

Evaluate tenderness and increased sensation from side to side, especially if there is a history of prolonged upper respiratory infection (Figure 13-12). It may be difficult for young school-age children to accurately determine increased pain or tenderness caused by sinus inflammation. The technique of transillumination of the sinuses is of questionable diagnostic value in children under middle-school age because of the limited sinus development.

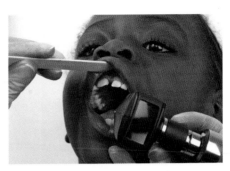

Figure **13-14** Inspection of teeth and gums in an older child.

Mouth

While inspecting the oral cavity, observe for the presence of any unusual odor or lesions. Inspect the lips for color, symmetry, lesions, swelling, dryness, and fissures. The color should be pink at rest and with feeding or crying. Note any asymmetry of movement or drooling that might indicate nerve impairment. Drooling during infancy from 3 to 15 months of age is normal, but drooling later may indicate nerve damage and loss of control of oral secretions. Young infants may have a callus or blister on the lip from vigorous sucking (Figure 13-13). Swelling of the lips may be caused by injury or allergic reaction. Cracked dry lips can be caused by harsh weather conditions, repeated lip licking or biting, mouth breathing due to nasal allergy, fever, or dehydration.

Note the *frenulum* under the inner surface of the upper lip, which extends to the maxillary ridge. It is prominent in the infant and disappears slowly in childhood with growth and development of the maxilla. Trauma to the upper lip and gum in the toddler often includes trauma to the frenulum. Inspect the buccal mucosa and gingivae for color, moisture, symmetry, and lesions (Figure 13-14). The mucosa normally is shiny, smooth, and moist throughout. The oral mucosa may appear bluish or pale in children with darkly pigmented skin, and pinker in Caucasian children. Use a tongue depressor or a gloved finger to move the tongue and lips to ensure all surfaces of the mucosa are inspected. *Epstein's pearls,* white pearly papules at the juncture of the hard and soft palates or on the anterior surface of the buccal mucosa, are common in newborns and resolve spontaneously. With a gloved finger, palpate unusual-looking areas for swelling and tenderness of the gum. If the mucosa of the gum appears inflamed or swollen, palpate for erupting teeth or hematomas. An *eruption hematoma,* a bluish blister-like swelling on the gum, may precede tooth eruption, particularly with the first and second molars.[3] Reddened, swollen, or friable gums can be an indication of poor oral hygiene, infection, or poor nutrition. Anticonvulsants may cause hyperplasia of the gums.

Candidiasis, appearing as bright white superficial lesions on the tongue and buccal mucosa of the cheeks, is often seen in the young infant or child after oral antibiotics have been taken or with chronic infection (Figure 13-15). The lesions of candidiasis can be differentiated from milk or formula residue by the bright white appearance and the fact that it does not scrape off with the side of the tongue depressor. *Petechiae,* pinpoint erythematous lesions, may be present on the soft

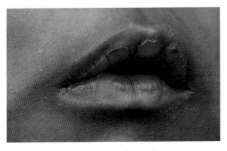

Figure **13-13** Sucking blister.

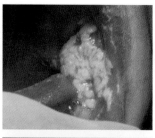

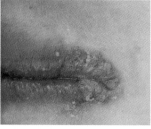

Figure **13-15** Candidiasis. (From Zitelli BJ, Davis HW: *Atlas of pediatric physical diagnosis,* ed 4, St Louis, 2002, Mosby.)

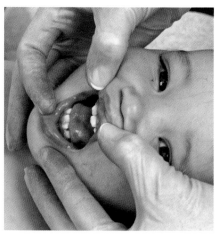

Figure **13-16** Inspection of primary teeth.

palate with streptococcal infections or may be indicative of a bleeding disorder.

Teeth

Inspect and note the number, color, size, and shape of the primary and permanent teeth and the pattern of eruption (Figure 13-16). *Natal teeth* are prematurely erupted primary teeth that are present at birth (Figure 13-17). The incidence of natal teeth is approximately 1 in 2000 births and is often seen in infants with cleft palate.[4] If the teeth are supernumerary, very loose, or cause feeding problems, extraction may be indicated. *Neonatal teeth* erupt in the first month of life, and 90% of neonatal teeth are lower primary teeth, or *mandibular incisors*. Precocious eruption of primary teeth has been associated with precious puberty.

Inspection of the teeth in infants and young children includes identifying any presence of plaque on the teeth. Evaluate dental hygiene practices. Check the primary teeth in the infant and toddler for "white spot" lesions or decalcifications and cavitations indicating the first sign of dental decay. White spots lesions

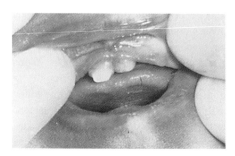

Figure **13-17** Natal teeth. (From Hardwick F, Ketchem L: *Oral pathologies in children: pediatric basics,* Fremont, Mich, Winter 1990, Gerber Medical Services, p 53.)

on the anterior surfaces can be a sign of *early childhood caries* (Figure 13-18). This infectious process of dental decay begins early and the bacterium *Streptococcus mutans* can be transmitted from parent or caretaker to the infant in the first few months of life.[2] The mandibular incisors are protected by the tongue and are therefore not prone to decay with prolonged bottle-feeding or breastfeeding. Daily oral hygiene using a damp cloth to gently rub the gums and teeth of the infant can prevent plaque development.

Maxillary permanent incisors may erupt widely spaced and protruding outward, and

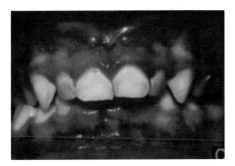

Figure **13-18** White spot lesions. *(Courtesy Dr. Francisco Ramos-Gomez, University of California at San Francisco School of Dentistry.)*

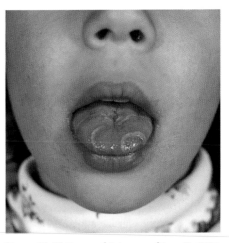

Figure **13-19** Geographic tongue. (From Zitelli BJ, Davis HW: *Atlas of pediatric physical diagnosis,* ed 4, St Louis, 2002, Mosby.)

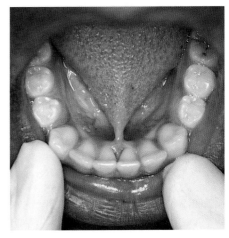

Figure **13-20** Ankyloglossia; short lingual frenulum. (From Zitelli BJ, Davis HW: *Atlas of pediatric physical diagnosis,* ed 4, St Louis, 2002, Mosby.)

mandibular incisors may erupt behind the primary incisors,[3] but align with normal development of the oral cavity unless there is a familial pattern of malocclusion or dental deformities. A slight overlap of the maxillary incisors to the mandibular incisors occurs with normal permanent dentition. *Bruxism,* or tooth grinding, a moderate wear on the surface of the canines and molars, may be noted on inspection. The peak incidence is during the developmental period of mixed dentition, and it rarely causes damage to the dentition. Children with special healthcare needs with moderate to severe bruxism should be referred to a pediatric dentist.

Tongue

Inspect the tongue, noting color, size, and movement. The dorsal surface should appear slightly rough but moist and pink to pale pink. There may be variation in the papillae, giving the dorsal surface a patterned appearance. *Geographic tongue,* a benign inflammation of the dorsal surface of the tongue, causes reddened areas with absent papillae and a surrounding whitish border (Figure 13-19).

The ventral surface appears thin with prominent vessels without hematomas. Connecting the ventral surface of the tongue to the floor of the mouth is the *lingual frenulum.* The lingual frenulum should allow movement of the tongue past the lips and to the roof of the palate. Observing the infant cry and the young child vocalize assesses movement of the tongue. Infants who are able to nurse or bottle-feed without difficulty have adequate movement of the tongue and no further assessment of *cranial nerve XII (hypoglossal)* is needed. A significantly shortened lingual frenulum, *ankyloglossia,* is caused by an anterior attachment of the frenulum to the tip of the tongue (Figure 13-20). Treatment for a shortened lingual frenulum remains controversial in infancy and beyond. It rarely causes problems but may in some cases interfere with adequate sucking in the newborn and later speech development. Surgical incision in the newborn is not recommended. *Macroglossia,* enlarged tongue, can be congenital or acquired and is associated with hypothyroidism, Down syndrome, and other congenital anomalies. *Pierre Robin* syndrome is associated with a malpositioned tongue, feeding and breathing difficulty, and a high-arched or cleft palate.

In the older child and adolescent, ask the child to stick the tongue out past the lips and move the tongue from side to side to test *cranial nerve XII (hypoglossal).* These maneuvers should be easy to perform without fasciculation of the tongue. The ability to curl the tongue is a familial trait and children often enjoy finding out whether they can curl their tongue. Any lesions, areas of tenderness, or swelling should be palpated to determine the size and depth.

Palate

Inspect the hard palate for patency or lesions. It should appear dome shaped but not deeply indented, whiter in appearance than the buccal mucosa and soft palate, and have transverse firm ridges. If the infant is jaundiced, the hard palate appears yellow in color. In darkly pigmented infants and children, it is a good place to evaluate jaundice. The hard palate is contiguous with the pinker soft palate that extends to the anterior pillars and the uvula. The soft palate should appear intact and rise symmetrically along with the uvula when the child vocalizes or says "ah." This movement tests for *cranial nerve X (vagus).* Movement of the soft palate is necessary for normal articulation.

The hard and soft palates should always be palpated in the newborn to determine whether there is any submucosal cleft not visible on inspection or congenital anomalies associated with cleft palate. A gloved finger can be placed on the infant's palate to determine whether the palate is intact. As the infant

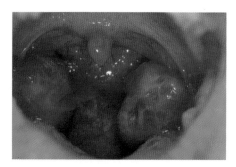

Figure **13-21** Large cryptic tonsils. (From Lemmi FO, Lemmi CAE: *Physical assessment findings multiuser CD-ROM,* St Louis, 2000, Saunders.)

sucks, evaluate the strength of the suck reflex and the palate surface. After the newborn period, palpation of the palate is not usually performed unless lesions, swelling, or erythema is noted.

Tonsils

Inspect the palatine tonsils for size, color, exudates, pitting or enlarged crypts, or membranous covering. Tonsils should appear equal in size and position, and should be rated on a scale of 1+ to 4+ during well visits and during periods of illness to evaluate change (see Table 13-3). Some children and adolescents have enlarged tonsils that extend all the way to the uvula and partially block air passage into and out of the oropharynx, requiring them to breathe with their mouth open to enlarge the air passageway. Chronically enlarged tonsils impact sleep patterns in children and adolescents and warrant referral to pediatric otolaryngology specialists. Dry lips are a hallmark of chronically enlarged tonsils in children.

The tonsils are normally the color of the buccal mucosa or slightly pinker. Dark pink tonsils that are larger than normal may indicate chronic respiratory allergies or infection. Exudate, white or yellow areas of material in the crypts of the tonsils, is often associated with bacterial *tonsillitis* or *infectious mononucleosis.*

Unequal size and color may indicate *peritonsillar abscess* that requires hospitalization or immediate antibiotic therapy and close follow-up. Pitting or enlarged crypts of the tonsils is often seen in children with history of recurrent infection or chronic allergies (Figure 13-21).

Vocalization

Vocalization and speech patterns in infants and children also should be assessed. A high-pitched cry may indicate increased intracranial pressure, and a hoarse cry may indicate *croup*. Prolonged hoarseness in children should be investigated to rule out vocal cord pathology. Prolonged unintelligible speech may indicate a speech articulation problem or hearing problem that should be evaluated. Intelligible speech is critical for success in school, and evaluation and therapy should not be withheld in hopes the child will "outgrow" the problem (see Chapter 3).

ABNORMAL CONDITIONS

Table 13-5 presents abnormal infectious conditions of the mouth and throat in infants, children, and adolescents.

CHARTING

Healthy Newborn

Nose, mouth, and throat: Nares patent bilaterally without flaring, clear nasal discharge. Strong suck. Mucous membranes pink, moist without lesions. Palate intact. Uvula and tongue midline, nonprotuberant, gag response intact, without natal teeth.

CHARTING

Adolescent

Nose, mouth, and throat: No nasal discharge, nasal septum midline, turbinates pink, moist. No facial swelling or tenderness over sinuses. Buccal mucous pink and moist without lesions. Gums pink, firm without bleeding. 32 teeth present in good repair without evidence of active decay. Pharynx pink, tonsils 1+ without exudate or pitting, uvula midline, sensitive gag response.

TABLE 13-5 ABNORMAL CONDITIONS OF THE MOUTH AND THROAT

Condition	Descriptions
Aptos ulcers	Round or oval ulcerations with an erythematous halo usually seen on buccal mucosa of cheeks
Diphtheria	A thin, tough membrane that becomes grayish-green and covers tonsils and pharynx; most common in children 5 to 14 years old living in crowded conditions
Epiglottitis	Edema and inflammation of epiglottis resulting in occlusion of trachea and acute respiratory distress; a medical emergency requiring intubation and radiographs for confirmation of diagnosis; avoid exam of oropharynx; incidence has decreased 80% to 90% with H flu vaccine
Gingivostomatitis (herpes simplex type I)	Vesicular lesions of lips, tongue, gingivae, oral mucosa resulting in swollen, painful, friable gums; most common 6 months to 3 years of age preceded by fever, headache, and irritability
Herpangina (coxsackievirus A and B)	Small vesicles on posterior pharynx, tonsils, soft palate that rupture to form ulcers; occurs in young children with onset of sore throat, fever, malaise
Mononucleosis	Enlarged tonsils, general malaise, fatigue, lymphadenopathy, splenomegaly caused by Epstein-Barr virus; confirmed by heterophil antibody testing
Parotitis or mumps	An acute contagious viral illness associated with fever, painful parotid enlargement; organ system involvement includes orchitis, testicular inflammation (in 15% to 25% of cases), deafness (usually unilateral); meningoencephalitis can be seen in 2.5% of cases; about 1500 cases occur annually
Streptococcal pharyngitis	Group A beta-hemolytic streptococcus: common bacteria in throat characterized by sudden onset of sore throat, fever, headache, exudate on tonsils, tender cervical adenopathy

REFERENCES

1. Bluestone CD, Stool SE, Alper CM et al: *Pediatric otolaryngology*, ed 4, Philadelphia, 2002, Saunders.
2. Ramos-Gomez F, Jue B, Bonta CY: Implementing an infant oral care program, *J Calif Dent Assoc* 30(10):752-761, 2002.

3. Muscari ME: *Advanced pediatric clinical assessment: skills and procedures*, Philadelphia, 2000, Lippincott.
4. Zitelli BJ, Davis HW: *Atlas of pediatric physical diagnosis*, ed 4, St Louis, 2002, Mosby.

CHAPTER 14

ABDOMEN

Laura J. Ohara

The assessment of the abdomen involves the evaluation of multiple organ systems and functions involving the gastrointestinal, renal, vascular, and female reproductive systems, liver, spleen, pancreas, and adrenal glands. The examiner should always keep in mind the holistic view of the child while examining the abdomen, which may help direct the exam or explain clinical findings.

DEVELOPMENT

The primitive gut forms during the fourth week of gestation from the dorsal section of the yolk sac. It begins as a hollow tube arising from the endoderm, which then forms the *foregut, midgut,* and *hindgut.* The *foregut* develops into the esophagus, stomach, upper portion of the duodenum (bile duct entrance), liver, biliary system, and pancreas. It is perfused by the celiac artery. The *midgut* develops into the distal duodenum and the remainder of the small intestine, cecum, appendix, the ascending colon, and most of the proximal portion of the transverse colon and is perfused by the superior mesenteric artery. The *hindgut* develops into the remaining transverse colon, the descending colon, the sigmoid colon, the rectum, and the superior portion of the anal canal and is perfused by the inferior mesenteric artery.

By the end of the sixth week of gestation, the gut herniates outside of the abdominal cavity, where it rotates 90 degrees counterclockwise and continues to elongate. By the tenth week of gestation, the gut returns to the abdominal cavity and rotates another 180 degrees counterclockwise. If a genetic or environmental insult disrupts the developmental process in the fetus, a defect in the abdominal wall, *gastroschisis,* can occur, causing herniation of the abdominal contents, usually the small bowel. With the normal intestinal rotation, the stomach and pancreas rotate into the left upper quadrant and are pressed against the dorsal abdominal wall to fuse into position. Up until the fourteenth week, the spleen is only a hematopoietic organ. Between weeks 15 and 18, the spleen then loses its hematopoietic function and transforms into an organ of the immune system.

The liver begins as a bud that develops on the distal part of the foregut and grows into the *septum transversum,* where it divides into two parts. The larger cranial part develops into the right and left lobes of the liver, and the second smaller division of the hepatic bud develops into the biliary system. Hematopoiesis begins at the sixth week of gestation and is responsible for the large size of the liver. It is approximately 10% of the total weight of the fetus. Bile begins to form at 16 weeks of gestation, giving meconium the dark green color. *Biliary atresia,* abnormal formation of the extrahepatic ducts, occurs early in fetal development, leading to biliary stasis and cirrhosis of the liver in the infant.

The pancreas arises from ectodermal cells from the most caudal part of the foregut and develops into dorsal and ventral buds. The dorsal bud is larger and becomes the major portion of the pancreas. The dorsal and ventral buds fuse to form the main pancreatic duct. Secretion of insulin begins around the twentieth week of gestation.

Development of the kidney begins with a primitive, transitory structure called the *pronephros,* or forekidney, which arises near the segments of the spinal cord. These segments appear early in the fourth week of gestation on either side of the nephrogenic cord. The pronephros itself soon degenerates but leaves behind its ducts for the next kidney formation, the *mesonephros,* or midkidney, to utilize. In the fifth week, the *metanephros,* or hindkidney, begins to develop and becomes the permanent kidney. By the eighth week, the hindkidney begins to produce urine and continues to do so throughout the duration of the fetal period.

The adrenal glands develop from the medulla, which originates from the neuroectoderm. At the seventh week of gestation, the medulla attaches to the fetal cortex, which develops from the mesoderm, and by the eighth week, the fetal cortex begins to encapsulate the medulla. The fetal adrenal gland is 20 times larger than the adult adrenal and is large compared to the kidneys. However, the adrenals rapidly decrease in size as the fetal cortex regresses and completely disappear by 4 years of age and are replaced by the adult cortex.

DEVELOPMENTAL VARIATIONS

The development of the abdomen is a complex process and errors can occur during the early stages of fetal life. Table 14-1 presents abnormal developmental variations in the abdomen and the resulting conditions.

ANATOMY AND PHYSIOLOGY

The abdomen is the area of the torso from the diaphragm to the pelvic floor and is lined by the *peritoneum,* a serous membrane covering the abdominal viscera. The membrane of the

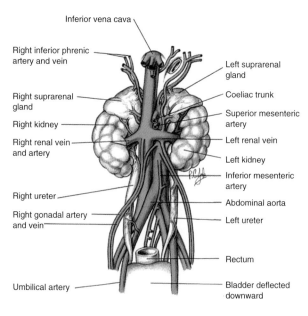

Figure **14-1** Posterior view of perfusion to the abdomen in the full-term neonate. Note the lobulated kidneys. (From Williams PM, Warwick R, Dyson M, Banister LH: *Gray's anatomy,* ed 38, 2005, Churchill Livingstone.)

Inferior vena cava

Right inferior phrenic artery and vein

Left suprarenal gland

Right suprarenal gland

Coeliac trunk

Superior mesenteric artery

Right kidney

Left renal vein

Right renal vein and artery

Left kidney

Inferior mesenteric artery

Right ureter

Abdominal aorta

Right gonadal artery and vein

Left ureter

Rectum

Umbilical artery

Bladder deflected downward

TABLE 14-1 ABNORMAL DEVELOPMENTAL VARIATIONS OF THE ABDOMEN

Condition	Developmental Variations
Bladder exstrophy	Incomplete midline closure of the lower part of abdomen; fissure includes anterior bladder wall
Choledochal cyst	Congenital anomalies of bile ducts with cystic dilations of the extrahepatic biliary tree and/or intrahepatic biliary radicles
Duplicated kidney	Complete or incomplete division of ureteric bud resulting in double kidney or divided kidney with two ureters
Hirschsprung's disease	Failure of ganglion cells of mesenteric plexus to migrate to a section of the colon; involves rectum and rectosigmoid, but extent can vary and may include total colon aganglionosis
Horseshoe kidney	Fusion of kidneys across midline
Hydronephrosis	Abnormal enlargement of kidney caused by acute ureteral obstruction or chronic kidney disease
Imperforate or ectopic anus	Anal canal ends blindly and may have an ectopic opening or fistula connecting to perineum (urethra in males, cloaca in females)
Omphalocele	Failure of intestinal loops to return to abdomen; encased in membranous sac formed by amnion
Meckel's diverticulum	Arises when proximal end of yolk stalk does not fully detach from gut at the end of the fifth week and persists as diverticula of ileum

Data from Moore KL: *Color atlas of clinical embryology,* ed 2, Philadelphia, 2000, Saunders; Sadler TW: *Langman's medical embryology,* ed 9, Philadelphia, 2004, Lippincott, Williams & Wilkins.

peritoneum creates a smooth, moist surface that allows the abdominal viscera to glide freely within the confines of the abdominal wall. There is some variation in the anatomical positions of the organs from one individual to another depending on the amount of contents within the intestines, the body type, and respiratory phase at the time of the exam.

The *liver* lies immediately below the right diaphragm and is the largest and heaviest organ in the body. It is composed of the right and left hepatic lobes and is an extremely vascular organ. The liver is perfused by the hepatic artery, which arises from the *abdominal aorta*. The abdominal aorta enters into the abdomen through the diaphragm at the level of the last thoracic vertebra and bifurcates into two common iliac arteries (Figure 14-1). The mesenteric arteries branch off the aorta to the spleen, kidneys, and adrenal glands superior to the bifurcation. The liver also receives blood from the portal vein, which delivers blood from the spleen, pancreas, and intestines. The hepatic veins return blood to the vena cava. The liver is responsible for metabolizing carbohydrates, fats, and proteins. It also breaks down toxic substances and drugs, stores vitamins and iron, produces antibodies, bile, prothrombin, and fibrinogen for coagulation, and excretes waste products.

Within the inferior surface of the liver lies the *gallbladder,* a saclike organ that excretes bile from the hepatocytes through the intrahepatic and extrahepatic ducts into the hepatic duct, which then is collected and stored in the gallbladder. Next the bile is secreted into the duodenum via the cystic duct and the common bile duct to aid in the digestion of fats.

Below the left diaphragm from posterior to anterior respectively, lie the spleen, pancreas, and stomach. The *spleen* is a concave organ made mostly of lymphoid tissue that lies around the posterior fundus of the stomach (Figure 14-2). The spleen filters and breaks down blood cells and produces white blood cells (lymphocytes and monocytes). It also stores blood that can be released into the vascular system during an acute blood loss. The *pancreas* is nestled between the spleen and stomach and crosses the midline over the major vessels. The pancreatic head extends to the duodenum and the tail reaches almost to the spleen. It is responsible for production of the pancreatic enzymes needed for the metabolism of proteins, fats, and carbohydrates;

theses enzymes are excreted into the duodenum via the pancreatic duct. The pancreas also produces insulin and glucagon, which are secreted directly into the bloodstream. The *stomach* is the most anterior organ in the left upper quadrant of the abdomen. It is connected proximally to the esophagus, which enters through the diaphragm at the *esophageal hiatus*. The stomach is a component of the gastrointestinal system and receives food from the esophagus through the lower esophageal sphincter. It secretes hydrochloric acid and digestive enzymes used to metabolize proteins and fats. When the stomach is distended, it is stimulated to contract and expel its contents through the pyloric sphincter into the *duodenum*, the first portion of the small intestine.

The *duodenum* is C-shaped and curls around the head of the pancreas. The pancreatic and bile ducts empty into the upper portion of the duodenum. The duodenum then transitions to the *jejunum*. The *jejunum* is responsible

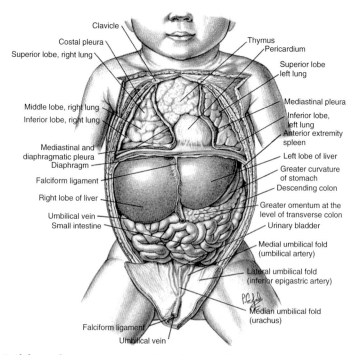

Figure **14-2** Abdominal organs in neonate. Note the size of the liver. (From Williams PM, Warwick R, Dyson M, Banister LH: *Gray's anatomy*, ed 38, 2005, Churchill Livingstone.)

for the majority of the absorption of water, proteins, carbohydrates, and vitamins. The *ileum* composes the last and longest part of the small intestine and absorbs bile salts, vitamins C and B$_{12}$, and chloride. The intestinal contents leave the ileum through the *ileocecal valve* and empty into the *cecum*, located in the right lower quadrant of the abdomen, which is the beginning of the large intestine. The *appendix*, a long, narrow tubular structure, arises from the base of the cecum. The large intestines lies anteriorly over the small intestines, ascends along the right anterior abdominal wall (*ascending colon*), traverses across the abdomen to the splenic flexure (*transverse colon*), and descends along the left lateral abdomen wall (*descending colon*) (Figure 14-3). At the level of the iliac crest, the colon becomes the S-shaped *sigmoid* colon. It descends into the pelvic cavity and turns medially to form a loop at the level of the midsacrum. The sigmoid colon connects to the *rectum*, which lies behind the bladder in males and the uterus in females. It stores feces until it is expelled through the *anal canal* and out the *anus*, which is located within a ring of nerves and muscle fibers. The anal canal and anus remain closed involuntarily by way of a ring of smooth muscle, the *internal anal sphincter* and voluntarily by a ring of skeletal muscle, the *external anal sphincter*.

The *kidneys* lie on either side of the vertebral column in the retroperitoneal space below the liver and spleen. The right kidney tends to be lower than the left because it lies below the right lobe of the liver. Kidneys have a lobulated appearance at birth, which disappears with the development of the glomeruli and tubules in the first year of life. The kidneys are perfused by the renal arteries and filter and reabsorb water, electrolytes, glucose, and some proteins. They regulate blood pressure, electrolyte and acid-base composition of blood, and other body fluids; actively excrete metabolic waste products; and produce urine. They are capped by the adrenal glands, which are pyramid-shaped organs. The adrenals synthesize, store, and secrete epinephrine and norepinephrine in response to stress and produce the corticosteroids, which affect the metabolism of glucose, proteins, fats, sodium, and potassium.

Urine is excreted from the kidney into the *ureters*, long, thin muscular tubules that transport urine to the bladder. The ureters connect to the superior pole of the renal pelvis. They descend posteriorly to the peritoneum and slightly medially in front of the psoas major muscle into the pelvic cavity and implant into the superior posterior wall of the *urinary bladder*. Urine normally is not able to reflux back into the ureters because of their oblique insertion through the bladder wall, which creates a one-way valvular mechanism. The urinary bladder lies anterior to the uterus in females and anterior to the rectum in males. When filled to its capacity, the bladder then contracts and releases urine through the bladder neck and out the *urethra*. The urethra is normally located at the tip of the penis in males and between the clitoris and vagina in females. Congenital misimplantation of the ureters into the bladder, known as *postureteral valves* or *ectopic ureteral implantation*, is a common cause of urinary reflux and urosepsis.

In nonpregnant females, the reproductive organs lie within the pelvis between the bladder (anterior pelvis) and the rectum (posterior pelvis). They include the *ovaries, uterine* or *fallopian tubes*, and *uterus*. Note the abdominal

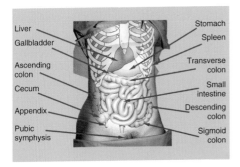

Figure 14-3 Internal abdominal structures in young adult female. (From Lemmi FO, Lemmi CAE: *Physical assessment findings multi-user CD-ROM*, St Louis, 2000, Saunders.)

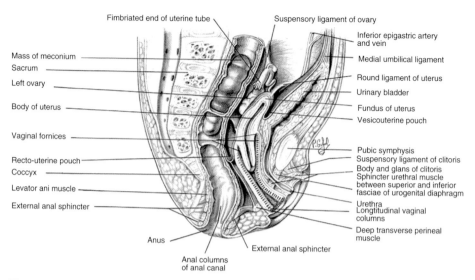

Fimbriated end of uterine tube

Suspensory ligament of ovary

Inferior epigastric artery
and vein

Mass of meconium

Medial umbilical ligament

Sacrum

Left ovary

Round ligament of uterus

Urinary bladder

Body of uterus

Fundus of uterus

Vesicouterine pouch

Vaginal fornices

Pubic symphysis

Recto-uterine pouch

Suspensory ligament of clitoris

Coccyx

Body and glans of clitoris

Sphincter urethral muscle
between superior and inferior
fasciae of urogenital diaphragm

Levator ani muscle

Urethra
Longtitudinal vaginal
columns

External anal sphincter

Deep transverse perineal
muscle

Anus

External anal sphincter

Anal columns
of anal canal

Figure **14-4** Midsagittal view of the pelvis in the full-term female neonate. (From Williams PM, Warwick R, Dyson M, Banister LH: *Gray's anatomy,* ed 38, 2005, Churchill Livingstone.)

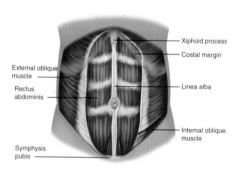

Xiphoid process

Costal margin

External oblique
muscle

Rectus
abdominis

Linea alba

Internal oblique
muscle

Symphysis
pubis

Figure **14-5** Abdominal musculature in adolescent.

position of the urinary bladder and uterus in the full-term neonate (Figure 14-4). These organs descend into the pelvic cavity during normal growth and development and ascend into the abdominal cavity during pregnancy, or with ovarian cysts or other abnormalities of the female reproductive system. Abdominal pain can be caused by obstetrical or gynecological conditions, so the reproductive system must always be considered in the differential diagnosis of abdominal pain (see Chapter 17).

Finally, a layer of fascia and then muscle covers the anterior abdomen. The *rectus abdominis* extends the entire length of the front of the abdomen and is separated by the *linea alba* in the midline. The *transverse abdominis, internal obliques,* and *external obliques* cover the lateral abdomen. The *umbilicus* lies in the midline usually below the midpoint of the abdomen (Figure 14-5).

SYSTEM-SPECIFIC HISTORY

Information gathering on the abdomen includes questions regarding the menstrual cycle in the prepubescent and adolescent female and sexual activity in adolescents, particularly with complaint of abdominal pain (see Chapter 17) (Table 14-2).

PHYSICAL ASSESSMENT

Equipment

In performing an abdominal exam in an infant or child, good lighting and a stethoscope may be all the equipment necessary.

TABLE 14-2 INFORMATIONAL GATHERING FOR ASSESSING THE ABDOMEN AT KEY DEVELOPMENTAL STAGES

Age-Group	Questions to Ask
Preterm and newborn	Any abnormal prenatal ultrasound findings (polyhydramnios, gastric bubble, intestine location, hydronephrosis)? Results of amniocentesis, genetics? Any maternal drug use, infection? Birth weight and gestational age? When was first meconium stool? Stooling and voiding patterns? Amount and type of feedings? Any vomiting? Constipation? Rectal tag?
Infant	Amount and type of feedings? Stooling and voiding patterns? Weight gain and growth pattern? Jaundice? Vomiting? Positive family history for chronic constipation?
Toddler and preschooler	Weight gain and growth pattern? Stooling and voiding patterns including toilet training? Constipation or stool withholding? Rectal bleeding? Nocturnal or diurnal enuresis? UTIs (frequency, dysuria, urgency)? Pattern of stool retention or withholding? Review 24-hour diet history.
School-age child	Weight gain and growth pattern? Nutrition? Stooling and voiding patterns? Constipation? Pattern of stool retention or withholding? Abdominal pain? UTIs? Rectal bleeding? Nocturnal or diurnal enuresis?
Adolescent	Stooling and voiding patterns? UTIs? Menstrual history? Abdominal pain? Sexual debut? Same-sex partners? History of STIs? Rectal bleeding?
Environmental risks	Water source? Exposure to waterborne bacteria or parasites? Recent travel to Mexico, Central America, Asia? Recent backpacking or camping trip? Exposure to contaminated food or milk products? Family members with chronic abdominal pain or diarrhea? Household lead exposure?

UTIs, Urinary tract infections; *STIs,* sexually transmitted infections.

Preparation

Initially the child can sit comfortably on the parent's lap directly facing the examiner. Inspection and auscultation of the abdomen can be done with the child sitting upright. For light and deep palpation, the examiner should be seated in a knee-to-knee position with the parent and the infant or toddler lying with head and torso in the parent's lap and the hips and legs in the examiner's lap.

The initial examination can occur with the child partially clothed; the diaper can be unfastened or pants and underwear pulled below the groin. If it is necessary to perform a rectal exam, then clothing below the waist can be removed or lowered below the knees at the time the exam is to be done. For a preschooler, school-age child, or adolescent, the abdomen should be assessed on the exam table.

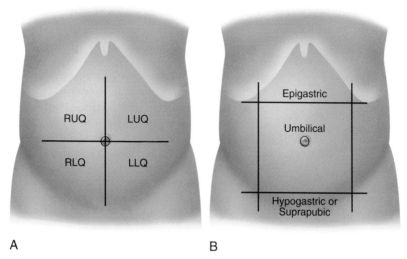

A   B

Figure **14-6 A,** Four quadrants of the abdomen. **B,** Nine regions of the abdomen.

Keep in mind that the abdomen is a three-dimensional space. Mentally visualize the anatomical location of the organs and their position relative to other organs in the abdomen. Adopt a mapping technique for the abdominal assessment. For general examination, the abdomen is divided into four equal quadrants, with the transverse and midsagittal planes intersecting at the umbilicus (Figure 14-6, *A*). For a child or adolescent who presents with abdominal pain or for other abdominal conditions, adopt the mapping technique with nine sections to accurately describe findings and for purposes of charting in the medical record (Figure 14-6, *B*).

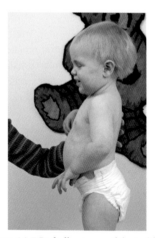

Figure **14-7** Potbelly stance of the toddler.

Inspection

Examination of the abdomen begins with the examiner's initial inspection of the child or adolescent's facial expression and color, attitude, activity level, and position of comfort to determine any distress.

Inspect the abdomen by noting its contours, symmetry, skin texture, color, and integrity. Note any lesions, rashes, pigment variations, or scars. Scars can indicate previous abdominal surgery and should always be explored during history taking. View the abdomen from the side and note the anteroposterior dimension. Infants and young children have less well developed abdominal musculature so the abdomen is more protuberant and round. A child up to 4 years of age will have a potbellied appearance while supine or standing (Figure 14-7). If the abdomen is scaphoid, it can indicate malnutrition or displaced abdominal organs as with a diaphragmatic hernia or intestinal atresia in a newborn. If the abdominal contour is distended, it can indicate an intestinal obstruction, a mass, organomegaly, or ascites. Fullness over the pubis symphysis can be seen in a thin child with a full bladder. Asymmetry may indicate a mass, organomegaly, or hollow organ distention.

Observe for any pulsations. It is normal to see pulsations in the epigastric area of a young infant or very thin child. Distended veins in the abdominal integument could indicate vascular compression or obstruction, hypertension, or intestinal obstruction. If an intestinal obstruction is suspected, note any obvious loops of bowel and observe for peristaltic waves on the surface by looking across the abdomen at eye level.

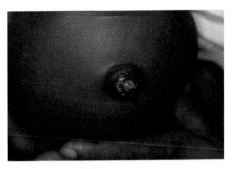

Figure **14-8** Umbilical granuloma. (From Clark DA: *Atlas of neonatology,* ed 7, Philadelphia, 2000, Saunders.)

Auscultation

Systematically listen to each quadrant or section of the abdomen with a stethoscope. In the infant and young child, auscultate the abdomen when completing the quiet parts of the physical exam during the cardiac and respiratory assessment. When attempting to identify areas of tenderness, use the diaphragm of a stethoscope to gently press on the abdomen during auscultation. In a newborn, bowel sounds are heard within the first few hours of life. Bowel sounds indicate peristalsis and movement of contents through the bowels. Normal bowel sounds are heard every 10 to 20 seconds. Hypoactive or absent bowel sounds indicate *paralytic ileus,* or inactivity of the intestines. Hyperactive bowel sounds indicate rapid movement through the intestines, usually associated with diarrhea, or a mechanical obstruction. There should not be any bruits. A newborn with *scaphoid* abdomen or signs of respiratory distress should be evaluated carefully for bowel sounds or decreased breath sounds in the chest. A *diaphragmatic hernia* may present in the neonatal period if not identified by prenatal sonography.[1]

Umbilicus

Inspect the umbilicus for any signs of drainage, infection, hernia, or mass. In the initial newborn exam, inspect the cord for the umbilical vessels, two arteries, and a single vein. The arteries are smaller and have a thicker vessel wall. Infants with a two-vessel cord may have other congenital anomalies and should be fully evaluated by a pediatric specialist. The majority of umbilical cords detach by the tenth day of life but can take up to 3 weeks to slough. A delayed separation longer than 3 weeks has been associated with neutrophil chemotactic defects and overwhelming bacterial infection.[1] Once the cord has detached, the stump should dry and heal within a few days. Occasionally, *umbilical granulomas* or granular tissue at the base of the umbilicus can be present and drain serous or seropurulent fluid or occasionally bleed (Figure 14-8). Careful attention to keeping the umbilical stump clean is important in preventing infection. For persistent umbilical granulomas, cauterization or surgical ligation of the stump may be needed. Any prolonged drainage should be investigated for presence of *urachal remnant* or *cyst.* If stool is noted coming from the umbilicus, an *omphalomesenteric duct remnant* is present, and the infant should be referred immediately to a pediatric surgeon. Any sign of infection in the umbilicus should be aggressively treated in the neonate. *Neonatal omphalitis* is a rapidly progressing, acute, and potentially fatal infection of the abdominal wall caused by a bacterial pathogen. Any infant with purulent discharge or sign of cellulitis should be treated with systemic

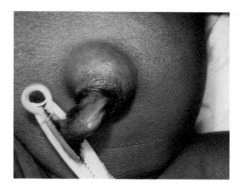

Figure **14-10** Umbilical hernia. (From Clark DA: *Atlas of neonatology,* ed 7, Philadelphia, 2000, Saunders.)

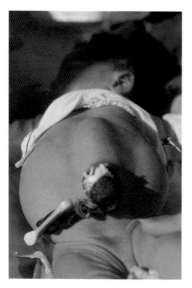

Figure **14-9** Diastasis recti. (From Clark DA: *Atlas of neonatology,* ed 7, Philadelphia, 2000, Saunders.)

antibiotics and referred immediately if the infection progresses.

Note any protrusion or mass in the umbilicus. Observe the midline of the abdomen of the infant or toddler when reclining or sitting. A wide bulging superior to the umbilicus is *diastasis rectus* (Figure 14-9), a common finding in children in whom the rectus abdominis muscles do not meet in the midline. Diastasis rectus does not create any functional problem for the child and will resolve or become less noticeable as the child grows. The separation of the abdominal wall musculature is noted with light palpation over the midquadrant.

The most common umbilical disorder is an *umbilical hernia* in which the intestine protrudes through the abdominal fascia, or *linea alba* (Figure 14-10). The umbilicus appears to protrude especially when the child is crying, stooling, or coughing, but generally can be easily reduced with the examiner applying light pressure with the fingertips to the umbilicus. Palpate the fascia below the umbilicus with the fingertips to determine the size of the defect. If the opening is larger than

the width of two fingers or the child is older than 3 years of age, surgical closure will most likely be necessary. Incarceration of an umbilical hernia is very rare. Most will spontaneously close by the time the child is 3 or 4 years of age. The most common umbilical mass is a *dermoid cyst.* It appears as a firm, skin-covered, nonreducible mass within the umbilicus that may have a slight discoloration and can be lobulated. Other cysts or an *umbilical polyp* should be referred to a pediatric surgeon for evaluation.

Check the groin area for a mass or *inguinal hernia.* Note any bulging or mass. Palpate to determine size and reducibility. If the bulge or *hernia* can be reduced, referral is indicated for elective surgery and repair. Scars from previous surgical hernia repairs also should be evaluated. An incisional hernia may be present and should be evaluated and referred.

Palpation

Palpation is the most important technique in assessing the abdomen and identifies areas of tenderness, masses, organomegaly, ascites, and signs of peritonitis. It should not be omitted even with a child who is having difficulty cooperating with the exam. If the child is supine, gently flex the knees and hips to relax the abdominal wall. Give infants a pacifier or bottle to suck to help relax the abdomen during the exam or distract toddlers in the parent's lap with a toy or favorite stuffed animal.

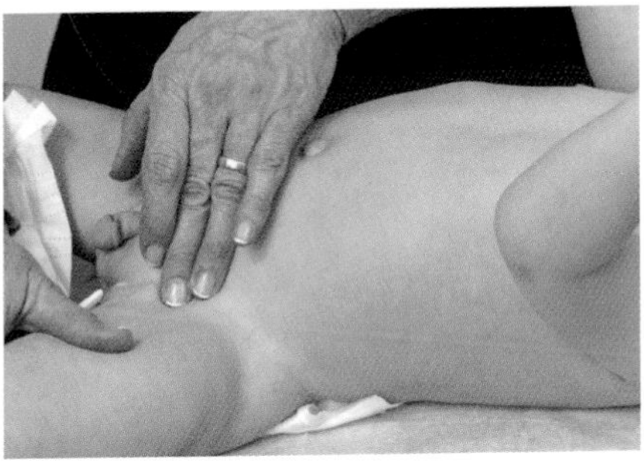

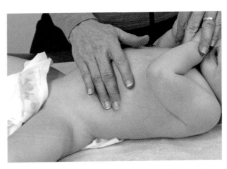

Figure **14-11** Palpating femoral pulses and lymph nodes.

Figure **14-12** Palpating the spleen in the toddler.

Begin with light palpation and observe the child's facial expression to note any signs of pain, discomfort, or areas of tenderness. If areas of tenderness are detected, examine those areas last when performing deep palpation. If the child is ticklish, place his or her hand under the examiner's hand and palpate the abdomen together. Distraction with conversation is also effective in eliciting cooperation throughout the exam. Press gently over each quadrant or section. Use a firm therapeutic touch. Massaging the abdomen should be avoided. Palpate any cutaneous lesions and note whether they are mobile, soft, firm, or reducible. Transilluminate to differentiate between a cyst and solid mass. A cyst will transilluminate; a mass will appear dark. All palpable masses should be handled carefully until malignancy is ruled out. Palpate the groin for femoral arterial pulses and lymph nodes (Figure 14-11). Skin *turgor* also should be evaluated during palpation by gently gathering a portion of the abdomen between the thumb and forefinger or second finger. Normal skin turgor is supple and adheres to adipose tissue. In children with poor skin turgor, the skin remains suspended or tented for a few seconds.[2]

An infant between the ages of 3 and 8 weeks of age with projectile, nonbilious vomiting may have *pyloric stenosis*. Examine the infant while the abdomen is relaxed and palpate in the upper abdomen, slightly right of the midline for a firm, olive-shaped mass. If a child presents with constipation, a sausage-shaped mass of stool may be palpated in the lower left quadrant or in the midline below the umbilicus or *rectosigmoid* colon.

The liver usually can be palpated in an infant or toddler 1 to 2 cm below the costal margin. Place the fingertips at the right midclavicular line a few centimeters below the rib cage at the costal margin, palpate toward the liver and feel for a firm nudge on inspiration. Move your fingers slightly up and inward until the sensation is felt beneath the costal margin. Note the distance between the location of the costal margin and liver tip. If it is more than 3 cm, hepatomegaly is suspected. Causes of an enlarged liver include infection, liver mass, storage disorders, biliary masses, intrahepatic vascular disease, or cardiac disease.

In a fashion similar to palpation of the liver, position the fingertips in the left midclavicular line below the costal margin and feel for a firmness on inspiration. The spleen can be felt in about 5% to 10% of children and should be slightly mobile (Figure 14-12). The spleen must be increased to 2 to 3 times its size to be consistently palpable.[1] An alternative technique in infants is to palpate the spleen between the thumb and forefinger of the right hand. If splenomegaly is suspected, an ultrasound can differentiate spleen enlargement from other masses that may arise in the left upper quadrant. Splenomegaly can be caused by infection, inflammation, blood dyscrasias, a mass, or vascular and oncological conditions. The spleen is a very vascular organ and should be *gently* palpated. If blunt trauma to the abdomen is suspected, do not deeply or frequently palpate the spleen or liver. If the liver or spleen is lacerated, a clot that may *tamponade* the laceration could be dislodged and cause further bleeding.

The kidneys in infants can sometimes be palpated. Place the left hand behind the right flank of the infant and using the tips of the right hand, palpate deeply in the right upper quadrant (RUQ), to the right of the midline. The right kidney may be "trapped" between the hands. Repeat the technique, placing the right hand behind the infant's left flank, and use the left fingertips to palpate the left kidney in the left upper quadrant (LUQ). The kidneys should be round, smooth, and firm. A distended bladder may be palpated in the midline above the pubis symphysis, which may indicate a vesicoureteral or bladder neck obstruction, acute bladder retention, or neurogenic bladder.

Percussion

Percussion of the abdomen can be done during palpation or separately. Percussion can help identify whether a distended abdomen is caused by air (tympany) or a mass or fluid (dull) (Figure 14-13). Tympany is common in

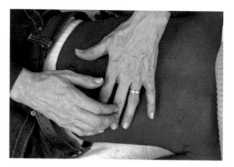

Figure **14-13** Percussion of the abdomen.

infants and young children because they swallow air when feeding and crying. Percussion also can delineate rough dimensions of solid masses and organs. To measure liver size, percuss superiorly between the ribs until no dullness is noted. The upper edge of the liver should be detected at the right midclavicular line near the fifth intercostal space. Mark this point and measure its distance from the lower edge of the liver. This technique identifies only the anterior surface of the liver and not the anteroposterior dimension. See Table 14-3 for the expected liver span in infants and children. Note the larger liver size in females until 3 years of age.

ABDOMINAL PAIN

When a complaint of abdominal pain is reported, the examiner must elicit a detailed

TABLE 14-3 LIVER SPAN IN INFANTS, CHILDREN, AND ADOLESCENTS

Age	Female	Male	Age	Female	Male
6 months	2.8 cm	2.4 cm	6 years	4.8 cm	5.1 cm
12 months	3.1 cm	2.8 cm	8 years	5.1 cm	5.6 cm
24 months	3.6 cm	3.5 cm	10 years	5.4 cm	6.1 cm
3 years	4.0 cm	4.0 cm	12 years	5.6 cm	6.5 cm
4 years	4.3 cm	4.4 cm	14 years	5.8 cm	6.8 cm
5 years	4.5 cm	4.8 cm	16 years	6.0 cm	7.1 cm

history of the pain. Information regarding the character of the pain, onset and duration, location, position of comfort, things that alleviate or worsen the pain, history of trauma, and any associated symptoms of fever, vomiting, anorexia, constipation, or diarrhea is important in narrowing the scope of the differential diagnosis. A detailed history can help in determining whether the abdominal pain is acute or chronic. Remember that abdominal pain can be referred from an extra-abdominal source or can be a condition associated with systemic disease. Abdominal pain is common in children with beta streptococcal pharyngitis, lower lobe pneumonia, sickle-cell anemia, cystic fibrosis, Henoch-Schönlein purpura, and many other conditions (Table 14-4).

⌿🔑 **Key Points**

A child's pain experience is usually limited, and the child may be unable to accurately describe the pain sensation. However, the crucial question to answer when a child presents with abdominal pain is, "Is this a surgical emergency?"

TABLE 14-4 COMMON CAUSES OF ABDOMINAL PAIN BY AGE

Age	Possible Cause of Abdominal Pain
Premature infant and neonate	Intestinal atresia
	Malrotation of the bowel
	Incarcerated hernia
	Ureteral obstruction
	Obstructing mass
	Hirschsprung's disease
	Imperforate anus
	Gastroesophageal reflux
	Food-induced (milk) colitis
	Meconium plug
	Necrotizing enterocolitis
Infant and toddler	Constipation
	Acute gastroenteritis
	Appendicitis
	Intussusception
	Abdominal mass
	Foreign body or poisonous ingestion
School-age child	Appendicitis
	Constipation
	Urinary tract infection
	Acute gastroenteritis
	Beta streptococcal pharyngitis/tonsillitis
	Lower lobe pneumonia
	Helicobacter pylori
	Lower lobe pneumonia
	Abdominal mass
	Chronic abdominal pain

Continued

TABLE 14-4 COMMON CAUSES OF ABDOMINAL PAIN BY AGE—CONT'D

Age	Possible Cause of Abdominal Pain
Adolescent	Appendicitis
	Lower lobe pneumonia
	Trauma
	Beta streptococcal pharyngitis/tonsillitis
	Inflammatory bowel disease
	Mass
	Henoch-Schönlein purpura
	Mesenteric adenitis
	Blunt abdominal trauma
	Mononucleosis
	Superior mesentery artery syndrome
Female adolescent	Urinary tract infection
	Ovarian cysts (rupture)
	Torsion of ovary
	Sexually transmitted infections
	Pelvic inflammatory disease
	Ectopic pregnancy
Male adolescent	Incarcerated hernia
	Testicular torsion
	Epididymitis
	Orchitis
Any age with prior abdominal surgery	Postsurgical adhesions

Assessing Abdominal Pain in Children

During the physical exam, note the child's position of comfort and ability to ambulate. If the child is rigid or prefers to keep the legs flexed, this can indicate diffuse peritonitis. Extend each leg and notice whether and where pain is sensed. Observe whether the child has difficulty climbing onto or off the exam table. Ask the child to hop or jump and note whether these movements elicit pain. Inspect the abdominal surface for signs of inflammation, distention, peristaltic waves, or asymmetry. Auscultate bowel sounds. Absent bowel sounds can be a sign of paralytic ileus or peritonitis. Hyperactive bowel sounds imply rapid movement through the intestines and along with diarrhea would indicate gastroenteritis.

Pediatric Pearls

If the child is old enough to understand, ask the child to use his or her index finger and with the eyes closed, point to the area of the abdomen that hurts the most. Examine the identified area last.

Carefully watch the child's facial expression to identify areas of tenderness as you lightly palpate the abdomen. Feel for organomegaly, masses, warmth, and rigidity. The child may resist palpation near or over areas of pain and inflammation. *Guarding* is an involuntary rigidity of the abdominal wall caused by peritonitis. If no acute areas of tenderness are noted on light palpation, progress to deep palpation. With deep palpation, *rebound tenderness* also can be assessed. An inflamed peritoneum may not elicit a pain response if the lining is gradually stretched, but when it is quickly retracted, the rebound will cause pain. To produce rebound tenderness, place fingertips at a 90-degree angle against the abdomen and gently but firmly press into the abdomen. Quickly release the fingers and note whether and where any pain is elicited. Ask the child if it hurts more when you press in or when you let go. Peritonitis is indicated if pain is worse with "letting go."

Rectal Examination

Whether to perform a rectal exam in a child is a hotly debated topic among practitioners and surgeons. If you are able to determine a diagnosis for the abdominal pain, a rectal exam is not necessary. Do perform a rectal exam if there is concern regarding anal or rectal patency, constipation or sphincter tone, or rectal polyps. Abdominal pain may be an indication for a rectal exam depending on the child or adolescent history. If you are examining an adolescent female, a rectal exam may be helpful to differentiate a gynecological diagnosis from appendicitis. If the abdominal exam and history are equivocal or the information obtained from a rectal exam would assist in the diagnosis, explain to the parent and child the need for the exam. Keep in mind a rectal exam is physically invasive and many children will no longer cooperate with a physical exam after a rectal exam has been performed. If it is necessary to perform a rectal exam, do so at the very end of the physical examination using the talk through-approach as presented in Chapter 1.

Position the child on the side with knees flexed (fetal position). An infant or toddler can lie supine with the hips and knees flexed. Gently insert a gloved, lubricated finger (usually the pinky finger) into the rectal vault and feel for any narrowing. Assess sphincter tones. Feel for any masses or pressure compressing the lumen of the rectum. Note whether there is stool in the rectum and whether it is hard or soft. If an explosive stool is elicited with the rectal exam, it may be a sign of a rectal obstruction such as *Hirschsprung's disease*. Gently press toward the right lower quadrant and observe whether it elicits a pain response. This can support a diagnosis of appendicitis. Alternately press in all directions and note any pain. If any stool is retrieved from the exam, guaiac test the specimen and assess for blood.

ABNORMAL CONDITIONS

Table 14-5 presents masses that can occur in the various areas of the abdomen.

TABLE 14-5   ABDOMINAL MASSES BY ANATOMICAL AREA

Abdominal Masses by Anatomical Area

Right Upper Quadrant	Midline	Left Upper Quadrant
Pyloric stenosis		Hydronephrosis
Intussusception		Splenomegaly
Hydronephrosis		Splenic cyst
Hepatomegaly		Left renal mass
Liver mass (hemangioma, cyst, tumor)		(Wilms' tumor)
Right renal mass (Wilms' tumor)		Left adrenal mass
Choledochal cyst		(neuroblastoma)
Right adrenal mass (neuroblastoma)		

Right Lower Quadrant	Midline	Left Lower Quadrant
Right ovarian mass (dermoid)	Full bladder	Stool
Lymphoma	Stool	Left ovarian mass
Abscess from previous rupture	Urachal remnant	(dermoid)
appendix	Hydrometrocolpos	
	Sacrococcygeal tumor	
	(internal)	
	Ureterocele	
	Pregnancy	
	Rhabdomyosarcoma	
	Bladder tumor	
	(hemangioma,	
	neurofibroma)	

CHARTING

1-Month-Old Term Infant

Abdomen: Abdomen symmetrical, soft, round, nontender without masses or organomegaly. Liver palpated 2 cm below right costal margin. Normal bowel sounds over all quadrants. Umbilicus clean, dry without hernia, mass, inflammation, or discharge. No lesions, scars, or skin discolorations. Skin warm, dry, with normal turgor and brisk CRT (capillary refill time). Regular epigastric pulsations. Percussion tones tympanic. No groin lymphadenopathy. Femoral pulses full and equal.

 CHARTING

12-Year-Old Female with Abdominal Pain

Abdomen: Position of comfort with hips flexed. Ambulates slowly, holding abdomen. Abdomen symmetrical, flat, tender with guarding and rebound tenderness noted in RLQ. Bowel sounds hypoactive especially in the lower quadrants. No masses or organomegaly. No skin lesions, scars, or discolorations. No lymphadenopathy. Femoral pulses full, equal, tachycardic.

REFERENCES

1. Behrman RE, Kleigman RM, Jenson HB: *Nelson textbook of pediatrics*, ed 17, Philadelphia, 2004, Saunders.

2. Hockenberry MJ, Wilson D, Winkelstien ML, Kline NE: *Wong's nursing and care of infants and children*, ed 7, St Louis, 2003, Mosby.

CHAPTER 15

MALE GENITALIA

Karen G. Duderstadt

The pediatric physical examination is not complete without a thorough evaluation of the developing genitalia. Many parents, children, and adolescents are concerned and anxious about the genitalia yet do not feel comfortable expressing those concerns. The review of systems and the routine genital exam offer an opportunity to the parent, child, or adolescent to voice concerns. The healthcare provider has a role in fostering dialogue between the parent and child regarding reproductive health. Establishing this dialogue early with families forms the basis for healthy discussions on reproductive health during puberty and in the developing adolescent.

Parental and family attitudes about sexuality vary widely both within cultures and among cultures. Sexual awakening first occurs in the preschool child with the discovery that the genitalia is a sensual organ. This initial experience and the parental attitude toward normal fondling and exploration may set the stage for either normal sexual development in a child or a feeling of shamefulness and an attitude in the child that fosters abnormal functioning throughout life. Often, cultural attitudes concerning sexuality and reproduction form the basis of conflict between parents and the preschooler or the maturing adolescent. Understanding and providing respect for cultural differences is a key part of the role of the healthcare professional. Mediating this difference between the adolescent and the parent may be the most important and difficult part of the professional role for the healthcare provider.

DEVELOPMENT

The differentiation of the sexual organs begins as early as the third week of embryonic development. The *mesoderm* is the embryonic layer that becomes smooth and striated muscle tissue, connective tissue, blood vessels, bone marrow, skeletal tissue, and the reproductive and excretory organs. As proliferation of the embryonic layers continues, maturation of the external genitalia in the fetus is established by the twelfth week. Urine production begins between the ninth and twelfth weeks and is excreted into the amniotic cavity through the *urethral meatus*. During development, the fetus continues the production and excretion of urine, which forms the amniotic fluid. Between the seventeenth and twentieth weeks, the *testes,* which develop in the abdominal cavity, begin to descend along the inguinal canal into the scrotum.[1] At birth, the infant's genitourinary system is functionally immature with limited bladder capacity, inability to concentrate urine sufficiently, and frequent voiding.

Growth of the fetus and differentiation of the sexual organs can be affected by placental function, hormonal environment during pregnancy, maternal nutrition, maternal infection, genetic factors or chromosomal abnormalities, and environmental factors. A fetal insult from intrinsic or extrinsic factors during the eighth or ninth week of gestation may lead to major abnormalities of the developing external genitalia.

ANATOMY AND PHYSIOLOGY

Penis

The *penis* consists of the shaft, meatus, prepuce, glans, and corona. The *shaft* is composed of strong connective tissue, muscle, and blood vessels. The interior of the shaft of the penis consists of the *corpus cavernosa*, which forms the dorsum and side of the penis, and the *corpus spongiosum*, the cylindrical structure in the shaft of the penis, which contains the *urethra*. The *corpus cavernosa* have erectile tissue and form the many fibrous columns of the penal shaft. The anterior portion of the corpus spongiosum forms the *glans penis*, the border or edge of which is called the *corona glandis*. The orifice, or *urethral meatus*, is the slitlike opening just ventral to the tip of the penis (Figure 15-1).

The *prepuce*, or *foreskin*, is the fold of skin at the head of the penis that covers the glans penis in the uncircumcised male and forms the secondary fold of skin from the urethral meatus to the neck of the penis called the *frenulum*. The skin of the penis is thin, does not contain subcutaneous fat and is loosely tied to the deeper layer of the dermis and fascia. Often, the skin of the shaft is more darkly pigmented. The skin of the glans penis contains no hair follicles but does have small glands and papillae that form in the epithelial cells to produce *smegma*, the cheesy white material found on the glans. Separation of the epithelial layers of the prepuce and the glans penis may be only partially complete at birth, and desquamation of the tissue layer continues the separation until the space between the prepuce and the glans penis is completely formed in early childhood and allows for retraction of the foreskin. Partial adhesions of the foreskin to the prepuce may produce smegma and it may persist throughout childhood.

Testes

The *scrotum* contains the *testes*, which are olive-size in the infant and young child. The *epididymis* is the thin palpable structure along the lateral edge of the posterior side of the testes. The *vas deferens* is the cordlike structure that is continuous with the base of the epididymis. The *spermatic cord* extends from the testes to the *inguinal ring* and is felt only on deep palpation of the *testicular sac*. The right spermatic cord is shorter in some males, which causes the right testis to hang higher than the left.

The *seminal vesicles* lay deep in the abdominal cavity alongside the vas deferens and secrete liquid into the *semen* as it passes from the testes. The opening of the seminal vesicles joins the vas deferens to form *ejaculatory ducts* and drains to the posterior urethra. The *Cowper's glands* are bulbar structures lying along the urethra that produce enzyme secretions that neutralize the acidic urethral secretions that could otherwise damage the semen. The *prostate gland* is the small, firm mass that lies

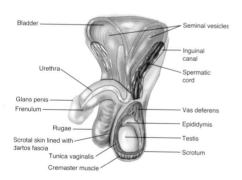

Figure **15-1** Internal and external genitalia.

TABLE 15-1 PHYSIOLOGICAL VARIATIONS OF THE MALE GENITALIA

Age	Variation
Preterm infant	Rugae absent on scrotum in low birth weight infant Testes undescended in ~20% of infants weighing <2500 g*
Newborn/infant	Rugae present from 37 weeks' gestation; testis: volume 1 to 2 ml; length of penis in term infant is 2.5 to 3.5 cm; note and evaluate any discoloration of scrotum at birth; shaft may appear short or retracted in obese infants with suprapubic fat pads, and size should be palpated during exam (Figure 15-2)
Toddler and preschooler	Foreskin partially retractable over glans penis; testes present in scrotal sac; initial sexual arousal and erection occur with normal sexual exploration or exposure of genitalia

*Data from Thureen PJ, Hall D, Deacon J, Hernandez JA: *Assessment and care of the well newborn,* ed 2, Philadelphia, 2005, Saunders.

within the pelvic cavity and surrounds the posterior urethra. It first becomes palpable on manual examination in the adolescent male.

PHYSIOLOGICAL VARIATIONS

Table 15-1 presents the physiological variations of the male genitalia in the pediatric age-group from the preterm infant to the preschool child.

Physiological Changes in Puberty

Puberty has a gradual onset and although it is initially marked by a growth spurt, it may be difficult to ascertain when the first changes begin in the transition to secondary sexual characteristics. In males, true gonadal activation begins with an increase in size of the genitalia, which is often difficult to determine. Testicular volume should be evaluated and is the most accurate measurement of the progression of puberty in the developing male. In some boys, this begins between 8 and 10 years of age and is complete in about 3 years, with the normal range extending to 5 years.[2]

It is the tempo of growth and maturation in male adolescents that is distinctly different than that in females. Males achieve peak

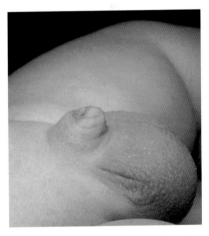

Figure **15-2** Suprapubic fat pad in infant. (From Zitelli BJ, Davis, HW: *Atlas of pediatric physical diagnosis,* ed 4, St Louis, 2002, Mosby.)

height velocity at Tanner stage 4 or 5 with 20% of boys in genital stage 5 at the time of peak height velocity (Figure 15-3).[2] Recent studies have provided evidence of earlier onset puberty in males, particularly in African Americans.[3] However, research has been unable to demonstrate an increased rate of progression to sexual maturity.

TABLE 15-2 DEVELOPMENTAL CHANGES IN PUBERTY

Sexual Maturity	Developmental Change
Tanner stage 1 Sexual maturity rating 1	Testes: volume <1.5 ml No pubic hair present Penis: unchanged from early childhood
Tanner stage 2 Sexual maturity rating 2	Period of increased testicular volume and growth of pubic hair Scrotum: enlarged, reddened, skin taut and thinner Testes: enlarged, volume 1.6 to 6 ml Penis: unchanged from Tanner stage 1 or slightly larger Small amount of light, downy hair along base of scrotum
Tanner stage 3 Sexual maturity rating 3	Testes and scrotum further enlarged Testes: volume 6 to 12 ml Penis: increased length and circumference Moderate amount of curly, pigmented coarse pubic hair extending laterally over symphysis pubis Voice changes occur, body odor appears
Tanner stage 4 Sexual maturity rating 4	Glans penis has become broader and larger Scrotum: further enlarged and darker Testes: volume 12 to 20 ml Penis: increased length and circumference Abundant pubic hair
Tanner stage 5 Sexual maturity rating 5	Pubic hair extends to medial surface of the thighs Penis and scrotum adult size Testes: volume >20 ml

Data from Neinstein LS: *Adolescent health care: a practical guide*, Baltimore, 2001, Williams & Wilkins.

During puberty, sexual development begins with testicular enlargement. Ejaculation usually occurs at Tanner stage 3 during the midpoint of sexual development. Fertility is established by Tanner stage 4 although sperm are present in some quantity with ejaculation during Tanner stage 3 (Table 15-2 and Figure 15-3).

SYSTEM SPECIFIC HISTORY

Table 15-3 presents the important information to gather for each age-group and developmental stage.

🔑 Key Points

Establishing whether the preschool or school-age child has experienced inappropriate touching of the genital area by any other person is a key component of the male genitourinary system history.

PHYSICAL ASSESSMENT

Although there is a tendency toward skipping assessment of the genitalia in the course of performing the physical examination, the

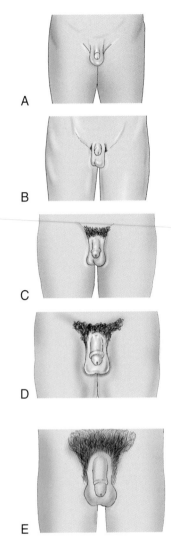

Figure **15-3** Tanner staging.

to the genital examination is required. The practitioner should proceed as with the rest of the physical examination, maintaining a firm and matter-of-fact approach, and yet using a technique that is sufficiently invasive to establish physical findings but is not traumatic for the child or adolescent.

As with all parts of the physical examination in pediatrics, it is important to "talk through" the examination when moving from one part of the male genitalia to another and verbalize findings as well as any concerns you may have when completing the examination. With the adolescent male, the talk-through exam is an integral part of a professional approach, establishes rapport, and validates feelings and concerns during and after the examination. There is often a hidden agenda with adolescents around issues of normalcy or reproduction. The healthcare provider must anticipate and be ready to discuss any issues involving reproduction in a supportive and professional manner. Maintaining confidentiality outside the examination room and with respect to the parents of an emancipated minor is a professional duty and is critical to building rapport with the developing adolescent (see section on confidentiality and teens in Chapter 4).

Positioning

During the first 4 to 6 months of life, infants are best positioned on the examination table for exam of the male genitalia. Beyond early infancy, it is easiest to exam the genitalia with the child lying on the parent's lap in a knee-to-knee position with the practitioner. The preschool child often is most comfortable sitting in the Taylor position on the exam table (Figure 15-4). The school-age child may be examined lying supine on the exam table or standing to enhance gravity of the testicles, as in the adolescent and young adult male (Figure 15-5). Respecting the need for privacy, particularly in the preschool child and the developing adolescent, establishes a good patient/provider relationship.

practitioner should be mindful that it is a critical part of evaluating a growing and developing body. If done regularly by the practitioner during pediatric well child visits, the genital examination then becomes simply a part of the routine physical that will be expected by the developing male in early, middle, and late adolescence. Reticence on the part of the child, adolescent, or parent is not a reason for omitting the examination of the genitalia. However, such a demeanor is an important indication that a careful approach

TABLE 15-3 INFORMATION GATHERING FOR MALE GENITALIA ASSESSMENT AT KEY DEVELOPMENTAL STAGES

Age-Group	Questions to Ask
Preterm and newborn	History of maternal hormone ingestion during pregnancy? Maternal alcohol abuse?
Newborn	History of maternal substance abuse or alcoholism? History of maternal infection? Significant neonatal infections? Significant family history of genital abnormalities?
Infant	Does infant have normal urinary stream? Stooling pattern?
Toddler or preschooler	Any history of urinary frequency, bedwetting, difficulty or pain on urination? Voiding pattern? Stooling pattern? Independent toileting achieved?
School-age child	Any history of urinary frequency, bedwetting, difficulty or pain on urination? Retractable foreskin in uncircumcised male? History of UTI? Family history of bedwetting? Any abnormality noted in growth pattern? Voiding pattern? Stooling pattern?
Adolescent	Any history of urinary frequency, bedwetting, difficulty or pain on urination? Family history of delayed puberty? Onset of growth spurt? Onset of puberty? History of inappropriate fondling, sexual molestation, or rape? Sexual debut? Inability to achieve erection? To ejaculate? Sexual activity with men, women, or both? Engaged in vaginal, oral, anal intercourse? Condom use? Age of sexual partners? Number of sexual partners? STI exposure? HIV exposure? History of trauma or witness to trauma?
Environmental risks	Maternal exposure to hazardous chemicals? Pesticides?

UTI, Urinary tract infection; *STI,* sexually transmitted infection; *HIV,* human immunodeficiency virus.

Inspection and Palpation

Examination of the male genitalia includes inspection and palpation of the penis, foreskin, and urethral meatus. In the newborn, the urethral meatus is normally on the tip of the glans penis. *Hypospadias,* abnormal placement of the urethral meatus on the ventral (underside) surface of the penis, or the meatus on the dorsal side, *epispadias,* is associated with fibrotic chordee and bladder anomalies. *Chordee,* fibrotic tissue causing ventral curvature of the erect penis, occurs as an isolated condition or with hypospadias.

Chronic irritation and ulceration of the meatus in circumcised males, particularly those in diapers, can lead to stenosis that causes urinary stricture. In the school-age and adolescent male, the urethral meatus is a slitlike opening on the ventral side of the glans penis. Examination in the adolescent male includes an inspection for erythema or discharge (Figure 15-6).

Mechanical retraction of the foreskin may cause trauma and put the newborn at risk for infection. In approximately 90% of uncircumcised males, the foreskin is retractable by

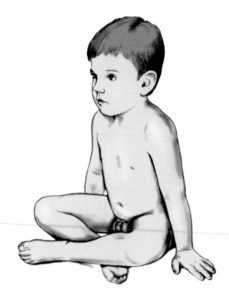

Figure **15-4** Preschooler sitting Taylor style in preparation for testicular exam.

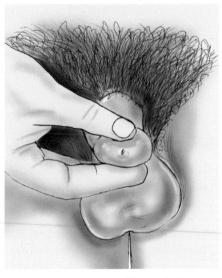

Figure **15-6** Examination of the urethral meatus in adolescent.

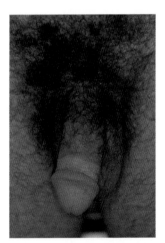

Figure **15-5** Adolescent male prepared for examination. (From Lemmi FO, Lemmi CAE: *Physical assessment findings multiuser CD-ROM,* St Louis, 2000, Saunders.)

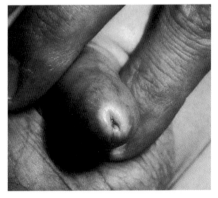

Figure **15-7** Phimosis. (From Lissauer R, Clayden G: *Illustrated textbook on pediatrics,* ed 2, St Louis, 2001, Mosby.)

5 years of age.[4] Good hygiene of the penis and foreskin can decrease the risk of developing infection or adhesions of the foreskin to the glans penis and should be reviewed regularly at well child visits during childhood.

Phimosis refers to a delayed separation of the prepuce, or foreskin, from the glans penis and may be the result of an incomplete retraction of the foreskin persisting after 5 years of age (Figure 15-7) or the result of chronic

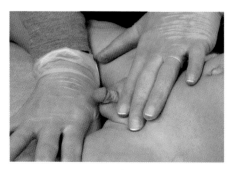

Figure **15-8** Trapping of testis in scrotum for examination.

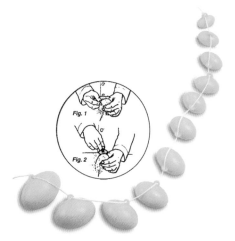

Figure **15-9** Orchidometer to evaluate testicular size. (Courtesy Accurate Surgical & Scientific Instruments Corp, Westbury, NY.)

inflammation causing a secondary phimosis. This condition requires referral if medical therapy is not successful. *Paraphimosis,* the inability to retract foreskin over the head of the penis, occurs in the uncircumcised child or adolescent, and can cause extreme congestion of blood flow to the glans penis. Medical therapy requires manual compression around the shaft of the penis to reduce swelling followed by reduction of the foreskin by manual downward pressure of the foreskin over the glans penis.

🔑 Key Points

Surgical intervention is rarely indicated in resolving phimosis. Do not forcibly retract! Medical therapy with betamethasone ointment 0.05% applied 3 times/day to tip of penis is indicated.

Before palpation of the scrotum in the infant and prepubertal male, the practitioner should apply pressure with the fingers at the base of the scrotum and penis over the inguinal canals to prevent passage of the testes into the abdominal cavity (Figure 15-8). The *cremasteric reflex* causes retraction of the testes and can be activated by cold, emotion, or touch, particularly in infancy and early childhood. If elicited, the cremasteric reflex can confuse findings of palpable testes in the scrotal sac during the physical examination in a normal male child. Trapping the testes in the scrotal sac before

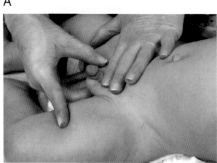

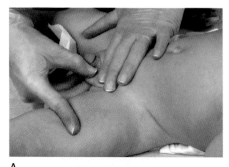

A

B

Figure **15-10** Palpation of scrotal sac.

attempting palpation will avoid abnormal findings. A test-size *orchidometer* can be used to evaluate testicular size in the growing and developing male (Figure 15-9).

TABLE 15-4 ABNORMAL FINDINGS OF MALE GENITALIA

Age	Examination	Abnormal Findings and Referral Criteria
Newborn and infant	Inspection of meatus, foreskin, penis	Abnormal position of urethral meatus ventral or dorsal to tip of penis Abnormal curvature of penis Microphallus: associated with syndromes and organ abnormalities
	Palpation of scrotum, testes, inguinal canal	Undescended or absent testes No testes visible on transillumination of scrotal sac with *hydrocele*
	Inspection of anus, rectum	Abnormal distance from scrotum to anus Abnormal rectal patency
Toddler and preschooler	Inspection of foreskin	Abnormal discharge, erythema (redness), swelling
	Palpation of scrotum, testes, inguinal canal	Undescended or absent testes
	Inspection of anus, rectum	Palpable lymph nodes in inguinal canal Inguinal hernia
School-age child	Inspection of foreskin	Phimosis: nonretractable foreskin
	Palpation of scrotum, testes, inguinal canal	Inguinal mass or hernia Testicular tenderness, pain, discoloration or swelling, palpable lymph nodes in inguinal canal
	Inspection for secondary sexual characteristics	Onset of puberty before 8 years of age in boys
Adolescent	Inspection of secondary sexual characteristics and skin	Absence or delay in Tanner staging Presence of skin lesions, vesicles, chancre, or lice
	Inspection of foreskin, meatus	Discharge from meatus, erythema or swelling of glans or penis
	Palpation of scrotum, testes, inguinal canal	Testicular tenderness, pain, discoloration or swelling, palpable lymph nodes in inguinal canal Inguinal or scrotal mass, inguinal hernia
	Rectal exam	Rectal polyps, hemorrhoids

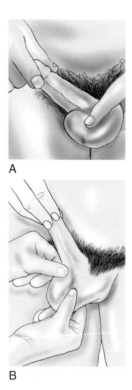

A

B

Figure **15-11** Positioning of the penis for inspection of scrotum.

While applying pressure at the base of the scrotal sac, gently palpate downward from the base with thumb and forefingers on the dorsal side and ventral side of the testis (Figure 15-10). Maintain a gentle downward motion on the inguinal ring to trap the testis for examination. This placement of the hand also allows the examiner to milk the testes into the scrotal sac if they are retractile. If the testis is not palpable and cannot be milked into the scrotal sac, then it is an *undescended testis. Cryptorchidism,* undescended testis or testicles, requires referral for evaluation between 6 and 9 months of age (Table 15-4). An undescended testicle also may be palpated along the inguinal canal. Bilateral nonpalpable testes in a term male raises concerns about virilizing adrenal hyperplasia. Inspection of the scrotum in the adolescent

male includes the assessment of the ventral side of the penis (Figure 15-11). Adult males with history of undescended testicle bilaterally have a 70% infertility rate and a 10% increased incidence of testicular cancer.[5]

A distended scrotal sac, which may be transient in the first year of life, indicates the presence of a hydrocele. A *hydrocele* is an enlargement of the scrotum that can be taut or firm and is nontender on palpation. The examiner is unable to palpate the testis when a hydrocele is present, but transillumination may reveal testes in the scrotal sac. Palpate the inguinal area for lymphadenopathy, an inguinal mass or hernia. A *hernia* is an inguinal mass or protrusion of tissue or bowel through muscle wall. The mass can be firm and reducible or hard and immobile, which requires immediate referral.

In the adolescent male, the examiner should palpate for the epididymis on the posterior surface. It can be felt on the lateral surface of the testes as smooth, discreet, and slightly irregular. The vas deferens can be palpated from the testes to the inguinal ring. *Testicular torsion,* swelling and tenderness of the scrotal sac, is a twisting of the testis and spermatic cord that results in venous obstruction, edema, and organ compromise, which causes testicular infarction. Testicular torsion is accompanied by acute onset of pain and an absent cremasteric reflex. The *Prehn sign,* decreased pain with elevation of the scrotum, is negative in a child or adolescent presenting with testicular torsion.[6] Testicular torsion also can occur in the fetus or neonate and may present as an *ecchymotic,* nontender testis caused by necrosis of the testis in utero. Referral to a pediatric urologist is indicated.

To examine the inguinal ring, advance the small digit or first finger into the slitlike opening of the inguinal ring by invaginating the skin from the scrotal sac (Figure 15-12). If cooperative, you can ask the preadolescent male to bear down or cough so any masses can be noted. If an inguinal mass is noted,

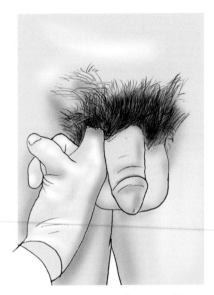

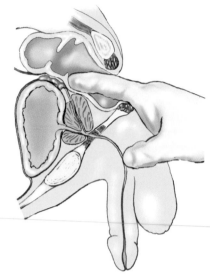

Figure **15-12** Examination for inguinal hernia.

Figure **15-13** Rectal examination technique in adolescent.

auscultation may occasionally be used to ascertain whether bowel sounds are present, although this technique has been replaced by the use of ultrasound in most instances.

⌐☞ Key Points

Males should begin genital self-examination by the time they reach puberty. The technique should be reviewed thereafter at every health maintenance visit or preparticipation sports physical.

Rectal Examination

Rectal examination in the infant and young child is indicated to assess tone, chronic constipation, rectal bleeding, fissures, hemorrhoids or other gastrointestinal concerns, and history of sexual abuse when indicated. The rectal examination is performed with the child supine with the legs flexed. Use the fourth digit, gloved and lubricated with a small amount

of gel. Press the pad of the finger against the anus. The anal sphincter should relax and allow the small digit to slip into the anal canal. Digital exploration of the rectal vault requires a gentle approach. Test any stool obtained on exam for blood using office fecal occult blood testing materials. This is not performed routinely unless symptoms or history warrant the examination. Note any sacral sinus, tufts of hair, or dimpling on the buttock. Inspect the anal area for fissures, rectal tears, hemorrhoids, any lesions, or inflammation. A discoloration around the anus may indicate heavy metal toxins.[7]

In the adolescent male, digital manipulation is performed with the adolescent positioned on his left side with knees flexed or standing with hips flexed and upper body supported with hands on the examining table. The first finger, gloved and lubricated, is used for the exam as above. Rotate the finger and palpate the anterior rectal wall to feel the prostate gland, which in the adolescent and young adult male should be firm and smooth and measuring about 2 to 3 cm (Figure 15-13). The rectal exam in the adolescent requires careful explanation of the purpose of the exam beforehand to avoid inflicting physical or psychological trauma.

CIRCUMCISION

Circumcision is the excision of the *foreskin*. In the newborn infant, the procedure is a matter of parental choice in consultation with the healthcare provider. Although circumcision has been associated with improved hygiene, routine circumcision performed merely to promote optimal hygiene of the penis is not required. However, current evidence indicates an association between an increased risk in males of urinary tract infection (UTI) and being uncircumcised during the first year of life.[8] A risk of penile cancer also has been noted in the uncircumcised male, although the risk is very low in adulthood.[4] The possible risk of both UTI and penile cancer in the adult male is not a sufficient reason currently to recommend routine neonatal circumcision. Newborns who are circumcised without analgesia experience pain; therefore the risks of analgesia should be reviewed with parents, and it should be explained that analgesia is necessary when proceeding with circumcision.

SEXUAL ABUSE

A complete physical examination including thorough evaluation of the genitourinary system is warranted with any indication or revelation of sexual misconduct on history taken either from parent or child or adolescent. Although no visible physical evidence is apparent in 40% to 60% of sexual assault cases, children and adolescents who are known or suspected victims of sexual assault require careful evaluation for any evidence that may be present.[5] Examination of the oral cavity as well as the genitals and anus requires careful inspection. Penis and scrotum should be evaluated for bruising or signs of external trauma, redness, swelling, or discharge. The anus and

rectum should be inspected for hemorrhoids, rectal fissures, or fistulas that would indicate trauma incurred as a result of intercourse. A digital exam should be performed with gloved lubricated finger to evaluate the sphincter tone and the rectal vault. A complete explanation of findings to the child or adolescent and family, referral, and follow-up is indicated.

AMBIGUOUS GENITALIA

As a primary care provider, the first step to diagnosis of the infant or child with ambiguous genitalia is to obtain a family history of previous spontaneous abortion, stillbirth, or any neonatal death of a male sibling that could be related to a family history of excess androgen and congenital adrenal hyperplasia or an autosomal *recessive genotype*. Perform a careful inspection of the genital area. The key finding of the genital exam is the presence or absence of gonadal or testicular tissue palpable in the scrotum, labioscrotal folds, or inguinal canal (Figure 15-14). Palpable gonads lead to the high probability that the infant is an XY male.[9,10] Referral and genetic karotyping is required to make a sex determination.

ABNORMAL CONDITIONS

Table 15-5 presents abnormal conditions of male genitalia in the infant, child, and adolescent.

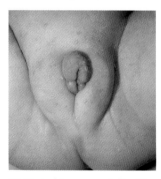

Figure **15-14** Ambiguous genitalia. (From Zitelli BJ, Davis, HW: *Atlas of pediatric physical diagnosis,* ed 4, St Louis, 2002, Mosby.)

TABLE 15-5 ABNORMAL CONDITIONS OF THE MALE GENITALIA

Condition	Description
Balanoposthitis	Redness, swelling, and extreme tenderness of prepuce and glans penis; yellowish discharge may be present
Epididymitis	Inflammation and swelling of epididymis from infection or trauma, often preceded by urethritis, generally associated with sexual activity; accompanied by pain in scrotum, inguinal area, or abdomen; occurs unilaterally, + Prehn sign: pain relief with elevation of scrotum
Epispadias	Abnormal placement of the urethral meatus on dorsal (top) surface of penis
Meatal stenosis	Recurrent inflammation of meatus from prolonged exposure to moist environment; prolonged urethral catheterization or trauma
Paraphimosis	Retraction of foreskin behind the corona or fornix of glans penis restricting blood flow, causing swelling and edema—**a urological medical emergency!**
Urethritis	Inflammation of urethral meatus, swelling, tenderness, occasionally yellowish discharge from meatus
Varicocele	Dilation of internal spermatic vein at venous plexus within spermatic cord; presents as soft mass on spermatic cord with associated pain; most common on left side

 CHARTING

Healthy 12-Year-Old Male

External genitalia: nl circumcised male, urethral meatus nl, no discharge noted, Tanner stage 2 with sparse amount of pubic hair over the symphysis pubis, testicular sac full, slightly vascular, and taut. Testes—increased volume descended bilaterally, palpable in scrotal sac, nontender, spermatic cord felt on deep palpation at base of the testes extending to inguinal canal, fingertip in canal revealed no hernia, without lymphadenopathy.

nl, Common abbreviation for *normal* in medical charting.

 CHARTING

Term Infant at 1 Month of Age

External genitalia: nl uncircumcised male, urethral meatus visualized at tip of penis with minimal retraction of the prepuce, no discharge noted, urinary stream normal, olive-sized testes descended bilaterally, palpable in scrotal sac, without hernia.

REFERENCES

1. Porth CM: Pathophysiology: concepts of altered health states, Philadelphia, 2004, Lippincott.
2. Reiter EO, Lee PA: Have the onset and tempo of puberty changed? *Arch Pediatr Adolesc Med* 155(9):988-989, 2001.
3. Herman Giddens ME: Secondary sexual characteristics in boys, *Arch Pediatr Adolesc Med* 155(9):1022-1028, 2001.
4. American Academy of Pediatrics Task Force on Circumcision: Circumcision policy statement, *Pediatrics* 103(3):686-693, 1999.
5. Hoekelman RA, Adam HM, Nelson NM, Weitzman ML, Wilson MH: *Primary pediatric care,* ed 4, St Louis, 2001, Mosby.
6. Adleman WP, Joffe A: The adolescent with a painful scrotum, *Contemp Pediatr* 17(3):111-127, 2000.
7. Muscari ME: *Advanced pediatric clinical assessment: skills and procedures,* Philadelphia, 2000, Lippincott.
8. Shaw KN, Gorelick MH: Urinary tract infection in the pediatric patient, *Pediatr Clin North Am* 46(6):1111-1124, 1999.
9. Anhalt H, Neely EK, Hintz RL: Ambiguous genitalia, *Pediatr Rev* 17(6):213-220, 1996.
10. Parker LA: Ambiguous genitalia: etiology, treatment, and nursing implications, *J Obstet Gynecol Neonaalt Nurs* 27(1):15-22, 1998.

CHAPTER 16

MALE AND FEMALE BREAST

Naomi A. Schapiro

Male and female breast development is similar until puberty; therefore the examination of both boys and girls will be included in this chapter, along with changes to expect during puberty for both genders. Making assessment of the breast part of the routine physical exam in preadolescents gives the parent and child an opportunity to voice any concerns and fosters a dialogue between parent and child about reproductive health. It is important to respect privacy in performing the examination of the breast in all children and adolescents.

DEVELOPMENT

A mammary ridge forms from the ectodermal layer on day 20 of embryonic life and extends from the forelimb to the hind limb. In the sixth week of fetal life, the nipple and areola form over a bud of breast tissue that is composed of the primary mammary ducts and a loose fibrous tissue or stroma. Fifteen to twenty-five secondary buds then develop and bifurcate into tubules, forming the basis of the duct system.[1] Each duct, as it develops, opens separately into the nipple.

PHYSIOLOGICAL VARIATIONS

At birth, the breasts of both male and female infants may be swollen because of the maternal estrogen effect (Figure 16-1). An unusual but normal finding in the newborn is the secretion of a milk-like substance, also known as "witch's milk," for 1 to 2 weeks[2] (Figure 16-2). Male and female breasts are similar until puberty, consisting of a small amount of breast tissue. Occasionally a prepubertal male or female develops an enlargement of one or both breasts, which involves a soft, mobile, subareolar nodule of uniform consistency.[1] Generally, the nipple and areola are not developed or pigmented with such an enlargement and no associated signs of puberty are present. This condition usually regresses spontaneously within weeks to months, and in the absence of other secondary sexual characteristics, a biopsy is not indicated.[1] If other signs of puberty appear, then these changes could be the first sign of *precocious puberty*, in which case referral and further diagnostic workup are indicated.

Supernumerary nipples may arise from the mammary ridge and be present at birth

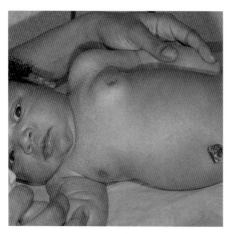

Figure **16-1** Estrogen effect in the newborn. (From Shah BR, Laude TA: *Atlas of pediatric clinical diagnosis*, Philadelphia, 2000, Saunders.)

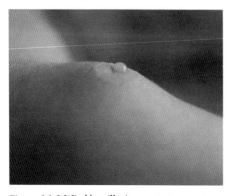

Figure **16-2** Witch's milk. (From Clark DA: *Atlas of neonatology*, ed 7, Philadelphia, 2000, Saunders.)

(Figure 16-3). They are often raised, generally require no treatment, and become imperceptible over time. There is a weak association between supernumerary nipples and renal and cardiovascular abnormalities in Caucasian newborns.[2] In females, supernumerary nipples will on rare occasion develop a small amount of breast tissue during puberty (see *polymastia* under Abnormal Breast Conditions) (Figure 16-3). Widespread nipples are defined as nipples being farther apart than 25% of the chest circumference and may be associated with congenital disorders such as Turner syndrome.[2]

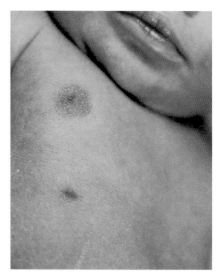

Figure **16-3** Supernumerary nipple. (From Mead Johnson & Company: *Variations and minor departures in infants*, Evansville, Indiana, 1999, Mead Johnson & Company.)

Physiological Variations in the Male Breast

At puberty, the ductal and periductal mesenchymal breast tissue of boys proliferates under the influence of estrogens, with later involution as testicular androgens rise to adult levels.[1] Male estradiol levels triple during puberty; androgens ultimately increase 30 times. If peak estrogen levels occur before androgen levels, the result is *gynecomastia*, a benign increase in glandular and stromal breast tissue in pubertal males (Figure 16-4). Most circulating estrogens are produced outside of the testes, and an increase in fatty tissue, as in obesity, may lead to an increase in estrogen levels and a higher incidence of *gynecomastia* (Box 16-1).

At 14 years of age, 64% of adolescent males have some degree of gynecomastia, with only 4% of adolescents having severe gynecomastia that persists into adulthood.[1] Approximately 50% of males with gynecomastia notice the onset at genital stage 2 of male development, with 20% noticing the change at genital stage 1 and 20% at genital stage 3, and 10%

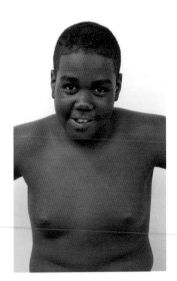

Figure **16-4** Gynecomastia.

beginning at genital stage 4 (see Chapter 15). Gynecomastia, although a normal variant, is also present in relation to hormone imbalances due to thyrotoxicosis, cirrhosis, adrenal and testicular neoplasm, primary hypogonadism, chromosome abnormalities such as Klinefelter syndrome, and severe malnutrition.[1] In addition, prescription medications such as cimetidine, ketoconazole, digoxin, spironolactone, phenothiazines, and illicit drugs, more notably marijuana and anabolic steroids but also amphetamines and opiates, can cause gynecomastia.

Box **16-1**   **Classifications of Gynecomastia**

- **Type I:** One or more subareolar nodules, freely movable
- **Type II:** Breast nodules beneath areola but also extending beyond the areolar perimeter
- **Type III:** Resembles female breast development stage 3 (see Table 16-1)

Data from Neinstein LS: *Adolescent health care: a practical guide,* ed 4, Philadelphia, 2002, Lippincott Williams & Wilkins.

Physiological Variations in the Female Breast

Thelarche, or the beginning of female breast development, is usually the first sign of puberty and occurs between 8 and 13 years of age (Table 16-1 and Figure 16-5). Full breast development marks the end of puberty in females. Breast development during puberty involves both multiple hormones and the binding of hormones to breast tissue. Estrogen, especially estradiol, influences ductal development, whereas progesterone influences additional lobular alveolar development.[1] Thyroxine and corticosteroids are also involved.

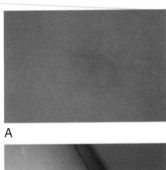

A

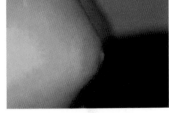

B

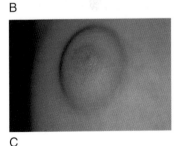

C

Figure **16-5** Female breast development. **A,** First stage of breast sexual maturity. **B,** Third stage of breast sexual maturity. **C,** Fourth stage of breast sexual maturity. (From Lemmi, FO, Lemmi, CAE: *Physical assessment findings multi-user CD-ROM,* St Louis, 2000, Saunders.)

TABLE 16-1 FEMALE BREAST DEVELOPMENT SEXUAL MATURITY RATING (SMR)

Tanner Stage/Sexual Maturity Rating (SMR)	Breast Findings	Areola and Nipple Findings
Tanner stage 1	Prepubertal; no glandular tissue	Conforms to general chest line
Tanner stage 2	Breast bud; small amount of glandular tissue	Areola widens
Tanner stage 3	Larger and more elevation; extends beyond areolar parameter	Areola continues to enlarge but remains in contour with breast
Tanner stage 4	Larger and more elevation	Areola and papilla form a mound projecting from breast contour (half of teens; in some cases persists into adulthood)
Tanner stage 5	Adult (size variable)	Areola part of breast contour, nipple projecting above areola

Data from Neinstein LS: *Adolescent health care: a practical guide,* ed 4, Philadelphia, 2002, Lippincott Williams & Wilkins.

Unlike testicular development in boys, breast development, an early sign of puberty in girls, is readily apparent to family members and peers, often eliciting unwanted comments as to presence or absence and size of breast tissue. Even minor comments can contribute to embarrassment and the teen's discomfort with the examiner's questions about breast development, as well as the breast exam itself. The examiner also should be mindful that sexual harassment is a major issue in today's middle schools, sometimes jeopardizing the teen's mental health and school performance.

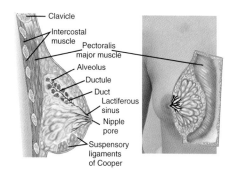

Figure **16-6** Anatomy of the breast.

ANATOMY AND PHYSIOLOGY

Mature female breast tissue extends from the second or third rib to the sixth or seventh rib, and from the sternal margin to the midaxillary line at stage 5 sexual maturity rating. The nipple is located centrally, surrounded by the areola. The breast is composed of glandular and fibrous tissue and subcutaneous and retromammary fat (Figure 16-6). Fifteen to twenty lobes radiate around the nipple, and each lobe is divided into 20 to 40 lobules of milk-producing acini cells that empty into lactiferous ducts.[1] These cells are small and inconspicuous in the nonpregnant, nonlactating woman. A layer of subcutaneous fibrous tissue provides support for the breast, as do the suspensory ligaments. The muscles forming the floor of the breast are pectoralis major, pectoralis minor, serratus anterior, latissimus dorsi, subscapularis, external oblique, and rectus abdominis. Vascular supply comes from the internal mammary artery and the lateral thoracic artery. The lymph system drains to the anterior axillary, subscapular and supraclavicular nodes.

CULTURAL VARIATIONS

African-American girls begin puberty about 1 to 1.5 years earlier than Caucasian girls and begin menstrual periods 8.5 months earlier. Breast development occurs at an average age of 8.87 years in African-American girls and at an average of 9.96 years of age in Caucasian girls.[3]

TABLE 16-2 INFORMATION GATHERING FOR MALE AND FEMALE BREAST ASSESSMENT AT KEY DEVELOPMENTAL STAGES

Age	Questions to Ask
Preadolescent girls and boys	Breast buds noted? At what age did breast development begin? Tenderness or pain in breast? Other signs of puberty noted? Concern about breast development?
Female adolescents	Contraceptive use? Last menstrual period? Previous pregnancy? Any pain noted in breast? Relationship of breast pain to menstrual cycle? Discharge from nipple? Any lump noted in breast or axilla? Redness on skin? Concerns about breast health or breast development? Doing breast self-exam?

SYSTEM-SPECIFIC HISTORY

Table 16-2 reviews the important information to be gathered for preadolescent and adolescent girls presenting for well care and screening questions for adolescents presenting with breast problems.

PHYSICAL ASSESSMENT

Inspection and Palpation

Prepubertal Breast

Prepubertal breasts are easily inspected and palpated while inspecting the chest to assess respiratory and cardiovascular status. The examiner should note any masses or pain, nipple discharge, or sign of premature thelarche, or breast development.

Adolescent Male

Pubertal breasts are inspected with the male adolescent supine with his hands behind his head. The examiner places the pads of the middle finger or the thumb and forefinger at opposing margins of the breast. As the examiner palpates the breast, the presence or absence of a firm rubbery mass or nodular tissue is appreciated. In conditions such as a *lipoma* or *dermoid cyst*, the mass is usually to one side of the areola.

Adolescent Female

There is some controversy about the age at which practitioners should perform routine breast exams in young women. While malignancies in adolescents are rare, routine exams in early to middle adolescence provide an opportunity for reassurance and education about normal breast findings and variations of normal. For teens whose close female relatives (mother, maternal aunts) have had premenopausal breast cancer, the exam can be an important forum for discussing breast cancer risk and protective factors.

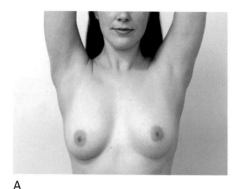

A

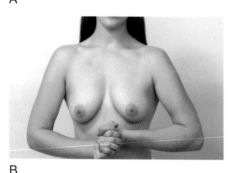

B

Figure **16-7** Inspection of the breast. **A,** Arms extended overhead. **B,** Hands pressed together.

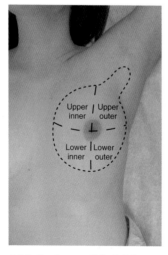

Upper inner | Upper outer
Lower inner | Lower outer

Figure **16-8** Quadrants of the left breast, tail of Spence.

Breast Examination

In a full adult breast exam, the breasts are initially inspected with the patient sitting, disrobed to the waist, in the following positions: arms extended overhead, hands pressed against hips or against each other, and leaning forward from the waist (Figure 16-7 *A, B*). These three positions are most helpful if a mass is palpated.[1] The practitioner will have to weigh the benefits of full inspection in this low-risk age group against the aversion most young teens have to being undressed in front of a provider.

While the breasts can be palpated with the adolescent sitting and supine, the preferred position for the adolescent is supine, with one arm under her head. With the adolescent supine, the breasts are in a more stable position, and touching of the breast with the nondominant hand of the examiner can be minimized.[1] For purposes of examination, the breast is divided into four quadrants and a tail that extends into the axilla (Figure 16-8).

The breasts should be palpated with the pads (not tips) of the middle three fingers, with the fingers rotating in either a clockwise or counterclockwise direction. There are three methods for covering the whole breast systematically, all of which are used in clinical practice (Figure 16-9). The examiner should include the *tail of Spence* in the axilla in addition to the supraclavicular and infraclavicular regions. When palpating the breast, the examiner should use the dominant hand, and stabilize the breast, if necessary, with the nondominant hand. Place the pads of the middle fingers at the margins of the breast to begin palpation, and note any masses, pain, nipple discharge, or sign of premature breast development. If firm rubbery tissue or a nodular mass is noted, fine palpation is required for accurate sizing and to distinguish among fatty tissue, cysts, and other nodular masses.

One technique that incorporates patient education into the breast examination is

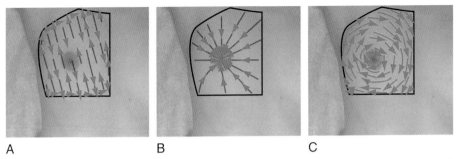

A   B   C

Figure **16-9** Methods of breast palpation. **A,** Palpation strip method. **B,** Palpation wedge method. **C,** Palpation circle method.

Pediatric Pearls

Asymmetrical breasts are common in early development.

that of demonstrating *breast self-exam* techniques to the adolescent before the actual exam of the breast begins, and then asking her permission to guide her hand onto her breast, pointing out landmarks and normal findings (as noted below) in the developing breast:

- Thicker ridge of breast tissue often found in the inferior aspect of the breast
- Nodularity of normal adolescent breast tissue (especially in the upper outer quadrant)
- Feel of the ribs underneath the medial border of the breast; this normal finding has been mistaken by some adolescents for breast lumps

Breast Self-Exam

Teaching *breast self-exam* (BSE) can assist the adolescent in accepting her body, increase comfort with the exam itself, and provide an opportunity to reinforce or correct information the adolescent may have received from health classes, teen magazines, or female relatives about breast health. The practitioner also should take into account the teen's developmental and temperamental readiness to learn the information (Box 16-2). Young adolescents often lack the future orientation needed to learn preventive self-care and are more receptive in the late adolescent years. The American Cancer Society continues to recommend BSE at age 20.

DEVELOPMENTAL BREAST CONDITIONS

The following are variations of normal that occur with stages of breast development:

- **Physiological swelling and tenderness:** Breast lobules undergo proliferative changes due to the normal menstrual cycle, leading to pain, swelling, and distinct masses that recede after menses.
- **Asymmetry:** In most women, one breast is slightly larger than the other, and this difference may be accentuated by asymmetrical breast development during puberty, which usually corrects by adulthood.
- **Proliferative breast changes:** Formerly called *fibrocystic disease,* many authorities now consider increased nodularity to be a variation of normal, occurring in more than 50% of women of reproductive age. Adolescents often have painless lumps, which may become tender 1 week

Box **16-2**   Breast Self-Examination

Breast self-exam (BSE) should be done once a month 2 or 3 days after the menses end. If periods are irregular or do not occur monthly because of oral contraceptive use, instruct the adolescent to perform the BSE on the first day of the month.

How to do BSE:

1. Inspect both breasts standing before a mirror. Note any dimpling, nodules, changes in the skin, or nipple discharge.
2. Clasp hands behind your head or in front of your waist and press your arms slightly forward. Note shape and contour of the breast.
3. Place hands on your hips and press down as you bow forward and pull your elbows and shoulders forward. Note any changes in the contour, shape, or smooth surface of the breast. Asymmetry in size often occurs during development.
4. With the left arm raised, palpate the contour of the left breast with the right hand extending from the axilla down and up over the entire surface of the breast in a vertical pattern, including palpation of the areola. Repeat with the right arm raised.
5. Check for nipple discharge by gently squeezing the nipples.
6. Lie down and place left hand under the head, raising the left shoulder slightly. Use a circular or vertical pattern to exam the breast with the right hand noted as above, moving from the outer edge to the mid-chest, including the axilla. Nodular lesions are often palpated in the upper outer quadrant of the breast. Note the borders of the ribs under the breast tissue. Repeat on the right breast.

---

before menses. Areas of nodularity may be a few millimeters to 1 cm in diameter.

- **Cysts:** Usually associated with few symptoms, cysts are well-circumscribed, small, and freely movable masses, commonly under 1 cm in adolescents.
- **Montgomery tubercles:** These tubercles arise from sebaceous glands associated with a lactiferous duct; they present as small, soft papules around the areola, with occasional thin, clear to brown discharge, and possibly a small lump under the areola. The condition usually resolves without intervention.

ABNORMAL BREAST CONDITIONS

Breast cancer in adolescents is extremely rare. Malignant lesions comprise only 0.9% of all surgically excised lesions in this age-group. Breast variations and benign tumors are presented in Table 16-3.

 CHARTING

14-Year-Old Male

Chest: Symmetrical, lungs clear to auscultation bilaterally, breast bud noted under L areola, warm and tender on palpation, R breast nl without swelling or tenderness.

 CHARTING

9-Year-Old Female

Chest: Symmetrical, lungs clear to auscultation bilaterally, breast bud noted under R areola, warm and tender to touch, nonerythematous, L breast nl without swelling or tenderness.

TABLE 16-3 NORMAL VARIATIONS AND ABNORMAL FINDINGS OF THE MALE AND FEMALE BREAST

Condition	Description
Polymastia	Breast tissue that develops around supernumerary nipples; although clinically insignificant, this tissue may become uncomfortably engorged postpartum
Fibroadenoma	Most common benign breast tumor excised during adolescence; firm, rubbery, mobile, nontender; ranges in size from <1 cm to 10 cm; usually discovered by the adolescent
Amastia	Absence of breast tissue. *Athelia*, absence of nipple; often connected to a chest wall defect or more extensive congenital anomalies
Breast atrophy	Most commonly caused by significant loss of fat and glandular tissue as a result of eating disorders but also may occur in premature ovarian failure, androgen excess (tumors or ingested steroids), and chronic diseases that lead to significant weight loss.
Macromastia	Exceptionally large breasts; definition of "normal" breast size is difficult to determine, but this condition is associated with obesity and a strong familial incidence; 80% of cases begin in adolescence with teens complaining of psychological effects as compared to the more common complaints of breast, shoulder, and back pain among adults
Virginal or juvenile hypertrophy	May be an abnormal response of the breast to normal estrogen levels, occurs perimenarchally; breasts may enlarge to as much as 30 to 50 lb
Nipple discharge	• Multicolored or sticky discharge may be caused by duct ectasia • Serous or serosanguineous discharge may be caused by intraductal papilloma, benign changes, duct ectasia, or rarely cancer • Milky discharge (galactorrhea) may be the result of hormonal imbalance, pregnancy, or past abortion; medications or illicit drugs such as marijuana; or pituitary tumors; or it may result from stimulation by sexual partners • Purulent discharge due to mastitis • Watery discharge due to papilloma or cancer

REFERENCES

1. Neinstein LS: Breast. In Neinstein LS, editor: *Adolescent health care: a practical guide,* Philadelphia, 2002, Lippincott Williams & Wilkins.
2. Thureen PJ, Hall D, Deacon J, Hernandez JA: *Assessment and care of the well newborn,* ed 2, Philadelphia, 2005, Saunders.
3. Reiter EO, Lee PA: Have the onset and tempo of puberty changed? *Arch Pediatr Adolesc Med* 155(9):988-989, 2001.

CHAPTER 17

FEMALE GENITALIA

Naomi A. Schapiro

Until recently, few healthcare providers were routinely taught to examine normal prepubertal female genitals. The refinement of the forensic colposcopic examination to detect the physical signs of sexual abuse in girls, and the need to testify accurately in court, have inspired the research of the last 20 years to document the range of "normal" in girls from birth through puberty.

With this knowledge of normal development of the female reproductive anatomy, the provider now can incorporate the routine examination of the genitals into well-child care. During the review of systems and genital exam, the provider can foster a dialogue between parent and child concerning reproductive health. For religious and cultural reasons, as well as personal preference, parents, children, and adolescents are more likely to request female providers for the breast and female genital exam. In nonemergent situations, it is important to honor this request, either within the practice setting or by referral, and to respect privacy and confidentiality in performing the examination and in giving results.

DEVELOPMENT

At 5 to 6 weeks of gestation, fetal gonads are bipotential, capable of differentiating either into a testis or into an ovary. Both male and female embryos have one pair of primary sex organs, or gonads, and two pairs of ducts, *Wolffian* ducts and the *Müllerian* ducts. During the sixth week, the primordial germ cells migrate into the primary sex cords and begin to differentiate. Leydig and Sertoli cells appear in male embryos, producing testosterone and anti-Müllerian hormone. In female embryos, the gonads do not produce testosterone, and the gonads develop into ovaries. The Wolffian ducts deteriorate, and the Müllerian ducts develop into the uterus, upper vaginal tract, and fallopian tubes. The external genitalia differentiate at between 8 and 12 weeks of gestation (Figure 17-1). Active mitosis continues and thousands of germ cells, *oocytes,* are produced. A newborn female may have 2 million primary oocytes at birth. However, after birth, no further oogonia occurs.

PHYSIOLOGICAL VARIATIONS

In preterm neonates, the *labia majora* may not cover the *labia minora,* and the *clitoris* will be prominent. Term newborns will have enlarged labia majora, which usually cover other external structures, a relatively large clitoris, and labia minora with dull pink epithelium, due to maternal estrogen effects (Figure 17-2). A creamy white or slightly blood-tinged discharge is normal for up to 10 days after birth.

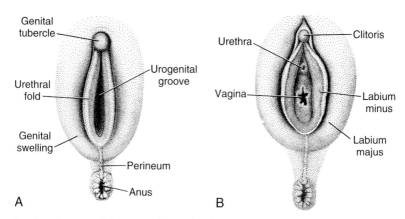

Figure **17-1** Development of the external genitalia. (From Sadler TW: *Langman's medical embryology,* ed 8, Philadelphia, 2000, Lippincott Williams & Wilkins.)

The *hymen* is relatively thicker, pink-white in color, and redundant and may remain so up until 2 to 4 years of age (Figure 17-3).

In the absence of congenital anomalies, all girl infants are born with hymens, which can present in a variety of configurations. Commonly, the hymen is fimbriated, *annular* or *crescentic* (Figure 17-4). Annular hymens are more common at birth, whereas crescentic hymens are more common in girls over 3 years of age. Hymen types that are rare include septate, cribriform, and imperforate (Figure 17-5).

in transverse diameter. Hymens in older but prepubertal girls are thinner, redder, and more sensitive to touch. With the onset of puberty, the hymen often shows an estrogen effect that makes it pinker and more redundant before the other secondary sexual characteristics appear.

The prepubertal *vagina* is rigid, nonelastic, and thin-walled, lined by columnar epithelium, which normally appears redder than the squamous epithelium lining the vagina of pubertal adolescents and adult women. Bacterial infections, such as *Streptococcus* and *Shigella*, can

ANATOMY AND PHYSIOLOGY

After the newborn period and before menarche, the clitoris is about 3 mm in length and 3 mm

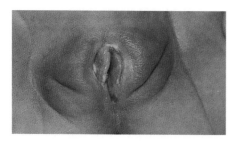

Figure **17-2** Newborn with estrogen effect. (From Zitelli BJ, Davis HW: *Atlas of pediatric physical diagnosis,* ed 4, St Louis, 2002, Mosby.)

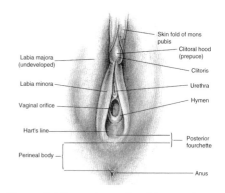

Figure **17-3** External genitalia of the prepubertal child. (Reprinted with permission from *Contemporary Pediatrics,* 16[1]:153, March 1999. *Contemporary Pediatrics* is a copyrighted publication of Advanstar Communications Inc. All rights reserved.)

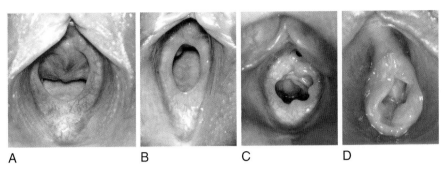

A   B   C   D

Figure **17-4** Variations in normal hymens. **A,** Crescentic; **B,** annular; **C,** fimbriated; **D,** redundant. (From McCann JJ, Kerns DL: *The anatomy of child and adolescent sexual abuse: a CD-ROM atlas/reference,* St Louis, 1999, Intercorp Inc.)

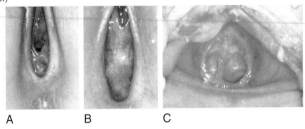

A   B   C

Figure **17-5** Abnormal hymens. **A,** Cribriform; **B,** fimbriated; **C,** septate. (**A** and **B** from McCann JJ, Kerns DL: *The anatomy of child and adolescent sexual abuse: a CD-ROM atlas/reference,* St Louis, 1999, Intercorp Inc. **C** from Lahoti SL, McClain N, Girardet R et al: Evaluating the child for sexual abuse, *Am Fam Physician* 63[5]:883-892, 2001.)

cause purulent or even bloody vaginal discharge. Sexually transmitted pathogens, such as *Neisseria gonorrhoeae* and *Chlamydia trachomatis,* infect the columnar epithelium of the vagina, rather than the *cervix.* The prepubertal vagina is hostile to yeast (Table 17-1), and vulvovaginal candidiasis is rare except in cases of diaper use, diabetes mellitus, recent antibiotic usage, and immunocompromise.

Adrenarche, the development of pubic and axillary hair, occurs at approximately the same time as *thelarche,* the development of the breast, occurring as early as 7 or 8 years of age, particularly in African-American girls, with a mean age of 9 to 10 years (Figure 17-6). Table 17-2 correlates development and *Tanner staging* or sexual maturity rating. The external genitalia and internal structures (labia majora, labia minora, hymen, vagina, ovaries, uterus) are changing under the influence of increasing estrogens all at the same time. The changes in the female genitalia have not been Tanner staged in the same manner as the development of male genitalia or development of the breast and pubic hair.

⌐☞ Key Points

Cultural variations: Development and amount of pubic and general body hair varies greatly with ethnicity: young women of Asian or Native American descent tend to have less body hair than young women of European or African descent, and pubic hair development may not correlate well with sexual maturity.

SYSTEM-SPECIFIC HISTORY

Table 17-3 reviews information gathering on preadolescent and adolescent menstrual history and adolescent sexual history.

TABLE 17-1 PUBERTAL CHANGES OF THE VAGINA

Vaginal Changes	Prepubertal Girls	Pubertal Adolescents
Vaginal pH	6.5-7.5 (alkaline)	< 4.5
Vaginal mucosa	Columnar epithelium (red)	Stratified squamous epithelium (pink); presence of columnar epithelium on ectocervix, surrounding the os
Vaginal mucous glands, discharge	Absent	Present; physiological leukorrhea usually begins at Tanner stage 2-3
Normal vaginal flora	Gram-positive cocci and anaerobic gram negatives; gonorrhea and chlamydia focally infect vagina	Lactobacilli; yeast part of normal flora; gonorrhea and chlamydia commonly infect cervix
Vaginal length	4-5 cm	11-12 cm
External genitalia	Thin labia, rigid, nonelastic, thin-walled vagina	Thicker labia; thicker, more elastic, wavy, or redundant hymen; more elastic vagina

Data from Jenny C: Sexually transmitted diseases and child abuse, *Pediatr Ann* 21(8):497-503, 1992.

P₁–Tanner 1 (preadolescent). No growth of pubic hair

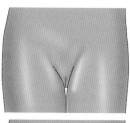

P₂–Tanner 2. Initial, scarcely pigmented straight hair, especially along medial border of the labia

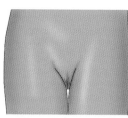

P₃–Tanner 3. Sparse, dark, visibly pigmented, curly public hair on labia.

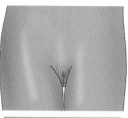

P₄–Tanner 4. Hair coarse and curly, abundant but less than adult.

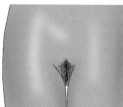

P₅–Tanner 5. Lateral speeding; type and triangle spread of adult hair to medial surface of thighs.

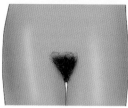

P₆–Tanner 6. Further extension laterally, upward, or dispersed (occurs in only 10% of women).

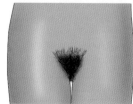

Figure **17-6** Biological maturity in girls.

TABLE 17-2 TANNER STAGING

Tanner Stage/ Sexual Maturity Rating (SMR)	Pubic Hair Development	Genital Changes Due to Estrogenization*
1	No growth of pubic hair	Thicker, more elastic labia minora and hymen, change from columnar (red) to squamous (pink) epithelium in vagina, T 1-2
2	Downy, scarcely pigmented straight hair, especially along medial border of labia majora	Physiological leukorrhea (T 2-3)
3	Sparse, visibly pigmented curly pubic hair on labia	Onset of menses (T 3-4)
4	Hair coarse, curly, abundant, but less so than adult; no extension onto medial thighs	
5	Lateral spreading, triangle distribution with some spread onto medial thighs	

Data from Neinstein LS: *Adolescent health care: a practical guide*, ed 4, Philadelphia, 2002, Lippincott Williams & Wilkins; Jenny C: Sexually transmitted diseases and child abuse, *Pediatr Ann* 21(8):497-503, 1992; Emans SJ, Laufer MR, Goldlstein DP, editors: *Pediatric and adolescent gynecology*, ed 4, Philadelphia, 1998, Lippincott Williams & Wilkins.
*Not part of classic Tanner staging, but important to note in exam findings and for anticipatory guidance.

TABLE 17-3 INFORMATION GATHERING FOR FEMALE GENITALIA AT KEY DEVELOPMENTAL STAGES

Age	Questions to Ask
Preadolescent and adolescent	*Menstrual history:* Age at menarche, regularity of cycles, any spotting or bleeding between cycles, dysmenorrhea, family history of menstrual problems? *For primary amenorrhea:* Age of thelarche and adrenarche, presence or absence of secondary sex characteristics? *For secondary amenorrhea:* Any weight loss attempts, including restriction, binging, purging?
Adolescent	*Sexual history:* Any prior sexual activity, including number and gender of partners, types of activity, use of contraception and/or barrier protection? Coerced or unwanted sexual activity? History of prior examinations, prior infections? Use of over-the-counter medications and cosmetic products or douches? Shaving or use of depilatories for pubic and thigh hair?

PHYSICAL ASSESSMENT

Examination of the Newborn

Inspection and Palpation

In the newborn, assess presence and size of the clitoris, patency of the vaginal orifice, presence and location of urethra, and distance between the posterior fourchette and the anus. The labia majora should be palpated for the presence of gonads or hernias, even in a normal-appearing female. Any palpable gonads are likely to be testes, because ovaries rarely descend below the inguinal ring.

Examination of Prepubertal Girls

Positioning

Most young children can be examined in the frog-leg position: supine, with knees apart and feet touching in the midline (Figure 17-7). For an apprehensive small child, the caretaker can sit in a chair or on the examination table in a semireclined position (feet in or out of stirrups) with the child's legs straddling her thighs (Figure 17-8). Older children can be placed in adjustable stirrups. In cases of suspected trauma or abuse, a foreign body in the vagina, or other suspected structural abnormalities, knee-chest position can be used in a child older than 2 years of age (Figure 17-9).

Have the child rest her chest on the exam table and support her weight on bent knees, which are positioned 6 to 8 inches apart. Her buttocks will be held up in the air and her back and abdomen will fall downward. In this position, using a penlight or an otoscope head for magnification and light, the examiner can visualize the lower vagina, and in prepubertal girls often the upper vagina. Lateral separation of the labia will be required to visualize the hymen (Figure 17-10).

Touching the hymen in prepubertal girls causes pain. Discharge for wet mounts,

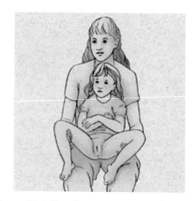

Figure **17-8** Frog-leg positioning with mother. (From Lahoti SL, McClain N, Girardet R et al: Evaluating the child for sexual abuse, *Am Fam Physician* 63[5]: 883-892, 2001. Used with permission by Maria Hartsock, MA, CMI, Medical Art Company, Cincinnati, Ohio, www.hartsock illustration.com.)

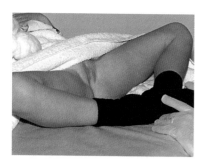

Figure **17-7** Frog-leg positioning. (From McCann JJ, Kerns DL: *The anatomy of child and adolescent sexual abuse: a CD-ROM atlas/reference,* St Louis, 1999, Intercorp Inc.)

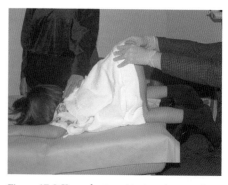

Figure **17-9** Knee-chest positioning. (From Gall JA, Boos SC, Payne-James JJ et al: *Forensic medicine,* London, 2003, Churchill Livingstone.)

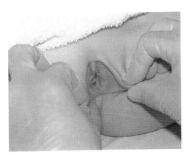

Figure **17-10** Anterior labial retraction. (From Gall JA, Boos SC, Payne-James JJ et al: *Forensic medicine*, London, 2003, Churchill Livingstone.)

potassium hydroxide (KOH) exams, Gram stains, or culture should be collected with a small Dacron-tipped swab moistened with saline. The child can be asked to take a deep breath for distraction and to open the hymen. If the examiner avoids touching the hymen, this procedure can be painless. If the examiner sees a foreign body, it may be removed by using a moistened cotton swab or by gently irrigating the vagina with normal saline.

Rarely, in cases of suspected abnormalities, a rectoabdominal examination may be performed by placing the gloved and lubricated index or little finger of one hand into the rectum and placing the other hand on the abdomen. The cervix and uterus may be felt as a "button," and ovaries are not palpable. As the examiner withdraws the finger, the vagina can be gently milked to elicit discharge, a foreign body, or (in rare cases) a polypoid tumor.

Key Points

There is no indication for a speculum exam in the prepubertal child; any invasive exams or procedures should be performed under anesthesia.

Examination of the Adolescent

Past recommendations indicated the first pelvic exam of an adolescent was to be performed after the onset of sexual activity and by age 18 to 20, if not sexually active before then. However, the recent developments listed below have impacted these recommendations:

1. The increased sensitivity and specificity of urine DNA amplification testing for gonorrhea and chlamydia over traditional methods (particularly for chlamydia).
2. The findings in some longitudinal studies indicate the majority of low-grade dysplasia noted as abnormal on Pap smears in adolescents reverts to normal over time, without treatment.
3. The accuracy of pelvic ultrasound in detecting abnormalities of the uterus, ovaries, and fallopian tubes

Table 17-4 reviews current indications for pelvic exams and alternatives to the recommended exam for adolescents who refuse or are unable to tolerate the pelvic examination.

This description of the pelvic examination should be considered a supplement to careful supervision and mentoring of the novice examiner by more experienced practitioners. Proper clean technique is more easily demonstrated, and specific procedures for collecting specimens for the Papanicolaou smear and testing of sexually transmitted infections (STIs) vary among clinics and laboratories.

Preparing for the Exam

Explain the pelvic exam carefully to the adolescent, including specific suggestions for positioning and relaxation. Some practitioners show the adolescent the speculum in advance, whereas others feel that this may increase anxiety. Although most adolescents have heard of the "Pap smear," many are not sure what it entails and have some anxiety about specimen collection. It may help to have an open sample of the Pap smear collection kit for demonstration purposes, so that the teen can feel the smooth edge of a spatula and the softness of a cytobrush. Many examiners provide the adolescent with a mirror, if desired, in order to observe the examination in progress. The adolescent should be encouraged to empty her bladder before the exam. If any specimens

TABLE 17-4 INDICATIONS FOR PELVIC EXAMS AND ALTERNATIVES

Indications	Recommended Exam	Alternatives to Recommended Exam
Sexually active adolescent, asymptomatic	Pap smear at age 21 or 3 years after the onset of coitus	Urine LCR screen for gonorrhea and chlamydia; vaginal swab for wet mount
Adolescent at age 21, asymptomatic, no history of sexual activity	Pelvic exam and Pap smear	
Sexually active adolescent, asymptomatic, desires start of hormonal contraception	Urine STI screen, urine β-hCG, weight and BP check	May defer STI screen and urine β-hCG if menstruating at time of visit
Adolescent desires start of hormonal contraception, no history of sexual activity	Urine β-hCG, weight and BP check	
Vaginal discharge without abdominal pain, no history of sexual activity	Vaginal swab for wet mount, KOH prep, STI screen if indicated by microscopic exam	Teen may insert vaginal swab, place in test tube with saline; wet mount, KOH prep
Vaginal discharge without abdominal pain, sexually active adolescent	Urine STI screen, vaginal swab for wet mount, KOH prep, speculum exam, Pap smear if due	Teen may insert vaginal swab, place in test tube with saline; wet mount, KOH prep
Adolescent with lower abdominal/pelvic pain; no history of sexual activity	Urine β-hCG, bimanual exam, speculum exam if indicated by history or presence of discharge or bleeding; ultrasound if results unclear	Urine β-hCG, urgent ultrasound
Sexually active adolescent with lower abdominal/pelvic pain	Pelvic exam, including speculum exam and bimanual, wet mount/KOH prep, and STI screening	Full exam essential; however, adolescent should not be examined against her will

Data from Saslow D, Runowicz CD, Solomon D et al: American Cancer Society guideline for early detection of cervical neoplasia and cancer, *CA Can J Clin* 52:342-362, 2002; Blake DR, Duggan A, Quinn T et al: Evaluation of vaginal infections in adolescent women: can it be done without a speculum? *Pediatrics* 102(4 Pt 1):939-944, 1998; Ricciardi R: First pelvic examination in the adolescent, *Nurse Pract Forum* 11(3):161-169, 2000; Shafer MA: Annual pelvic examination in the sexually active adolescent female: what are we doing and why are we doing it? *J Adolesc Health* 23(2):68-73, 1998.

LCR, Ligase chain reaction; *STI,* sexually transmitted infection; β-*hCG,* beta human chorionic gonadotropin; *BP,* blood pressure; *KOH,* potassium hydroxide.

are needed, such as for urine pregnancy test, urinalysis, or urine for DNA amplification, they can be collected at this time. The adolescent should be informed that she may change her mind about the exam at any point, and the exam should never be forced or coerced. Younger teens may want to have a parent present for the pelvic examination. With sufficient preparation and explanations, most adolescents are able to tolerate the examination well. However, adolescents who have been sexually abused, have suffered other trauma, or are particularly anxious may be helped by specific visualization and relaxation techniques.[1]

Positioning

Adjust stirrups appropriately for the leg length. The adolescent can leave socks on to make the stirrups more comfortable. Move the buttocks forward to the very edge of the exam table, while the feet are in the stirrups. Although many adolescents are uncomfortable with this position, it is necessary for proper manipulation of the speculum. Avoid touching or pulling the teen, encourage her to move on her own. Most adolescents prefer to have a sheet draped over their abdomen and thighs, but the drape should be positioned so that the examiner can maintain eye contact with the adolescent. The knees should be abducted as far as possible. In order to have the teen's active participation, encourage her to push her knees apart as if she were doing a dance or aerobics stretch in order to avoid any references that could remind her of unwanted sexual activity. The adolescent should be encouraged to take slow, even breaths, to avoid tensing her abdominal muscles, and to keep her buttocks down on the exam table.

Pediatric Pearls

A Valsalva maneuver, or bearing-down sensation, can facilitate speculum insertion in the teen.

Inspection

Note the condition of the clitoris, urethra, labia majora, labia minora, hymen, and

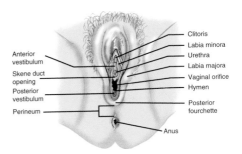

Figure **17-11** External female genitalia.

introitus, including any swellings or lesions (such as inflamed pubic hair follicles or condyloma, venereal warts), any clitoral hypertrophy, presence or absence of estrogenization, and any inflammation or discharge (Figure 17-11). The external structures can be visualized more completely if the examiner places the palms of both hands adjacent to the labia majora and gently separates them.

Palpation

Palpation of the labia, the Skene's glands, and the Bartholin's glands is usually avoided in the adolescent, unless the teen complains of pain or swelling or the examiner notes abnormalities upon inspection (Figure 17-12).

Speculum Exam

Choosing the Speculum

The correct size speculum should be selected, and the speculum warmed, if possible, before insertion. Although many clinics use plastic specula, that type is not offered in the size range that is available in metal, and their open position is often too wide to be used for an anxious adolescent.

- A Huffman (Huffman-Graves) speculum, ($\frac{1}{2} \times 4\frac{1}{2}$ inches) should be used if the hymenal opening is small, as in virginal teens.
- A Pedersen speculum ($\frac{7}{8} \times 4\frac{1}{2}$ inches) and rarely a Graves speculum ($1\frac{3}{4} \times 3\frac{3}{4}$ inches) are used for a sexually active teen (Figure 17-13).

- *Light source:* Some plastic specula have a built-in light source. Otherwise, angle the light over the examiner's shoulder to illuminate the introitus. Warn the patient that the light may feel warm. If the lamp needs readjustment after speculum insertion, remember to change gloves before touching the neck of the light.

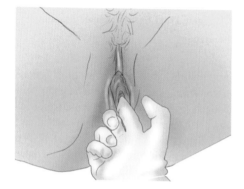

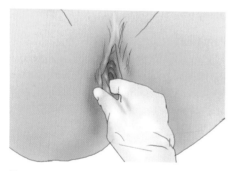

Figure **17-12** Examination of the Skene's and Bartholin's glands.

- *Inserting the speculum:* The examiner should double glove. In anxious patients, and patients with a small hymenal opening, one finger, moistened with water, can be inserted into the vagina to palpate the cervix and then withdrawn, in order to facilitate easy insertion of the speculum. Using the fingers of one hand to separate the labia and press down on the *fossa navicularis,* the examiner should use the other hand to gently insert the speculum, angled toward

the sacrum, with slight downward pressure to avoid irritating the urethra. Be careful not to pinch the labia minora or to catch pubic hair in the speculum bills.

- Avoid pressure on the hymen in virginal teens.
- An alternate method of speculum insertion is to use the second and middle fingers to separate the labia, then press in gently on either side of the lower introitus, in order to relax the fourchette tissues without direct pressure.
- Have the teen take in a deep breath or perform a Valsalva maneuver to help relax the introitus.
- If the cervix does not come into view, use a slight side-to-side motion to find the cervix; if still not visualized, it may cause less discomfort to withdraw the speculum and use one finger to locate the cervix than to move the speculum excessively.
- Once the speculum is in place, secure the speculum in the open position, and remove the first glove on the hand that separated the labia; then proceed with specimen collection. Some practitioners hold the plastic speculum in place because the fully open position of the speculum is too wide for some teens (Figure 17-14).

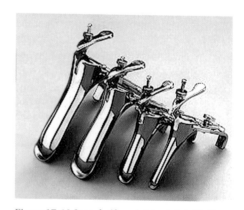

Figure **17-13** Specula (from left to right): Medium Graves, small Graves, Pederson, Huffman. (Courtesy Spectrum Surgical Instruments Corp, Stow, Ohio.)

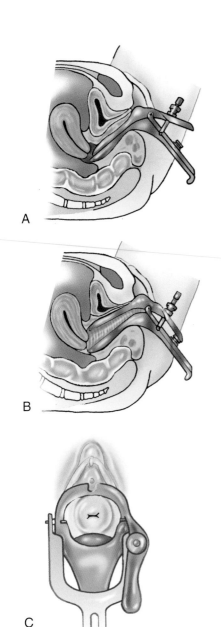

A

B

C

Figure **17-14** Female genital examination.

Inspection of the Cervix

Carefully inspect the cervix for color, lesions, and any discharge at the cervical os. Variations of normal include Nabothian cysts (small, white or yellow, raised, round areas) and

ectropion (visible ring of reddened columnar epithelium surrounding the os). The os in a nulliparous woman is round, but may be slit-like in a parous adolescent. Inspect the walls of the vagina, and note the presence, color, and consistency of any discharge.

Specimen Collection

In adolescents, sexually transmitted infections (STIs) are far more prevalent than high-grade cervical dysplasia, or cancer of the cervix. If the examiner is using cervical swabs for STI testing, these should be collected first.

- If not using urine for DNA amplification, collect a cervical swab for chlamydia and gonorrhea (or DNA amplification swab for chlamydia and culture for gonorrhea).
- Use a moistened cotton-tip swab or wooden spatula to collect some vaginal secretions for wet mount and KOH preparations.
- Use a spatula and cytobrush for Pap smear collection (following laboratory instructions for either a traditional Pap smear or the newer Thinprep, in which the cells are collected in a liquid medium). Be sure to sample the squamocolumnar junction, which may be on the ectocervix in some adolescents.

Make sure to close the speculum before withdrawal and to not pinch the cervix in closing the speculum bills. Testing vaginal pH is often a valuable adjunct to the wet mount and KOH prep exams, and vaginal discharge adhering to the speculum bills can be collected for testing before the speculum is discarded or placed in cleaning solution. Alternately, a swab of vaginal secretions can be applied to the pH tape or strip.

The Bimanual Exam

The purpose of the bimanual exam is to assess the cervix, the corpus of the uterus, and the adnexa. The adolescent should be encouraged, again, to relax abdominal muscles by breathing slowly and steadily. The examiner inserts the middle and index fingers of a gloved hand, using lubricant, into the vagina (Figure 17-15). In virginal adolescents, it may only be possible to insert one finger. Having the teen take a deep breath or perform a Valsalva maneuver may facilitate insertion of the examiner's fingers.

- **Assess the cervix:** Note consistency (usually firm and shaped like the tip of a nose), presence of any bumps (such as Nabothian cysts, 3 to 8 mm smooth, non-tender firm lumps on the cervix, which result from blockage of endocervical gland ducts).

- **Assess the uterus:** Press down on the abdomen with the other hand, while supporting the cervix. Assess the size, shape, consistency, mobility, and tenderness of the uterus and any palpable masses. The position of the uterus varies from anteverted, anteflexed, midposition, and retroverted to

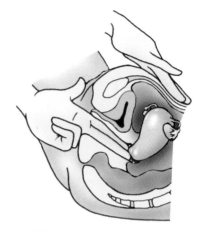

Figure **17-15** Bimanual exam.

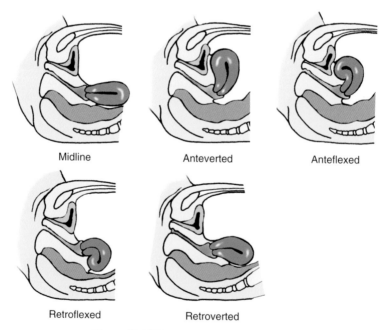

Midline   Anteverted   Anteflexed

Retroflexed   Retroverted

Figure **17-16** Various positions of the uterus.

retroflexed (Figure 17-16). The normal uterus is shaped like an upside-down pear and is approximately 7.5 cm long and 2.5 cm thick (or the size of a lime).

- **Assess cervical motion tenderness:** Wiggle the cervix side to side and forward and back with the examiner's fingers. The sensation in a normal exam is unusual for an adolescent, so ask her to distinguish between pain and slight discomfort or a "strange" feeling. Tenderness or pain on exam is a symptom of pelvic infection.
- **Assess the adnexae:** Place the examining fingers in the vagina first at the right lateral fornix, then at the left, posteriorly and high. Begin with the opposite hand on the abdomen just below and medial to the iliac crest and move diagonally toward the symphysis pubis. Apply a firm, steady sweeping motion with the hand on the abdomen as you palpate briefly. Normal ovaries are smooth and almond-shaped, slightly tender to deep palpation, and approximately 3 cm by 1.5 cm by 1 cm. Tenderness or fullness of the adnexae is abnormal and may indicate infection, ectopic pregnancy or endometriosis.
- **Rectovaginal exams:** This exam is usually omitted in adolescents, unless there is a suspicion of abnormality or an extremely retroflexed uterus. It is performed with the index finger in the vagina, the middle finger in the rectum and the opposite hand on the abdomen. The rectovaginal septum should be thin, pliable, and free of masses. The teen should be reassured that although she may feel the urge to defecate, she will not.
- **Sizing an intrauterine pregnancy:** Recognizing a pregnancy in the adolescent can aid in the swift diagnosis of the cause of complaints ranging from fatigue and nausea to secondary amenorrhea, abdominal fullness, or a mass. The provider should maintain a high index of suspicion for pregnancy, even in the youngest adolescents who deny a history of sexual activity: the teen may be reluctant to disclose early or unwanted sexual activity. Point of care urine testing for β-hCG is invaluable. The weeks of pregnancy are counted from the first day of the last menstrual period, even though ovulation generally occurs 2 weeks after the beginning of menses (Box 17-1). Fundal height provides a guide for estimating uterine size (Figure 17-17).

Box **17-1** Sizing an Intrauterine Pregnancy

Nulliparous uterus: 7.5×2.5 cm (size of small lime on bimanual exam)

Eight-week uterus: 9-11 cm $\times$ 5 cm (size of orange on bimanual exam)

Twelve-week uterus: 12-14 cm $\times$ 7 cm (size of grapefruit, very soft, sometimes difficult to palpate on bimanual exam); just palpable, abdominally at level of symphysis pubis

Sixteen-week uterus: Palpate abdomen, felt halfway between symphysis pubis and umbilicus

Twenty-week uterus: Palpate abdomen, felt at umbilicus

Over twenty-weeks: Measure from symphysis pubis to height of fundus (number of cm = approximate number of weeks)

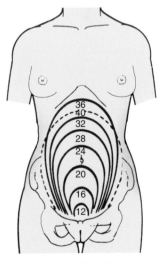

Figure **17-17** Fundal height.

Wrapping Up the Examination

The adolescent should be handed some tissues, so she may wipe off the lubricant used. The examiner should stay in the room long enough to ensure that the teen does not feel dizzy upon sitting up, and then leave while she dresses. Results of the exam should be given while the teen is dressed, and any abnormalities should be thoroughly explained. To ensure confidentiality, present and discuss results with the adolescent alone.

SUSPICION OF SEXUAL ABUSE

In cases of suspected child sexual abuse, the history and behavioral observations are crucial. Any history of abuse disclosed to the healthcare provider that occurred within the previous 72 hours (up to 120 hours in some locales) requires immediate referral for a forensic examination with possible collection of evidence. Most sexually abused prepubertal girls will have normal physical exams because of the following:

- Delays in disclosure
- Rapid healing of genital and anal tissue in prepubertal children
- Predominance in this age-group of sexual abuse involving fondling or oral-genital contact, which does not leave physical signs

The following physical findings in prepubertal girls should raise suspicion of sexual abuse and prompt referral for an exam by specially trained practitioners:

- Hymenal irregularities or absence (notches, transections or thin, rounded edges), particularly posterior (from the 3 to 9 o'clock position with the child supine); should be confirmed in knee-chest position, because an apparent notch may be a fold in a redundant hymen
- Acute trauma to the hymen, posterior fourchette, or laceration of vaginal mucosa (particularly extending to the rectal mucosa)
- Confirmed sexually transmitted infection (including human papillomavirus [HPV] infection in a child ≥2 years)

TABLE 17-5 ABNORMAL FINDINGS ASSOCIATED WITH PELVIC EXAM

Findings	Descriptions
Vulvar and vaginal abnormalities	Imperforate hymen, hematocolpos, vaginal agenesis or signs of a transverse vaginal septum (caused by congenital incomplete fusion of upper and lower vagina), external condyloma, signs of trauma, erythema, and discharge
Cervical abnormalities	Reddened, friable (bleeds with insertion of cotton swab into os), visible condyloma, petechiae ("strawberry spots" rarely seen with trichomoniasis), erosions, double cervix (associated with uterus didelphys), absence of cervix
Pelvic masses	Masses resulting from intrauterine or ectopic pregnancy, from pelvic infection (salpingitis or tuboovarian abscess), adnexal torsion secondary to cyst (which presents with twisting sensation, intermittent bouts of severe pain separated by generalized aching, can be surgical emergency), functional, corpus luteal or dermoid or other complex ovarian cysts, endometriosis Uterine tumors (such as leiomyomas) are rare in the adolescent; ovarian cancers comprise approximately 1% of all childhood cancers, but they are the most common genital tract cancer in adolescents All adnexal masses should be imaged, first with ultrasound, then (if needed) with computed tomography or magnetic resonance imaging

Other possible findings include increased erythema, irritation, and vaginal discharge, which may be signs of sexual abuse, but may have other causes (Table 17-5). The examiner should keep the possibility of sexual abuse in mind whenever other nonvenereal infections, chemical irritation, foreign bodies, and/or poor hygiene are included in the differential diagnosis. Failure or delay of fusion of the median *raphe* between the posterior fourchette and the anus is often mistaken for trauma or sexual abuse

ABNORMAL CONDITIONS

Table 17-6 presents abnormal findings of the genitalia in the prepubertal and pubertal female.

TABLE 17-6 ABNORMAL CONDITIONS OF THE FEMALE GENITALIA

Condition	Description
Labial adhesions	Adherence of labia minora or majora, primarily seen in girls 3 months to 6 years of age; adhesion may persist until puberty, or may separate spontaneously; treatment is controversial if opening is large enough for normal urinary flow and vaginal drainage
Labial abscesses	Usually caused by *Staphylococcus aureus* and *Streptococcus pyogenes*
Labial lipoma	May be initially mistaken for a hernia
Clitoral lesions	Edema of clitoris, with hypoproteinemia, in conditions such as nephrotic syndrome Hypertrophy of clitoral hood and clitoris, caused by neurofibromatosis, rhabdomyosarcoma, increased androgens Hemorrhages around clitoris caused by lichen sclerosis or trauma (see below)
Urethral prolapse	Presents with bleeding and friable, red-blue doughnut-like annular mass that may be visible in perineum ("hemorrhagic cranberry")
Lichen sclerosis	Uncommon; presents with atrophic, hypopigmented, parchment-like friable skin around vulva and anus, often in an "hour-glass" configuration, with inflammation and subepithelial hemorrhages
Vulvar irritation	Often results from irritants such as bubble bath, poor hygiene, candidal overgrowth caused by antibiotics or diaper occlusion; rarely scratching can occur secondary to pruritus from a pinworm infestation
Vulvovaginitis	Vaginal discharge may be caused by bacteria (e.g., *Streptococcus, Shigella*) or overgrowth of normal flora; foreign body in vagina (typically toilet paper); poor hygiene; sexually transmitted infection (STI)
Straddle injuries to vulva	Straddle injuries (as in playground falls) generally cause trauma to anterior vulvar structures and rarely cause trauma to posterior portion of hymen or posterior fourchette; in addition, injury is usually somewhat asymmetrical and not penetrating in nature

Female Circumcision

Female circumcision, or female genital mutilation, is prevalent in many parts of the world, particularly sub-Saharan Africa, and is considered a rite of passage and a prerequisite for marriage in some cultures.[2] The procedure is not legal in the United States or Canada, but immigrant girls and adolescents may have had the procedure performed previously in their country of origin. Complications include infection, hemorrhage, tetanus, lower urinary tract disturbances, sexual dysfunction, and infertility.[3] According to the World Health Organization, there are three types:

- Type I, or "sunna" circumcision, involves removal of all or part of the clitoris
- Type II involves excision of the clitoris and some of the labia minora
- Type III, "pharonic" circumcision or infibulation, involves excision of the clitoris, the labia minora and the medial aspect of the labia majora, with suturing of the

CHARTING

Charting on a Sexually Active Female Teen

External genitalia: Pink, no discharge noted, without lesions. Tanner stage 4 to 5 pubic hair distribution. **Vaginal exam:** Cervix pink without lesions, scant blood at os from menses, scant mucoid discharge in vault. **Bimanual:** No pain on deep palpation or with movement of cervix. Uterus midposition. Adnexae nontender, nonthickened. **Rectal:** No fissures, lesions, or hemorrhoids; stool brown, guaiac neg.

remaining labia minora in the midline (Figure 17-18).

Abnormal Congenital Conditions

Table 17-7 presents abnormal congenital conditions most often noted at birth.

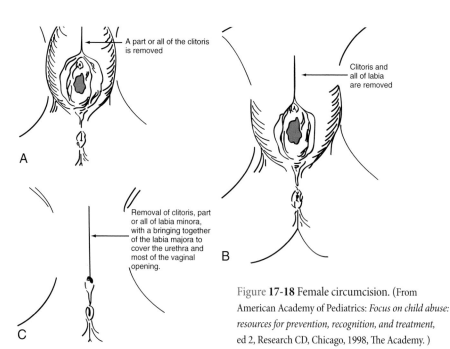

Figure **17-18** Female circumcision. (From American Academy of Pediatrics: *Focus on child abuse: resources for prevention, recognition, and treatment,* ed 2, Research CD, Chicago, 1998, The Academy.)

TABLE 17-7 ABNORMAL CONGENITAL CONDITIONS OF FEMALE GENITALIA

Condition	Description
Ambiguous genitalia	Partially fused labia, enlarged clitoris; hypospadias, bilateral cryptorchidism in an apparent male are signs of a possible intersex condition (see Chapter 15)
Hydrocolpos	Vaginal secretions collecting behind an imperforate hymen at birth may appear as small cystic mass between labia
Vaginal agenesis	Congenital absence of or hypoplasia of fallopian tubes, uterine corpus, uterine cervix, and proximal portion of vagina; occurring in approximately 1 in 5000 births; in approximately 10% of these births, there is a rudimentary or functional uterus Commonly diagnosed at puberty when child presents with primary amenorrhea; however, can be recognized at birth; should be diagnosed before onset of puberty

REFERENCES

1. Hennigen L, Kollar LM, Rosenthal SL: Methods for managing pelvic examination anxiety: individual differences and relaxation techniques, *J Pediatr Health Care* 14(1):9-12, 2000.
2. Morris R: The culture of female circumcision, *ANS Adv Nurs Sci* 19(2):43-53, 1996.
3. Strickland JL: Female circumcision/female genital mutilation, *J Pediatr Adolesc Gynecol* 14(3):109-112, 2001.

MUSCULOSKELETAL SYSTEM

Karen G. Duderstadt and Naomi A. Schapiro

Growth and movement, such a natural part of a normal childhood, require a strong musculoskeletal system. The musculoskeletal system is one of the most challenging to assess because of the variation in growth and development and the normal range of rotational changes in the extremities in infants, children, and adolescents. Early identification and treatment of common abnormal musculoskeletal conditions can avoid permanent disabilities that would impact a child throughout life.

DEVELOPMENT

Bone Growth

The rudimentary skeletal system forms as early as the fourth week of gestation when the upper extremities begin as buds on the fetus. Bone growth begins with the formation of cartilage arising from the primary centers of *ossification* in the long bones. As early as the seventh week of gestation, embryonic vascular growth progresses toward the center of the *osteoblasts* in the long bone, which forms cartilage and establishes the primary ossification centers. At birth, the *epiphyses* of the long bone are composed of hyaline cartilage. Shortly after

birth, the secondary ossification centers begin to replace the cartilage along the *epiphyseal plate*. The replacement of cartilage by bone is known as endochondral *ossification*. The epiphyseal plate ossifies becoming the *diaphysis*, or the shaft of the long bone. Growth along the epiphyseal line continues until closure of the growth plate occurs in young adults (Figure 18-1).

During early periods of rapid growth, ossification occurs in secondary sites throughout the body: the ends of the long bones, the vertebrae, the flat bones in the clavicle and the skull. Bone growth in children occurs in two ways. Longitudinal growth of the bone occurs in the ossification centers. Changes in width and strength of the bone occur as *intramembranous* ossification, where new bone builds or is laid down upon newly formed bone in the long shaft. The bone composition continues to change and model the skeletal system from childhood through adolescence (Figure 18-2). The thickness of the bones and the health of the marrow are influenced by nutrition, hormonal factors, and mechanical forces during the process of growth. Nutritional factors such as adequate protein in the diet, the amount of calcium intake, and adequate intake of vitamin D, particularly in breastfeeding infants, impacts

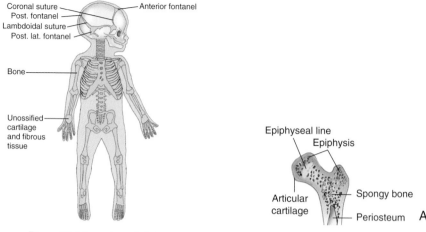

Figure **18-1** Immature skeleton.

Figure **18-2 A,** Mature bone.

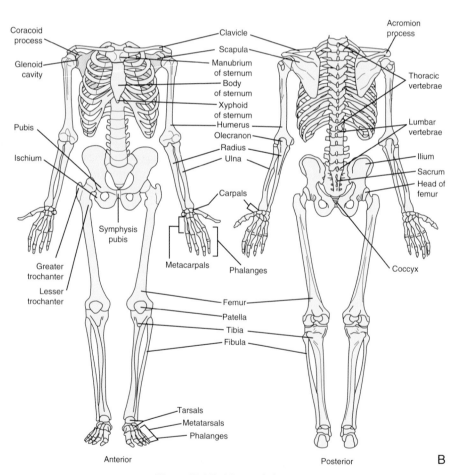

Anterior

Posterior   **B**

Figure **18-2 B,** Mature skeleton.

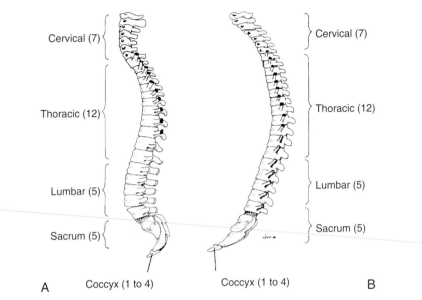

Cervical (7)

Thoracic (12)

Lumbar (5)

Sacrum (5)

A   Coccyx (1 to 4)

Cervical (7)

Thoracic (12)

Lumbar (5)

Sacrum (5)

Coccyx (1 to 4)   B

Figure **18-3 A,** Immature spinal column. **B,** Mature spinal column. (From Alexander MM, Brown MS: *Pediatric physical diagnosis for nurses,* New York, 1974, McGraw-Hill.)

the overall growth and development of the musculoskeletal system. Many abnormalities of the skeletal system are genetic in origin. However, recent evidence includes environmental insults as a contributing factor to some malformations.

ANATOMY AND PHYSIOLOGY

Growth of Spine and Extremities

The infant has a C-shaped spinal curve at birth in comparison to the double S curvature that is present in late adolescence. Thoracic and pelvic curves are present at birth, and the secondary cervical curve is present by 3 to 4 months of age when the infant begins to hold up his or her head. The lumbar curvature appears later as the child begins to walk. Toddlers often have an exaggerated thoracic-lumbar curvature and a protuberant abdomen until they enter the preschool years, when gait and balance become more normal (see Chapter 14). The *sacrum,*

the final section of the spinal column, is composed of five separate bones at birth and by 18 to 20 years of age is fused into one large bone. The *coccyx* consists of three or four small vertebrae that begin to ossify between the first and fourth years and become fused into one bone by 25 years of age (Figure 18-3).

The hipbone contains three distinct parts in childhood, which are later fused in adulthood. The *ilium* is the superior, broad, flat surface of the hipbone; the *ischium* is the strongest portion of the hipbone and contains a portion of the *acetabulum,* which forms the attachment at the hipbone for the femur, and the *foramen,* an opening; the *pubis* contains the medial portion of the acetabulum and joins medially to form the complete pelvic girdle.

The *femur,* the longest and strongest bone in the body, begins ossification during the seventh week of fetal life. The head of the femur becomes ossified sometime during the first year of life, but the shaft does not become completely ossified until 14 years of age.

The long bones of the extremities continue to grow at the site of the epiphyseal cartilage throughout childhood and adolescence; peak bone mass is achieved by young adulthood.

The *patella* is the small triangular bone that forms the kneecap and lies over the junction of the *femur* and the *tibia*. The health of the patella during growth and development depends not only on strong bone growth but also on the strength of the ligaments and tendons supporting the patella.

The hand at birth consists of many carpal bones that are cartilaginous. A radiograph of a child's hand at 2½ years of age illustrates ossification of only the *capitate* and *hamate* bones. Development and ossification continue until 11 years of age when all of the carpal bones are ossified except for the small *pisiform* bone that develops by 12 years of age. Limb abnormalities such as *polydactyly,* the presence of supernumerary digits, are common (Figure 18-4). Other abnormalities such as *syndactyly,* webbing or fusion between adjacent digits of the hands or feet, may be indicative of profound developmental delay.

The foot of the infant also undergoes a dramatic formation during the first year of life. The *calcaneus* ossifies at the sixth month of fetal life. The ossification of the foot follows the normal developmental gross motor milestones. The *talus* is ossified by the seventh month of life to form the ankle, and the remaining *metatarsal* bones continue to form during the latter half of the first year of life. The *phalanges* continue the ossification process until adolescence.

The limbs go through a continuous process of rotational change until about 8 years of age, a process that begins in infancy as the child progresses from sitting position to pulling up, to crawling, then standing, cruising, and finally walking with an exaggerated gait and a wide base of support. During growth, bone has the remarkable capacity to remodel itself. Bone is deposited in areas subjected to stress and reabsorbed in areas where there is little stress. This concept forms the basis for the ability of children to remodel residual deformity after fractures and explains the biological plasticity in growing bones. The rate of bone growth is greatest in the lower extremities before the onset of puberty; the *distal* extremities reach adult size in early puberty, which is reflected in shoe size in preadolescents. The trunk and *proximal* extremities exhibit the dominant growth during puberty and into young adulthood. Bone growth is completed at age 20, and peak bone mass is achieved by age 35.

Monitoring Growth

Monitoring the velocity of growth or obtaining and analyzing past growth record information is critical to evaluating the child with slow growth or delayed onset of puberty. *Bone age* radiographs of the secondary ossification centers at the end of the long bones are used to

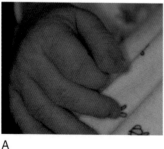
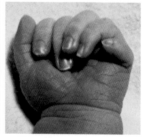

A   B

Figure **18-4 A,** Syndactyly. **B,** Polydactyly. (**A** from Lemmi FO, Lemmi CAE: *Physical assessment findings multi-user CD-ROM,* St Louis, 2000, Saunders. **B** from Zitelli BJ, Davis, HW: *Atlas of pediatric physical diagnosis,* ed 4, St Louis, 2002, Mosby.)

assess growth rate in children who lag behind in height velocity compared to the norm or who have delayed onset of puberty.

Key Points

Cultural and ethnic diversity impact the growth rate of bone and must be considered when evaluating growth curves in the primary care setting. A growth parameter that falls outside of the accepted two standard deviations (SD) above or below the mean may be normal when the parental stature is considered.

Muscle Development

Muscle structures, including the tendons, ligaments, cartilage, and joints, originate from the embryonic *mesoderm*. Muscle fibers are developed by the fourth or fifth month of gestation and increase in size along with muscle growth that occurs throughout childhood. The rate of

muscle growth increases rapidly beginning at age 2 years, with the greatest increase in muscle cell size occurring during puberty. Girls' muscle size increases at a greater rate than that of boys in early and middle childhood up until puberty; then boys' muscle mass and cell size begins to exceed that of girls (Figure 18-5).

PHYSIOLOGICAL VARIATIONS

Table 18-1 reviews developmental changes in the musculoskeletal system from the neonatal period through adolescence.

CULTURAL VARIATIONS

African-American infants often have advanced musculoskeletal development and achieve developmental milestones earlier. Asian-American infants often have increased hypotonia at birth and may have an increased abduction of the hips bilaterally on examination in early infancy.

TABLE 18-1 PHYSIOLOGICAL VARIATIONS OF THE MUSCULOSKELETAL SYSTEM AT KEY DEVELOPMENTAL STAGES

Age-Group	Variation
Preterm infant and newborn	Lower extremities in external rotation and flexion at hips; upper femur is anteverted and knees are flexed; tibias are internally rotated; feet are dorsiflexed
Infant	Tibias gradually rotate externally to about 20 degrees toward midline by 12 months of age; flat feet and bowed legs until walking is firmly established
Toddler	Stance with wide base of support, hyperflexion of hips and knees with disjointed (toddling) pattern when walking; arms held abducted and elbows extended; normal arm swing and heel-toe walking generally begin by 18 months of age; toeing-in is common beginning at 15 months; longitudinal arch not present in toddler but begins to develop by 2½ years of age
Preschooler	At 3 years of age, children exhibit mature pattern of motion and muscle action; resolution of toeing-in and marked torsion of lower extremities normally disappear by school entry; normal longitudinal arch develops in preschooler
School-age child	*Knock-knee* is present until 7 years of age; by 8 to 10 years of age, femur rotates to position of about 14 degrees toward midline from average of 45 degrees at birth
Adolescent	Hormonal changes impact ligaments and tendons; laxity of knees is particularly common in adolescent females, making them vulnerable to injury

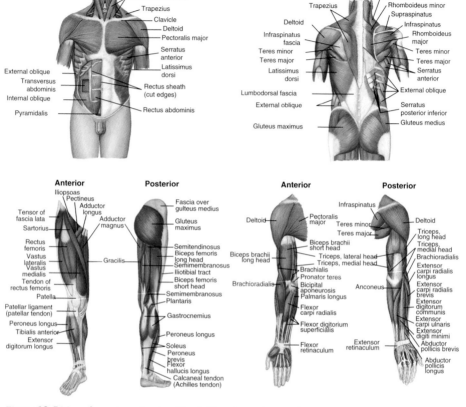

Figure **18-5** Muscular system, front and back. (From Mourad LA: *Orthopedic disorders,* St Louis, 1991, Mosby.)

SYSTEM-SPECIFIC HISTORY

Table 18-1 reviews important information to be gathered for assessing the musculoskeletal system from birth through adolescence.

PHYSICAL ASSESSMENT

Preparation for the Examination

For a thorough and complete assessment of the musculoskeletal system, infants must be undressed except for the diaper, and children must be undressed except for underwear. A young child cannot be thoroughly assessed when wearing socks and shoes or when gowned. In preadolescence and adolescence, maintaining modesty and still obtaining an accurate

🔑 Key Points

An accurate history of achievement of developmental milestones is key to determining significant delays and to timely diagnosis of abnormal conditions.

assessment of the spine can be challenging, particularly in girls. Maturing females must be in underwear and gown to obtain a thorough evaluation of the spine.

Inspection and Palpation

Initial inspection of the musculoskeletal system in the child from birth to adolescence includes inspection of skin for color and temperature; inspection of palmar creases; noting of scars,

TABLE 18-2   INFORMATION GATHERING FOR ASSESSMENT OF THE MUSCULOSKELETAL SYSTEM AT KEY DEVELOPMENTAL STAGES

Age-Group	Questions to Ask
Preterm infant	History of hypoxia in early neonatal period? Intraventricular insult? Any maternal alcohol or substance abuse? When did prenatal care begin?
Newborn	History of maternal infection while in utero? Any trauma sustained at birth? Need for resuscitation or ventilation in immediate newborn period? Presentation at birth? Breech or shoulder? Family history of skeletal deformities or genetic disorders?
Infant	Family history of bone or joint disorders? Any delay in achieving gross motor milestones? Does infant roll over? Sit without support? Crawl? Stand alone? Walk without support? Any evidence of toe-walking? Any evidence of widening of wrist joints?
Toddler	Any clumsiness/bumping into objects? Any limp when walking? Toeing-in or toeing-out when walking or running? Any pronounced bowing of legs? History of trauma or falls? Evidence of unintentional injury? History of chronic conditions?
Preschooler	Does child sit in "W" or TV squat position while playing or watching videos? Frequent falls or history of unintentional injury?
School-age child	Involved in organized/competitive sports? Any complaint of pain when walking/running or pain that awakens child at night? History of joint stiffness or swelling? Weight of school backpack? History of prolonged steroid use with chronic conditions?
Adolescent	Involved in organized/competitive sports? Any limited range of motion of joints? Is gait normal and erect? History of fractures, sprains, or trauma? Weight of school backpack? Any evidence of habitual slouching? Family history of skeletal deformities? Start of menstrual periods?
Environmental risks	Contact with chemical cleaning agents, hazardous smoke, or chemicals? Exposure to toxic pesticides? History of elevated lead level?

bruises, unusual pigmentation or lesions, swelling or erythema; observation of posture, proportion of extremities, or obvious gait deformities; and evaluation of muscle strength and symmetry. Erythema, swelling, tenderness, or temperature changes should be noted over joints or extremities. Palpation for bone or joint tenderness, any unusual prominence, thickening, and/or indentations in the bony skeleton should be noted. Assessment of the range of motion of extremities and inspection, palpation, and assessment of mobility of the spine is included in a thorough and complete assessment.

Position of the Extremities

Terms to describe the position of the extremities include the following: (1) *flexion*—a decrease in the angle of the resting joint in the upper or lower extremities; (2) *extension*—an increase in the joint angle; (3) *hyperextension*—an increase in the angle of the joint beyond the usual arc; (4) *abduction*—movement away from the midline; (5) *adduction*—movement toward the midline; (6) *rotation*—movement around a central axis; (7) *circumduction*—rotation or circular movement of the limbs; and (8) *dorsiflexion*—backward rotation (Figure 18-6).

Joints

Assessment of the extremities includes evaluating the mobility of the joints. Joints have a slightly moveable to freely moveable motion throughout the period of growth and development. The *hinge joint*, between the humerus and the ulna, permits motion in one plane, whereas the *pivotal joint*, between the radial-ulnar joint, allows rotation only. The *condyloid joint* in the wrist allows flexion, extension, adduction, abduction, and circumduction. *Saddle joints*, such as in the thumb, have a similar motion to the condyloid joint in the wrist except that the joint forms a concave-convex

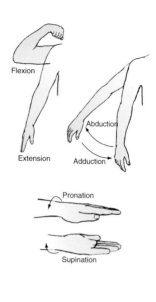
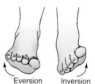

Figure **18-6** Skeletal positions.

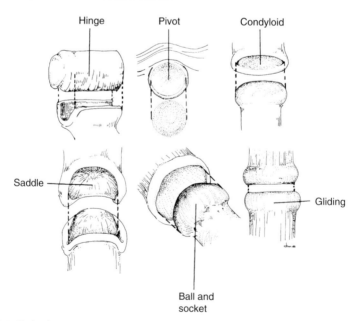

Figure **18-7** Skeletal joints. (From Alexander MM, Brown MS: *Pediatric physical diagnosis for nurses*, New York, 1974, McGraw-Hill.)

fit to achieve motion. The hip and shoulder joints are examples of ball-and-socket joints. Finally, the gliding joints allow a gliding motion between two flat surfaces, such as in the vertebrae and carpal joints in the hands and feet (Figure 18-7).

Upper Extremities and Clavicle

In the newborn infant, the clavicles must be palpated fully to detect a fracture associated with a traumatic delivery. Localized tenderness at the proximal end of the clavicle shortly after birth often leads to a palpable bony prominence as the fracture heals.[1] A full range of motion of the upper extremities, including the elbows and wrists must be evaluated to determine any trauma that may have affected the shoulder during the birth process. In *Erb's palsy,* injury to the fifth and sixth cranial nerves, no spontaneous abduction of the shoulder muscles or flexion of the elbow is found. The arm is adducted and internally rotated, but normal grip in the hand is present.

In the toddler and young child, the radial-ulnar joint is particularly vulnerable. *Subluxation,* or partial dislocation, of the radius from the humerus is common in children from 2 to 4 years of age. Often there is no clear history of trauma. In cases of a subluxation, the child usually refuses to use the affected arm. Passive range of motion is possible except for *supination* (palm facing upward). Dislocation of the shoulder can occur in the preschooler and is marked by swelling, pain, and a limp arm.

Trauma to the upper extremities is common in children and adolescents. Strains, sprains, or fractures can occur with strenuous activity, falls, motor vehicle or pedestrian injuries, or participation in competitive sports. Careful assessment is warranted in the growing child when any history of trauma is obtained.

Lower Extremities

Inspection of the lower extremities includes flexion/extension, adduction/abduction, and internal/external rotation. Leg length is evaluated with the infant or child supine, with knee and hip joints extended and legs aligned. A discrepancy in length or asymmetrical appearance may indicate an abnormality in hips, long bones, or knees.

Inspect the *malleoli* to evaluate the presence of torsion in the lower extremities. The medial *malleolus* lies at the distal end of the *tibia* forming the medial ankle, and the lateral *malleolus* forms the lateral ankle at the distal end of the *fibula.* In the infant, the medial and lateral malleoli are parallel when examining the infant supine. A rotation of up to 20 degrees occurs in the lateral malleoli during the normal growth and development of the musculoskeletal system.

At birth, the infant has significant torsion in the lower extremities related to the fetal position in utero. Bowleggedness, or *genu varum,* is a normal condition until 2½ to 3 years of age (Figure 18-8). It is the most common cause of toeing-in in children less than 3 years of age, and normally resolves with growth. Observation of gait, particularly watching the toddler walk from the rear, is important in evaluating the impact of *genu varum* on motor

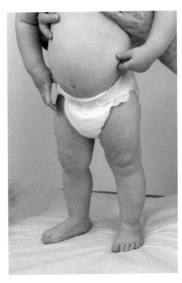

Figure **18-8** Genu varum (bowleggedness).

development and performance. *Genu varum* that is severe can be the result of nutritional deficiencies. If bowing is severe after 2 years of age, referral is recommended because pathological conditions should be considered.

Tibial torsion, a curvature or twisting of the tibia, is the term used for the condition of bowleggedness, particularly after 3 to 4 years of age (Figure 18-9). Intrauterine positioning may be a contributing factor. To evaluate the toddler, preschooler, or school-age child for *tibial torsion*, the child should be examined

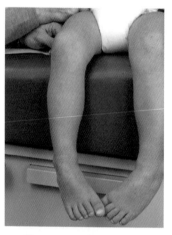

Figure **18-9** Tibial torsion.

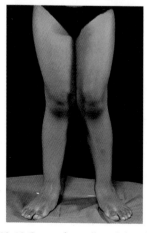

Figure **18-10** Genu valgum (knock-knee). (From Chaudhry B, Harvey D: *Mosby's color atlas and text of pediatrics and child health,* St Louis, 2001, Mosby.)

wearing only underwear and be seated with the legs dangling freely from a chair or exam table. The provider places a thumb and forefinger on the lateral and medial malleoli with the knee facing forward to determine the degree of rotation and flexibility of the tibia. The forefoot and hindfoot should be in line with the knees. On inspection, only the anterior edge of the lateral malleolus should be in the midline. The torsion generally resolves with growth; therefore reassuring the parent is an important component of management.

Genu valgum, knock-knee, is present if the medial malleoli are more than an inch apart and the knees are touching. This condition is normal until 7 years of age, when the rotational development of the lower extremities is nearly complete (Figure 18-10).

Feet

Assessment of the feet in the infant includes the position and alignment of the forefoot and heels and the range of motion of the ankle and plantar arch. Limited dorsiflexion, or a fixed position of the hindfoot, is abnormal in the newborn, as is adduction of the forefoot (Figure 18-11). Decreased range of motion or pain should be noted on exam. With the infant

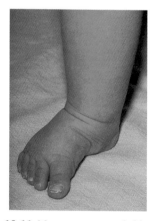

Figure **18-11** Metatarsus varus (adduction of the forefoot). (From Chaudhry B, Harvey D: *Mosby's color atlas and text of pediatrics and child health,* St Louis, 2001, Mosby.)

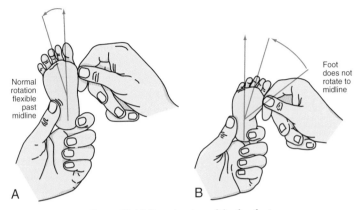

Figure **18-12** Examination of the forefoot.

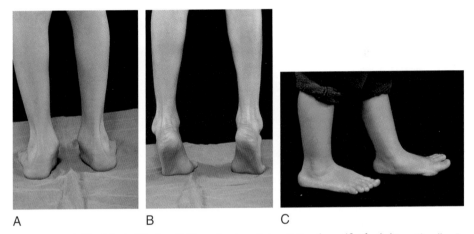

Figure **18-13 A,** Physiological flat feet. **B,** Normal arch on tiptoe. **C,** Pes planus (flat foot). (From Chaudhry B, Harvey D: *Mosby's color atlas and text of pediatrics and child health,* St Louis, 2001, Mosby.)

supine and the knees flexed to 90 degrees, inspect the thigh-foot angle and evaluate any adduction of the forefoot past the midline (Figure 18-12). A foot that is rigid on range of motion requires immediate orthopedic evaluation. Management begins with manipulation and serial casting. The goal of correction is to produce a supple foot that assumes a normal angle to the tibia. A mild deformity with a flexible foot requires passive stretching, which consists of supporting the heel at a right angle to the leg and rotating and stretching the forefoot laterally. Infants and toddlers do not develop a longitudinal arch until the second or third year of life. Older children may have physiological flat feet due to laxity of the ligaments (Figure 18-13). True *pes planus* or flat foot in children is rare.[2] Lack of development of a longitudinal arch in the preschooler may indicate a generalized laxity of the ligaments and a thorough assessment of muscle tone is warranted.

Examination of the Hip

The examination of the hip in the newborn and growing infant is performed with the infant in the supine position with the knees flexed bilaterally and supported by the thumb and forefinger of the examiner, with the pad of the second finger on the bony prominence of the greater trochanter and the thumb near the lesser trochanter (Figure 18-14, *A*). With abduction of the thighs, pressure to the greater trochanter causes the hip to move from an unreduced to a reduced position if it is unstable. *Ortolani's sign*, the presence of a *clunk* during the maneuver, is a positive sign for dislocation of the hip (Table 18-3). *Barlow's test* also assists in detecting the unstable, dislocatable hip. With the infant supine and the knees flexed,

the thigh is grasped and adducted while applying downward pressure (Figure 18-14, *B*). With pressure on the acetabulum, the hip goes from a reduced position to a dislocated position. A dislocation of the femoral head is a positive *Barlow's*. A *click* can occur during the maneuvers that may radiate the knee or ankle and is considered benign. With the knees flexed to 90 degrees, inspect for symmetry. The knees should be equally aligned. Any asymmetry of the knees is abnormal and may indicate a subluxed or dislocated hip that requires further evaluation. With the infant prone, inspect for the symmetry of the thigh folds (Figure 18-14, *C*). Asymmetry should be noted, but is not a high correlate with hip abnormality.[1]

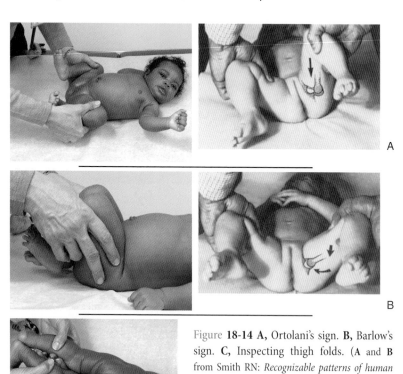

Figure **18-14 A,** Ortolani's sign. **B,** Barlow's sign. **C,** Inspecting thigh folds. (**A** and **B** from Smith RN: *Recognizable patterns of human deformations*, Philadelphia, 1981, Saunders.)

TABLE 18-3 MUSCULOSKELETAL SCREENING

Age-Group	Techniques	Referral Criteria
Newborn and Infant	*Ortolani's sign* *Barlow's test* *Galeazzi's or Allis' sign* *Foot alignment*	Presence of a clunk on abduction of hips Any instability of hip joints Knees when flexed are unequal in height Rigid foot with limited range of motion Rigid in-turning, inability of foot to assume normal angle to leg
Toddler and preschooler	*Trendelenburg sign*	When child bears weight, note any asymmetry in level of iliac crests With leg lifted, iliac crest drops, indicating hip abductor muscles on weight-bearing side are weak
School-age child and adolescent	*Forward bend test*	Asymmetrical elevation of scapula or rib hump; unequal shoulders or iliac crests, uneven waistline A spinal rotation of 5 to 7 degrees should be evaluated
Newborn to adolescent	*Flexion of neck* *Brudzinski sign* *Kernig sign*	*Nuchal rigidity*—Resistance or pain when neck is flexed when lying supine Involuntary flexion of knees or legs when neck is flexed when lying supine Resistance to or pain on straightening knees or legs from flexed position when lying supine

Data from Chin KR, Price JS, Zimbler S: *Contemp Pediatr* 18(9):77-103, 2001.

Key Points

Predisposing factors for unstable hips:
Mother is a primipara
Infant is female
Positive family history
Breech presentation
Other congenital anomalies

EXAMINATION OF THE KNEE

The symmetry and range of motion of the knee should be assessed. Congenital dislocation of the knee, or *patella,* is rare and manifests as limited knee motion in the newborn. Children and youth with a history of knee pain or laxity, as well as those who are unable to fully squat and perform a duck walk during the screening exam, merit a more complete examination of the knee. The examiner is looking for swelling, obvious deformity, incomplete range of motion, as well as signs of *ligamentous* laxity or *meniscal* damage.

The knee is a common site for both overuse and sudden traumatic injury in the young athlete, particularly an adolescent female. A common complaint of adolescent athletes is medial or anterior patellar pain with exercise or prolonged sitting, and pain or buckling when ascending or descending the stairs. Pain may be elicited on exam, or findings may be relatively normal. The following maneuvers may help the practitioner identify specific problems in the knee. They should be performed bilaterally because there is a natural variation from person to person in the laxity of the joints (Figure 18-15).

Anterior/Posterior Drawer

- With the child supine, the hips flexed to 45 degrees, the knees flexed to 90 degrees and

the feet stabilized on the exam table, place both hands above the calf on the lower leg, and try to pull the leg forward (anterior drawer test) and backward (posterior drawer test). Excessive movement in the knee is unexpected. Laxity suggests rupture of the anterior or posterior cruciate ligament.

- Tests for anterior or posterior cruciate ligament damage.

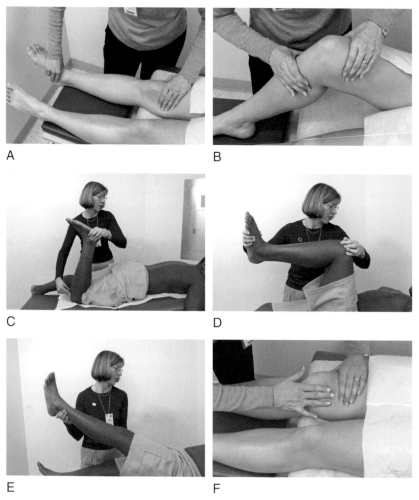

A

B

C

D

E

F

Figure **18-15** Examination of the knee. **A,** Varus/valgus stress test with knee extended. **B,** Varus/valgus test with knee flexed. **C,** Apley test. **D,** McMurray test. **E,** Bragard test for nerve root irritation. **F,** Testing for excess fluid in the knee.

Varus/Valgus Stress Test

- With the child supine and the knee flexed to 30 degrees, stabilize both the femur and the ankle. Apply both gentle varus and valgus stress to the knee and repeat with a gentle rocking motion. Laxity or opening in the joint space suggests a tear of the medial collateral or lateral collateral ligament.
- Tests for damage to medial collateral or lateral collateral ligaments of knee.

Mcmurray Test

- With the child lying supine, flex the knee completely with foot on the examining table near the buttocks. Maintain flexion and stabilize the knee with thumb and forefinger. Using the other hand, rotate the lower leg to a lateral position while extending the knee to 90 degrees. Any clicking, pain, or lack of extension is a positive finding and indicates a meniscal injury. Repeat with the lower leg rotated medially.
- Tests for damage to medial, lateral, posterior meniscus.

Ballottement and Bulge

- Ballottement sign—With the knee extended, the examiner applies downward pressure on the suprapatellar pouch to force fluid between the patella and the femur and then pushes the patella downward against the femur. Patella floats back to position if fluid is present. A palpable click on patella striking the femur is positive for knee joint effusion.
- Bulge sign—With the knee extended, the examiner uses the ball of the hand to milk fluid distally from the suprapatellar pouch several times and then presses behind margin of the patella. If swelling reappears in the suprapatellar pouch, it is positive for knee joint effusion.
- Tests for effusion or the presence of excess fluid in the knee joint.

Apley Compression Test

- With the child or adolescent in the prone position on exam table, flex the knee to 90 degrees. While supporting the leg, apply pressure to the heel firmly and compress the tibia into the femur, rotating the tibia internally and externally on femur. Presence of pain, clicks, or resistance indicates positive finding.
- Test to determine the presence of a meniscal tear.

EXAMINATION OF THE SPINE

The spine should be inspected and palpated to note any congenital abnormalities such as hair tufts, dimples, a sacral sinus, or hemangiomas that could indicate spinal abnormalities. Inspection of the spine begins with the child or adolescent standing facing away from the examiner. Assess for the contour of the back, the symmetry of the shoulders, the shape and/or prominence of the scapula and ribs, the symmetry of the waistline and the iliac crests (Figure 18-16, *A*, *B*, and *C*). The head should be aligned directly over the sacrum because any deviation from the midline may indicate a spinal deformity.[3] Range of motion of the spine is evaluated by asking the child or adolescent to bend to the side, flex, and extend. An elevated scapula, an uneven waistline, or the presence of a rib hump indicates a positive finding (Figure 18-17) (Table 18-3). More than five café au lait spots or the presence of axillary freckles suggest *neurofibromatosis.*

Beginning at the toddler age, children develop a normal curvature of the spine with *lordosis* of the neck and lumbar region and *kyphosis* of the thorax. An exaggerated *lordosis* is normal in the toddler. Viewing the child or adolescent from the side allows the examiner to evaluate normal alignment. Evaluation of *Tanner stage* is key to determining skeletal and spinal maturity.

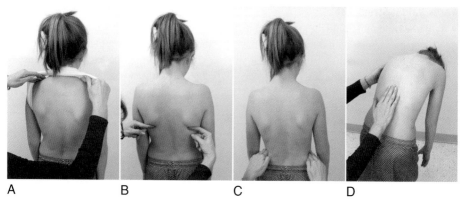

Figure **18-16** Assessment of the spine. **A,** Testing shoulder symmetry. **B,** Scapular symmetry. **C,** Iliac crest symmetry. **D,** Beginning Adam's forward bend test.

Adam's Forward Bend test

- Child or adolescent should bend forward and touch the toes if possible with hands dangling or in a diving position (Figure 18-16, *D*). Observe for alignment of spine, any curvature, asymmetry, or rib hump from the rear and sides. A level ruler or *scoliometer* can be used to assess the angle of trunk rotation. Place the scoliometer on the trunk at the peak of the curvature to evaluate alignment. A rotation of 5 to 7 degrees should be evaluated further.[4]
- Tests for scoliosis.

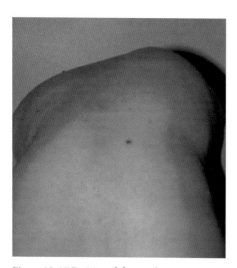

Figure **18-17** Positive rib hump. (From Lemmi FO, Lemmi CAE: *Physical assessment findings multi-user CD-ROM,* St Louis, 2000, Saunders.)

PREPARTICIPATION SPORTS PHYSICAL

Preparticipation Sports History

The young athlete deserves special consideration to ensure protection from trauma and promote continued healthy growth and development of the muscles, tendons, ligaments, and bones throughout the body. The primary purpose of the preparticipation sports physical exam is to exclude or restrict the young athlete with a temporary or permanent contraindication from participation in competitive sports. Additionally, the practitioner can help match the athlete to the appropriate type and level of sport and can help prevent injury by recommending the appropriate stretching or strengthening exercises. The sports physical is often the healthy adolescent's only regular contact with the healthcare provider; therefore the encounter should incorporate regular health maintenance and a confidential psychosocial screening. It is important to uncover any hidden risks related to sports participation.

Box **18-1** Focused History for Preparticipation Sports Examination for the School-Age Child and Adolescent

Current Medical History	Past Medical History	Family History	Dietary History
• Sport youth intends to play, including position and weight class if relevant • Any medications used by the youth, including diet supplements, creatine, anabolic steroids and their analogs, *macrolide* antibiotics, *tricyclic* antidepressants, *neuroleptics* • Any chronic illnesses, including asthma, how controlled, and any exacerbations during exercise	• Any previous experience in the same or other sports, including previous injuries, especially injuries requiring exclusion for >1 week • Any history of shortness of breath, syncope, or chest pain during exertion • History of seizures, including type, frequency, controlling medication, and past complications • *For young women:* Age of menarche, regularity of menses, and any prior disturbances of menses during sports	• Family history of cerebrovascular accident (CVA) or myocardial infarction (MI) before age 50 • Any family history of sudden, unexplained death in adolescent or young adult relative • Family history of hypertrophic cardiomyopathy (HCM), prolonged QT syndrome, Marfan's syndrome, or other cardiac/circulatory abnormalities	• Are you happy with current weight? Want to gain or lose for sport? • *Weight loss methods:* Ask explicitly: any binging, purging, restricting? • Fruits/vegetables daily? Milk or calcium intake? • Fluids for hydration (water, sports drinks, sodas, caffeine intake)? • Supplements, medications for weight loss, weight gain, muscle gain?

TABLE 18-4　REVIEW OF SYSTEMS FOR PREPARTICIPATION SPORTS FOR SCHOOL-AGE CHILD AND ADOLESCENT

System	Disorders
HEENT	Otitis externa, frequent otitis media (OM), allergic rhinitis?
Respiratory	Shortness of breath (SOB), wheezing with exercise?
Cardiovascular	SOB, chest pain, dizziness, syncope with exertion, palpitations with exertion?
Gastrointestinal	Pain or reflux with exercise? Current/chronic problems with diarrhea, constipation?
Genitourinary	*For males:* History or symptoms of hernias, lumps or masses in groin or testicles? *For females:* Menstrual history (menarche, length, regularity of cycles, missed cycles during sports)? Last menstrual period (LMP)?
Musculoskeletal	Instability of any joints (especially shoulder, knee, ankle)? Leg or foot pain with exercise? Swelling of joints? Any weakness?
Neurological	Headaches, dizziness, seizures, recent concussions, recent injuries, weakness, difficulties with balance or gait?
Dermatological	*Lesions:* Recent history of herpes, fungal infections, bacterial infections? Extent of acne and usual treatments? Eczema, reaction of skin to perspiration or athletic equipment?

HEENT, Head, eyes, ears, nose, and throat.

TABLE 18-5　MEDICAL CONDITIONS AND LEVEL OF SPORTS PARTICIPATION

Condition	Level of Sports Participation and Rationale
Bleeding disorder	Qualified yes*
Cardiovascular disease	
Carditis (inflammation of the heart)	No May result in sudden death with exertion
Hypertension (high blood pressure)	Qualified yes*
Congenital heart disease (structural heart defects present at birth)	Qualified yes* Those with mild forms may participate fully; moderate or severe forms or those who have undergone surgery need evaluation

TABLE 18-5   MEDICAL CONDITIONS AND LEVEL OF SPORTS PARTICIPATION—CONT'D

Condition	Level of Sports Participation and Rationale
Dysrhythmia (irregular heart rhythm)	Qualified yes* Those with symptoms (chest pain, syncope, dizziness, shortness of breath) or evidence of mitral valve regurgitation (leaking) need evaluation; all others may participate fully
Heart murmur	Qualified yes* If innocent, full participation is permitted; otherwise, the athlete needs evaluation.
Cerebral palsy	Qualified yes*
Diabetes mellitus	Yes Blood glucose concentration should be monitored every 30 minutes during continuous exercise and 15 minutes after completion of exercise
Diarrhea	Qualified no* Unless mild, no participation is permitted, may increase risk of dehydration
Eating disorders Anorexia nervosa Bulimia nervosa	 Qualified yes* Qualified yes*
Fever	No Increases cardiopulmonary effort, reduces maximum exercise capacity, makes heat illness more likely, and increases orthostatic hypertension during exercise
Hepatitis/HIV	Yes All sports may be played that athlete's state of health allows; skin lesions should be covered properly, and universal precautions used when handling blood or body fluids with visible blood
Musculoskeletal disorders	Qualified yes*
Neurological disorders History of serious head or spine trauma, severe or repeated concussions, or craniotomy	Qualified yes* Research supports conservative approach to management of concussion

Continued

TABLE 18-5 MEDICAL CONDITIONS AND LEVEL OF SPORTS PARTICIPATION—CONT'D

Condition	Level of Sports Participation and Rationale
Seizure disorder	
Well-controlled	Yes
	Risk of seizure during participation is minimal
Poorly-controlled	Qualified yes*
	Archery, riflery, swimming, weight or power lifting, strength training, or sports involving heights should be avoided because occurrence of a seizure may pose risk to self or others
Obesity	Qualified yes*
Organ transplant recipient	Qualified yes*
Respiratory conditions	
Pulmonary compromise, including cystic fibrosis	Qualified yes*
Asthma	Yes
	Only most severe asthma requires modified participation
Acute upper respiratory infection	Qualified yes*
	Individual assessment required for all but mild disease
Sickle cell disease or trait	Qualified yes*
	Carefully condition, acclimatize, and hydrate to reduce any possible risk
Skin disorders	Qualified yes*
Boils, herpes simplex, impetigo, scabies, molluscum contagiosum	While contagious, participation in gymnastics with mats; martial arts; wrestling; or other collision contact or limited-contact sports is not allowed

Adapted from American Academy of Pediatrics, Committee on Sports Medicine and Fitness: medical conditions affecting sports participation, *Pediatrics* 107(5):1205-1209, 2001.
*Patient needs evaluation.

The preparticipation physical exam is also an opportunity for the examiner to uncover risky health practices directly related to or exacerbated by a sport, particularly unhealthy weight loss or weight gain (Box 18-1). Sports such as wrestling, boxing, and martial arts are graded by weight class, which creates significant pressure on the young athlete to maximize body strength and bulk. There are equally powerful pressures on dancers and gymnasts to keep their weight low. By contrast, youth playing positions such as linebacker in football may be trying to increase their weight, even if their body mass index (BMI) is already over the 95th percentile for age. Each athlete should be asked directly about satisfaction with or concerns about weight and about practices such as severe food restriction, binging or purging, or weight loss or muscle-enhancing supplements, including medications containing *ephedra, creatine,* and anabolic steroids or their analogs. Tables 18-4 and 18-5

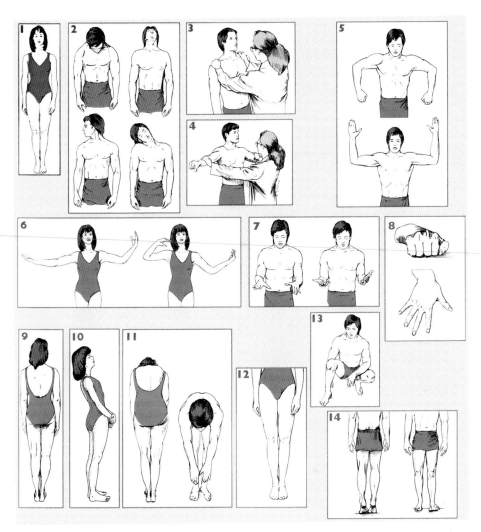

Figure 18-18 14-step orthopedic examination. (From American Academy of Family Physicians, American Academy of Pediatrics, American College of Sports Medicine, American Medical Society for Sports Medicine, American Orthopedic Society for Sports Medicine, American Osteopathic Academy of Sports Medicine [2005]. *Preparticipation Physical evaluation, ed 3*, Minneapolis, McGraw-Hill Healthcare Information.)

present a review of systems and medical conditions for the preparticipation sports examination. The preparticipation screening examination includes a 14-step orthopedic exam (Figure 18-18).[5,6] The young pubertal female athlete should be in shorts and sport bra and young males should be in shorts for the preparticipation physical to ensure the joints and muscles can be examined easily. The 14-step orthopedic exam assesses the athlete's musculoskeletal health as follows:

1. With the young athlete standing, assess for frontal symmetry of trunk, shoulders, and extremities.
2. Assess neck flexion, extension, lateral flexion side to side, and rotation to evaluate range of motion of cervical spine.
3. Assess trapezius strength by having the young athlete shrug shoulders against resistance from the practitioner.
4. Assess deltoid strength by having the young athlete abduct the shoulders against resistance from the practitioner.
5. Assess internal and external rotation of shoulder to evaluate range of motion of the glenoid/humeral joint.
6. Assess range of motion of elbow by having young athlete perform flexion and extension of the arms.
7. Assess range of motion of wrist and elbow by observing pronation and supination of the forearm.
8. Assess range of motion of the hands and fingers by having young athlete clench the fist and spread the fingers.
9. Assess symmetry from the rear with young athlete standing.
10. Have the young athlete stand with knees straight and then flex forward and bend backward to assess any discomfort of the lumbar spine.
11. Perform Adam's forward bend test as described earlier in the chapter.
12. To assess for symmetry of leg musculature, have the young athlete stand facing the practitioner with quadriceps flexed.
13. Assess hip, knee, and ankle range of motion, strength, and balance by having the young athlete duck walk four steps.
14. Assess calf strength, symmetry, and balance by having the young athlete stand on heels and then toes.

Cardiac Preparticipation Sports History

Although it is not clear how many sudden cardiac deaths in young athletes could have been prevented with proper screening, the American Heart Association recommends a preparticipation history and physical examination for all competitive athletes. Some form of preparticipation physical examination is mandated by 49 of the 50 states, but exact requirements vary from state to state. In young athletes, the leading cause of sudden death is *hypertrophic cardiomyopathy*, a cardiovascular condition manifested by an asymmetrical

---

Box **18-2** Cardiac Guidelines for Exclusion from Sports

CRITERIA FOR REFERRAL TO A CARDIOLOGIST

History

- Family history of sudden death before age 50
- Palpitations, chest pain, dizziness, syncope during exercise
- Dyspnea with exercise disproportionate to level of exertion

Physical Examination

- Diastolic murmur
- Systolic murmur 3/6 or greater
- Murmur ↑ with Valsalva
- Weak femoral pulses
- Significant hypertension
- Stigmata of Marfan's syndrome (tall, thin with high-arched palate, long metacarpals, and lens dislocation)

Data from Lyznicki JM, Nielsen NH, Schneider JF: Cardiovascular screening of student athletes, *Am Fam Physician* 62(4):765-774, 2000.

TABLE 18-6   CLASSIFICATION OF SPORTS BY CONTACT

Contact or Collision	Limited Contact	Noncontact
Basketball	Baseball	Archery
Diving	Bicycling	Badminton
Field hockey	Cheerleading	Bowling
Football	Canoeing and kayaking	Curling
Ice hockey	Fencing	Dancing
Lacrosse	Field events*	Field events*
Martial arts	Floor hockey	Golf
Rodeo	Gymnastics	Power lifting
Rugby	Horseback riding	Race walking
Ski jumping	Racquetball	Riflery
Soccer	Skating	Rope jumping
Team handball	Skiing	Running
Water polo	Skateboarding	Sailing
Wrestling	Snowboarding	Scuba diving
	Softball	Swimming
	Squash	Table tennis
	Ultimate Frisbee	Tennis
	Volleyball	Track
	Surfing	Weight lifting

Adapted from American Academy of Pediatrics, Committee on Sports Medicine and Fitness: medical conditions affecting sports participation, *Pediatrics* 107(5):1205-1209, 2001.
*High jump and hurdles—limited contact; javelin, discus, and shot put—noncontact.

hypertrophied, nondilated left ventricle. Generally no evidence of cardiac disease is present prior to sudden death. Symptoms of dyspnea, angina, sudden fatigue with exertion, or syncope should be carefully evaluated (Box 18-2). Other related cardiac conditions include anomalous coronary arteries, *Marfan's syndrome*, prolonged QT interval, and cardiac *dysrhythmias*.

SPORTS INJURIES

Sports injuries can be classified as traumatic (*macrotrauma*), usually from collision or

contact sports such as basketball, football, or soccer, or as overuse (*microtrauma*) (Tables 18-6 and 18-7). The examiner should screen youth who play high-contact sports for previous history of concussion, fractures, and ligament damage. Youth who play lower-contact sports that involve repetitive motion, such as running or swimming, should be screened for overuse injuries to the shoulder, knee, elbow, or shin (tibia). Because injuries may recur from season to season, athletes with, for example, a history of frequent ankle sprain should be given strengthening exercises at the time of the sports physical to help prevent future injury.

TABLE 18-7 CLASSIFICATION OF SPORTS BY STRENUOUSNESS*

	A. Low Dynamic	B. Moderate Dynamic	C. High Dynamic

I. Low static	Billiards
	Bowling
	Cricket
	Curling
	Golf
	Riflery
		Baseball/Softball[†]
		Fencing
		Table tennis
		Volleyball
			Badminton
			Cross-country
			  skiing (classic
			  technique)
			Field hockey[†]
			Orienteering
			Race walking
			Racquetball/squash
			Running (long
			  distance)
			Soccer[†]
			Tennis

II. Moderate
  static
	Archery
	Auto racing[†,‡]
	Diving[†,‡]
	Equestrian[†,‡]
	Motorcycling[†,‡]
		Fencing
		Field events
		  (jumping)
		Figure skating[†]
		Football (American)[†]
		Rodeoing[†,‡]
		Rugby[†]
		Running (sprint)
		Surfing[†,‡]
		Synchronized
		  swimming[†]
			Basketball[†]
			Ice hockey[†]
			Cross-country
			  skiing (skating
			  technique)
			Lacrosse[†]
			Running
			  (middle distance)
			Swimming
			Team handball

III. High static	Bobsledding/
	  Luge[†,‡]
	Field events
	  (throwing)
	Gymnastics[†,‡]
	Martial arts[†]
	Sailing
	Sports climbing
	Waterskiing[†,‡]
	Weight lifting[†,‡]
	Windsurfing[†,‡]
		Body building[†,‡]
		Downhill skiing[†]
		Skateboarding[†,‡]
		Snowboarding[†,‡]
		Wrestling[†]
			Boxing[†]
			Canoeing/kayaking
			Cycling[†,‡]
			Decathlon
			Rowing
			Speed skating[†,‡]
			Triathlon[†,‡]

Adapted from Mitchell JH, Haskell WL, Snell P et al: Task force 8: Classification of Sports, *J Am Coll Cardiol* 45(8):1364-1367, 2005.
*Classification of sports is based on peak dynamic and static components during competition.
†Danger of bodily collision.
‡Increased risk if syncope occurs.

Pediatric Pearls

Ligaments are stronger than bones until adolescence; therefore injuries to long bones and joints in the preadolescent are more likely to cause fractures rather than sprains.

The athlete's sexual maturity rating (SMR or Tanner stage) is also relevant to injury prevention. Rapid growth during adolescence, particularly during Tanner stage 3 in females and Tanner stage 4 in males, results in decreased strength in the growth plates, leading to greater potential for injury. The relative muscle strength and cartilaginous physes of Tanner 3 predispose the athlete to physeal (growth plate) fractures. For most adolescents, including adolescents with chronic conditions, the physical and social benefits of carefully monitored sports participation outweigh the risks.

Female Athlete Triad

Young women should be screened for "female adolescent triad": *anorexia, amenorrhea,* and *osteopenia.* This triad in young female athletes begins with disordered eating that leads to amenorrhea (absence of menses), and eventually leads to osteoporosis (loss of bone mass), in some cases by the late teens or early 20s. This is a preventable condition and yet it is increasing in frequency because of the lack of understanding on the part of coaches, parents, and athletes regarding the triad symptoms. A strong competitive environment contributes to this serious safety issue. The examiner also should be aware that some long-distance runners and swimmers may have irregular menses during their sports seasons without necessarily having an eating disorder.

ABNORMAL CONDITIONS

Table 18-8 presents the most common abnormal orthopedic conditions seen in infants, children, and adolescents by the pediatric healthcare practitioner.

 CHARTING

A Healthy Toddler

Extremities and back: nl ROM (range of motion), mild tibial torsion and toeing-in bilaterally R > L, spine straight with mild lordosis.

TABLE 18-8 *ABNORMAL MUSCULOSKELETAL CONDITIONS*

Condition	Description
Clubfoot	Rigidity of foot and inability of foot to right itself from fixed medial position
Talipes equinovarus	Inversion of forefoot, plantar flexion and heel inversion
Talipes calcaneovalgus	Eversion and dorsiflexion of forefoot
Metatarsus adductus	*Varus* abnormality of forefoot at the tarso-metatarsal junction; ankle and hindfoot are normal; lateral border of foot is curved rather than straight, usually shaped like a "kidney bean"; line drawn medially from heel often intersects third toe

Continued

TABLE 18-8 ABNORMAL MUSCULOSKELETAL CONDITIONS—CONT'D

Condition	Description
Pes planus (flat feet)	Flattening of longitudinal arch in school-age child when standing erect with full weight bearing on feet bilaterally; flat feet in toddler are developmentally normal and often are accentuated by fat pad on ventral surface
Tibial torsion	Inward twisting or bowing of tibia and fibula, often a variation of normal rotational development; intrauterine position may be contributing factor; most common cause of toeing-in children <3 years of age; resolves with normal growth; continued reassurance to parent is important
Slipped femoral capital epiphysis	Proximal femoral epiphysis slips in a posterior and inferior direction over neck of femur; presenting symptoms are limp, knee or hip pain, particularly with strenuous activity; occurs more commonly between 8 and 16 years of age during rapid growth periods
Legg-Calvé-Perthes	Blood supply to femoral capital epiphysis is disturbed and produces avascular necrosis of femoral head; affects children 3 to 12 years of age, with peak incidence in males 4 to 8 years old; children may present with diffuse pain in hip, knee, or the upper thigh; may have history of intermittent limp; early diagnosis and management are key to preventing long-term sequelae
Femoral anteversion	Increased forward rotation of femoral head in relation to knee; may be exacerbated by child sitting in "W" position when playing, watching TV, or sleeping; common cause of toeing-in after 3 years of age; evaluate child when undressed and lying in prone position; note internal rotation of hip; resolution usually occurs after 7 years of age
Osgood-Schlatter syndrome	Inflammation of tibia causing swelling and tenderness at insertion of infrapatellar tendon into tibial tubercle; presents with knee pain after vigorous activity; common finding in adolescent athletes, especially 9 to 15 years of age
Developmental dysplasia of the hip	Condition in which femoral head has abnormal relationship to acetabulum: unstable, subluxated, or dislocated; incidence of unstable hip 1/100 and 1 to 1.5/1000 for dislocation, incidence higher in girls; management ranges from observation of unstable hip to reduction and stabilization of dislocated hip with *Pavlik* harness

TABLE 18-8 ABNORMAL MUSCULOSKELETAL CONDITIONS—CONT'D

Condition	Description
Idiopathic scoliosis	Lateral bending of spine and associated rotation of vertebral bodies; lateral curvature of >10 degrees indicates scoliosis; scoliometer reading of 7 degrees correlates with 20 degrees radiological curvature; 30% have positive family history*

Data from American Academy of Pediatrics, Committee on Quality Improvement: clinical practice guideline: early detection of developmental dysplasia of the hip, *Pediatrics* 105(4 Pt 1):896-905, 2000.
*Data from Killian JT, Mayberry S, Wilkinson L: Current concepts in adolescent idiopathic scoliosis, *Pediatr Ann* 28(12):755-761, 1999.

REFERENCES

1. Ganel A, Dudkiewicz I, Grogan DP: Pediatric orthopedic physical examination of the infant: a 5-minute assessment, *J Pediatr Health Care* 17(1): 39-41, 2003.
2. Chaudhry B, Harvey D: *Mosby's color atlas and text of pediatrics and child health,* St Louis, 2001, Mosby.
3. Taft E, Francis R: Evaluation and management of scoliosis, *J Pediatr Health Care* 17(1):42-44, 2003.
4. Chin KR, Price JS, Zimbler S: A guide to early detection of scoliosis, *Contemp Pediatr* 18(9):77-103, 2001.
5. Andrews JS: Making the most of the sports physical, *Contemp Pediatr* 14(3):183-205, 1997.
6. Smith DM, Kovan Jr BSE et al: *Preparticipation physical evaluation,* ed 2, Minneapolis, 1997, McGraw-Hill.

CHAPTER 19

NEUROLOGICAL SYSTEM

Karen G. Duderstadt

The nervous system contains the most complex and delicate pathways in the body and is the center of all vital bodily functions. The balance of these pathways provides the vital motor, sensory, and cognitive functions that sustain human life and comprise human behavior. For the healthcare practitioner, monitoring the development of the nervous system is one of the most important aspects of the physical examination. The challenge for the practitioner is to assess not only the progress of gross motor development in children but also the fine motor function and any subtle deficits that may impact learning behavior.

DEVELOPMENT

The formation of the neurological system begins during cell differentiation in the third week of fetal life. The *notochord* develops during this period; it forms the neural plate and neural folds. Closure of the neural plate is complete by the fourth week of embryonic development and the neural tube is formed. Any fetal insults that occur during this period can result in defects in the brain and spinal cord, such as *spina bifida*. During the fifth week of fetal development, brain growth proceeds at a rapid

pace and secondary growth of the skull bones occurs.

By 24 weeks' gestation, the fetus has developed all of the nerve cells, or neurons, needed for the formation of the neural pathways. The *neuron* is the basic unit of the nervous system, and each neuron contains numerous dendrites and one axon (Figure 19-1). Dendrites are the protoplasmic branches of the cell body. Neural impulses enter the cell body through the dendrites and leave through the single axon. They then connect by a series of synapses with another dendrite of the next axon. *Myelin*, a lipoid material surrounding cell fibers, covers some of the axons whereas others are not covered. *Myelination*, the deposit of the protective fatty substance around the axons, continues in the brain throughout the first 2 years of life, and in the preterm infant continues into third year of life.

At birth, the brain of the term infant weighs an average of 325 g and by the end of the first year, the weight of the brain has tripled.[1] As brain growth and neurological maturation continue, the myelination of the nerves proceeds from head to toe, *cephalocaudal*, and from midline to fingertips, *proximodistal*. The most rapid growth of the brain occurs in the

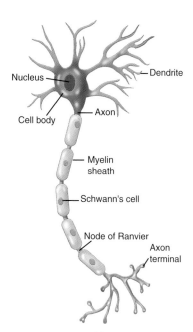

Nucleus

Dendrite

Cell body

Axon

Myelin sheath

Schwann's cell

Node of Ranvier

Axon terminal

Figure **19-1** The neuron.

postnatal period between 4 and 5 months of age when the neurons mature and inter-connectedness of the dendrites and axons increases.[1] Head circumference is the best indication of brain growth. Normally, in the term infant, the head circumference increases sixfold in the first year of life.[1] Half of the post-natal growth of the brain is achieved by 1 year of age.

CULTURAL VARIATIONS

Cultural practices also may affect the progress of developmental milestones. Infants who are swaddled on a mother's back for the first year may stand and begin walking at a later age. Increased muscle tone is normally seen in African-American infants, with an equal bal-ance between increased flexor and extensor tone. Decreased tone is common in Asian infants and is usually unbalanced, with more extensor tone throughout movement.

PHYSIOLOGICAL VARIATIONS

Table 19-1 reviews the physical, developmen-tal, and cognitive variations that occur during childhood.

ANATOMY AND PHYSIOLOGY

Central Nervous System

Brain

The brain is covered by protective layers that cushion and lubricate the outer surface. The *dura mater* lies just beneath the skull bone and periosteum and consists of layers of fibrous connective tissue. Adjacent to the dura mater is the *arachnoid,* the avascular, weblike mem-brane that cushions the cortex. The dura mater is separated from the arachnoid by the *subdu-ral* space. The *pia mater* is the highly vascular area of the cortex that attaches directly to the gray matter or irregular surface of the brain. The subarachnoid area and a cushion of cere-brospinal fluid separate the arachnoid from the pia mater (Figure 19-2).

The *cortex,* the outermost part of the brain, is often referred to as the "gray matter" because the neurons are unmyelinated, which makes them appear gray rather than white. The *cerebrum,* which includes the cortex, is the largest structure in the skull. It is divided into two hemispheres, with the left hemisphere being dominant in 95% of individuals.[2] The hemispheres are connected

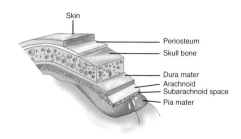

Skin

Periosteum

Skull bone

Dura mater

Arachnoid

Subarachnoid space

Pia mater

Figure **19-2** The meningeal layers.

TABLE 19-1 PHYSIOLOGICAL VARIATIONS DURING DEVELOPMENT

Age-Group	Physical Variations	Developmental Variations	Cognitive Variations
Preterm	Head lag persists for 6 months; myelination of brain continues until 3 years of age	Increased extensor tone in lower extremities; with marked stiffening and toe pointing	Sensorimotor reflexive response to stimulus
Newborn	Brain surface initially smooth at birth; cerebral cortex is half the adult thickness	Exhibits primitive reflexes until 3 to 4 months; requires strong stimulus to elicit response	Innate knowledge of environment, evokes survival response such as sucking
Infant	Head circumference increases sixfold in first year; in term infant, important myelination of brain continues until 2 years of age	*Plagiocephaly,* asymmetrical head, shape, is common; most often related to sleeping position; normally, resolves by 3 months	Develops mental image of hidden object; imitates sounds by 6 months
Toddler	Proprioception, awareness of spatial/body positions begins; increased movement and sphincter control	Develops basic self-control and ability to separate from attachment person; body exploration and realization of sexuality	Parallel play; independence increases; attention span develops
Preschooler	Slowed growth, minimal change in head circumference; increased connectivity between neurons to initiate complex thought	Hand preference established; rapid fine motor development; gross motor athletic ability	Egocentric; aggressive behavior; one-dimensional understanding; magical thinking
School-age child	Brain reaches 90% of adult size by 7 years of age; deepening of sulci in brain, increasing complex thought	Transmission of nerve impulses improves, thereby enhancing fine motor and gross motor development	Consequential understanding; concrete operations and objective thought
Adolescent	Neurological development continues into adolescence	Defines self-concept; role diffusion causes conflict	Develops abstract thinking ability

by the *corpus callosum,* which controls and integrates motor, sensory, and higher intellectual functions. The hemispheres are divided into four lobes, each controlling particular bodily functions and behavior (Figure 19-3).

- **Frontal**: Initiates voluntary musculoskeletal movement. Broca's area mediates motor speech.
- **Parietal**: Controls processing and interpretation of sensory input—visual, auditory, smell, taste, and touch sensations, including pain, temperature, and pressure.
- **Occipital**: Primary center for receiving and interpretation of visual data.
- **Temporal**: Primary center for the perception and interpretation of sound. Wernicke's area is related to language comprehension.

The surface of the brain is composed of fissures and grooves, or *sulci.* The young infant has fewer convolutional surfaces, or sulci, in the cortex and a more pliable skull. These characteristics decrease the incidence of bruising and tearing of the cerebral cortex in the young infant with minor head trauma. However, severe shaking in small infants causes acceleration and deceleration of the delicate brain tissue within the periosteum, and subarachnoid and subdural hematomas occur as a result, which can be fatal. Throughout childhood, the sulci of the brain deepen.

Completion of brain growth occurs in early adolescence.

The *cerebellum* maintains the body's equilibrium, coordinates movement, and relays signals to the muscles from the cerebrum. It is the portion of the brain that processes the sensory input from the musculoskeletal system as well as from the visual, auditory, and touch receptors. Research indicates that the cerebellum plays an important role in cognitive functions.[3]

The brain and spinal cord are lubricated by *cerebrospinal fluid,* normally a clear liquid, which is formed in the ventricles of the brain. It flows from the lateral ventricles to the third and fourth ventricles through a series of foramens. The fourth ventricle, which lies in the medulla, contains three openings that allow the cerebrospinal fluid to pass into the subarachnoid space.

Brainstem

The *brainstem* is in the central core of the brain and includes the *pons, medulla oblongata, midbrain,* and the *diencephalon* (Figure 19-4). The *pons* acts as the neural transmission center, supporting ascending and descending nerve fibers. The *medulla oblongata,* which lies between the pons and the cerebellum, is a continuation of the spinal cord. It transmits impulses along the spinal cord and aids in the life centers of respiration and circulation. It controls the

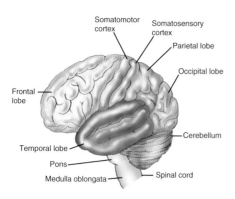

Figure **19-3** Brain and brainstem.

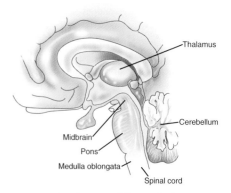

Figure **19-4** Regions of the cerebral cortex.

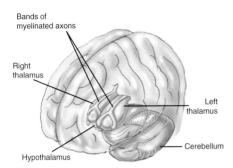

Bands of myelinated axons

Right thalamus

Left thalamus

Cerebellum

Hypothalamus

Figure **19-5** The diencephalon.

involuntary reflexes such as coughing, sneezing, and yawning. The *diencephalon* is the extension of the brainstem that lies embedded in the cerebral cortex and contains the *thalamus* and *pineal body* (Figure 19-5). The *hypothalamus, pituitary gland,* and parts of the third ventricle arise from the diencephalon and the nuclei of the cranial nerves. The *midbrain* contains the neural fibers that come from the spinal cord and merge into the thalamus and hypothalamus.

- *Thalamus*—Acts as the brain's relay station and receives input from the sensory and motor systems of the body and dispatches input to the appropriate region of the cerebral cortex.
- *Hypothalamus*—Regulates body temperature, metabolic processes, and involuntary response activity.
- *Pituitary gland*—Responsible for hormonal control of growth, lactation, and metabolism.

The *limbic system* is the group of subcortical structures in the diencephalon including the *hypothalamus* and the *hippocampus.* This system regulates emotion and motivation and organizes memories. Aggression and fear also are regulated by the limbic system. Disruption that occurs during the development of the limbic system causes distorted perceptions and aggressive behavior. Exposure to cocaine early in gestation can disrupt the migration of neurons up the cortical wall, and later prenatal exposure causes disruption of neuronal

synapses.[3] Children exposed to cocaine in utero have disturbances in memory, learning, attention span, and behavior.

Spinal Cord

The spinal cord is an extension of the medulla oblongata and is composed of gray and white matter extending to the lumbar region. The gray matter runs laterally along the spinal cord and protects the myelinated and unmyelinated fibers of the white matter. *Proprioceptors,* the specialized nerve endings in muscles, tendons, and joints, are located in the white matter and are sensitive to changes in the tension of muscles and tendons. Temperature, pain, touch, and equilibrium are transmitted through the proprioceptors to the brainstem.

Upper and Lower Motor Neurons

Upper motor neurons are located within the central nervous system and convey impulses from the motor areas of the cerebral cortex to the *lower motor neurons* in the spinal cord. They can influence the function of the lower motor neurons as evidenced in conditions such as *cerebral palsy.* The lower motor neurons are located primarily in the peripheral nervous system and provide pathways for nerve fibers to translate movement of the muscles into action. Muscle wasting can be the result of dysfunction in the anterior horn cells of the upper motor neurons. Dysfunction in the lower motor neurons can cause wasting of localized muscle groups and a soft rather than firm tone to the muscle mass. Acquired atrophy of the muscles accompanied by a wide-based gait and muscle weakness when arising from a sitting position is characteristic of *muscular dystrophy,* a developmental muscle wasting condition with onset in early childhood.

Peripheral Nervous System

The *spinal nerves* originate in the spinal cord and exit from the intervertebral spaces. They contain sensory and motor fibers, and with the cranial nerves and visceral fibers of the *autonomic nervous system* compose the pathways of the *peripheral nervous system.* The autonomic nervous system carries impulses to and from the central nervous system. It is divided into the *sympathetic* and *parasympathetic nervous systems* and is made up of unmyelinated nerves. The sympathetic nervous system activates in times of stress and provides increased energy for needed bursts of activity. The parasympathetic system balances the activities of the sympathetic by restoring stability and maintaining reserve energy for daily bodily functions such as digestion and elimination.

Spinal Nerves

There are 31 pairs of *spinal nerves* that innervate the torso and extremities (Figure 19-6). The body surface that is innervated by the plexus of a spinal nerve is called a *dermatome.* Although dermatomes map specific segments of the body surface, spinal nerve sensation can be transmitted to adjacent dermatomes (Figure 19-6). The sensory pathways of the spinal nerves carry sensations of touch, temperature, and pain; the motor fibers activate reflexes and impulses that control skeletal muscles and the involuntary muscles of the viscera. The spinal nerves function as part of the lower motor neurons and become dysfunctional in the presence of spinal cord lesions.

Reflex Arc

Reflex behavior provides the major assessment of brainstem function. The *reflex arc* operates outside the level of conscious control and is the basic defense mechanism of the nervous system. Reflexes help the body maintain appropriate muscle tension and permit a brisk reaction to painful or harmful stimuli. A stimulus creates an impulse transmitted instantaneously outward by the motor neuron of the spinal cord via the spinal nerve and peripheral nervous system to produce a brisk contraction (Figure 19-7).

Cranial Nerves

The twelve *cranial nerves* originate in the cranium and supply motor and sensory function primarily to the head and neck area. The *vagus nerve,* cranial nerve X, is the exception because it innervates part of the cardiac and abdominal viscera. Both the spinal and cranial nerves are myelinated nerves. The cranial nerves function by way of impulses conveyed from the motor and sensory pathways and the parasympathetic nervous system to the cortex.

SYSTEM-SPECIFIC HISTORY

Table 19-2 presents important information to be gathered when reviewing the neurological system from birth to adolescence.

☞ Key Points

An accurate history of fine and gross motor milestones is key to determining developmental delays in the infant and young child. Any loss of a previously acquired skill indicates need for referral for further neurological assessment and diagnosis.

PHYSICAL ASSESSMENT

Box 19-1 presents a pediatric neurological assessment checklist for the practitioner.

Evaluation of Motor Function

Assessment of muscle tone and strength is a key component of evaluating the development of the neurological system. *Muscle tone,* the normal degree of tension maintained by muscles while at rest, changes over time as myelination extends and the cortex takes over control of the motor functions. The assessment of muscle tone begins in the young infant by observing the resting posture. In the term infant at birth, arms and legs are in a semiflexed position with the hips slightly abducted (Figure 19-8).

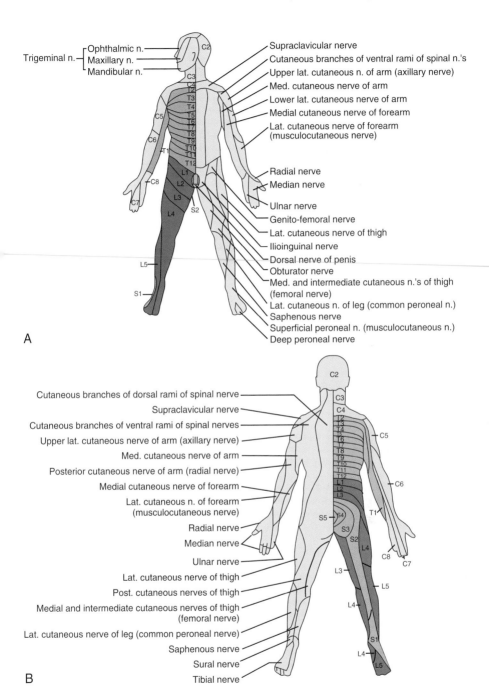

Figure **19-6** The spinal nerves and dermatomes.

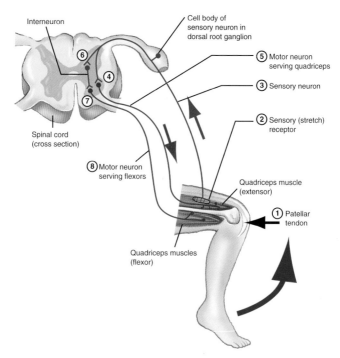

Figure **19-7** Reflex arc.

TABLE 19-2 INFORMATION GATHERING FOR NEUROLOGICAL ASSESSMENT AT KEY DEVELOPMENTAL STAGES

Age-Group	Questions to Ask
Preterm infant	History of hypoxia in early neonatal period?
	Intraventricular insult?
	Maternal alcohol/substance abuse?
	Exposure to TORCH viruses?
Newborn	Vaginal or cesarean birth? History of birth injury? Shoulder presentation? Need for resuscitation/ventilation in immediate newborn period?
	Maternal infection or toxemia? Fetal movement during pregnancy? Age of mother and father at time of infant's birth?
	Appropriate gestational age? Apgar scores? Jaundice? Neonatal meningitis? Congenital abnormalities?
Infant	Difficulty feeding? Protuberant tongue or tongue thrust?
	Any delay in achieving gross motor milestones? Does infant roll over? Sit without support? Crawl? Stand alone? Walk without support?
	Cooing, babbling?
	Any evidence of toe-walking?
	Any loss of developmental milestones?

TABLE 19-2   INFORMATION GATHERING FOR NEUROLOGICAL ASSESSMENT AT KEY DEVELOPMENTAL STAGES—CONT'D

Age-Group	Questions to Ask
Toddler	Hand dominance? Feeds self?
	Any loss of developmental milestones?
	Any stumbling, limping, poor coordination?
	History of seizures/spasms, staring spells, daydreaming?
	Speech development?
Preschooler	Ability to dress independently?
	Independent toileting achieved?
	Attention span? Completion of tasks?
School-age child	Visual and auditory perceptions?
	Learning difficulties/delays?
Adolescent	Headache history?
	Sports-related concussions?
Pediatric	Maternal exposure to potential irritants?
environmental	Location of housing in relation to hazardous exposures?
risks	History of housing and lead exposures? Contact with chemical cleaning agents, hazardous chemicals, smoke?
	Pesticide exposures?

TORCH, Toxoplasmosis, other (congenital syphilis and viruses), rubella, cytomegalovirus infections, and herpes simplex virus.

Box **19-1**   Pediatric Neurological Assessment Checklist

- Infant reflexes at <1 year of age
- Fontanels at <18 months
- Level of alertness or consciousness
- Motor and sensory function
- Cranial nerves
- Deep and superficial reflexes
- Coordination

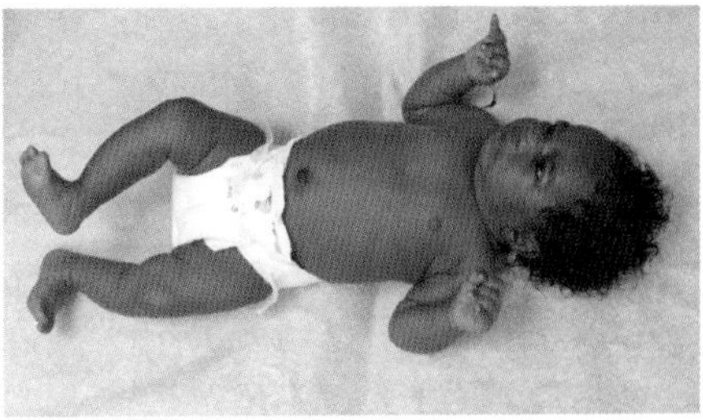

Figure **19-8** Normal flexion in term infant.

Tone in the neck and trunk is evaluated by *gently* pulling the infant to a sitting position. Significant head lag or inability of the young infant to exhibit strength when pulled to sitting indicates muscle weakness. In the 4- to 6-month-old, strength in the extremities and trunk is evaluated by *gently* pulling the infant from the sitting to standing position. Premature infants are known to have increased extensor tone in their lower extremities but decreased truncal tone during their first year of life. Infants who have poor muscle tone initially may later develop spasticity as the cortex matures. Asymmetry in muscle tone may not be identified early because of lack of volitional control in the cortex. With toddlers, assess balance and agility while the child walks, pivots, and turns holding the parent's hand. It is important to observe normal gait and balance with the child undressed except for diapers. In the toddler who is fearful or refuses to walk as requested, gently pick up the child and direct him or her to toddle toward the parent.

Abnormal muscle tone and abnormal positioning or posturing of the extremities in the young infant indicates neurological dysfunction. Hips positioned in external rotation or in a "frog-leg" position may be a sign of a floppy infant. Persistent abnormal positioning of the head and/or persistent asymmetrical extension of the arm with hand extended indicates neurological dysfunction. If the infant exhibits *opisthotonos*, persistent arching of the back and extension of the neck, serious neurological compromise is indicated. Delays can occur in any area of development—gross motor, fine motor, language, cognitive—but are usually first manifest in gross motor abilities. Paying careful attention to neonatal primitive and postural reflexes will help the practitioner detect any evidence of delayed maturation of sensory and motor function and prompt early referral for evaluation and therapy.

Primitive Reflexes

The *primitive reflexes* are controlled at birth by the brainstem and are involuntary. They diminish by 3 to 4 months of age and disappear altogether in the normal term newborn by 4 to 6 months of age as the cerebral cortex develops during the first year of life (Table 19-3). The primitive reflexes should always be symmetrical and are considered abnormal if asymmetrical, absent, or persistent after 6 months

(Figures 19-9 through 19-12). They may provide the earliest indication of central nervous system dysfunction. All primitive reflexes will be diminished if the infant is very sleepy, irritable, or satiated after feeds.

Postural Reflexes

The appearance of the postural reflexes predicts normal development (Table 19-4). As the primitive reflexes disappear, the postural reflexes appear between 5 and 6 months and progress in a cephalocaudal direction from head control to grasping objects. When evaluating tone in a young infant, the infant's head must be kept in the midline position when supine to eliminate eliciting the *asymmetrical tonic neck reflex* (Figure 19-13). Holding the infant firmly suspended prone in the examiner's hand, the infant should lift the head and extend the spine and lower extremities (Figure 19-14).

Involuntary Motor Function

Tremors, coarse repetitive shaking, can be observed intermittently in the term newborn in the first few days after birth and are generally considered within normal limits. Persistent tremors in the newborn period and beyond are abnormal and require further diagnostic evaluation. *Clonus*, rhythmic tonic-clonic movements of the foot, in the newborn can be normal. Clonus can be elicited by the examiner's firm touch on the sole of the foot with the finger. With sustained clonus beyond the newborn period, the examiner should suspect upper motor neuron dysfunction. *Tics*, involuntary muscle contractions and/or audible sounds or words, are abnormal neurological signs and can be the result of emotional upset, severe anxiety in the child related to language or learning difficulties or the onset of *Tourette's syndrome*.

Evaluation of Sensory Function

Touch, deep pressure, pain, temperature, and vibration are all characteristics assessed in sensory function. Tactile sensation can be tested in the verbal child by gently touching different

TABLE 19-3 PRIMITIVE REFLEXES

Reflex	How Initiated	Response
Asymmetrical tonic neck	With infant on flat surface turn head 90 degrees to surface	Arm and leg extend on same side infant is turned toward, arm and leg on opposite side flex
Moro	Support infant at 30-degree angle above flat surface with examiner's hand; allow head and trunk to drop back to surface supported by examiner's hand; or pull infant up by hands to 30-degree angle above examining table; gently drop infant back to surface quickly and release arms	Arms extend and abduct, hands open, fingers fan out, thumb and forefinger form a C; then arms flex and adduct, knees clench, hips flex, eyes open, infant may cry
Palmar grasp	With infant's head midline, touch palm of infant's hand on ulnar surface with examiner's thumb	Fingers clasp examiner's thumb
Placing	Hold infant upright under arms over edge of table; touch dorsal surface of foot to table edge	Flexion of knees/hips, foot lifts as if stepping up on table
Plantar grasp	Touch infant on plantar surface of foot at base of toes	Toes curl downward
Rooting	Touch or stroke cheek	Infant's head turns toward stimulus and mouth should open
Stepping	Hold infant upright under the arms above exam table; palmar surface of feet should be allowed to just touch table surface	Stepping-like motion with alternate flexion and extension of legs
Sucking	Gently stroke the lips	Infant's mouth opens, sucking begins; gloved finger inserted into mouth evaluates strength of suck reflex
Truncal incurvation or Gallant's reflex	Hold infant firmly suspended in prone position with examiner's hand supporting chest; with opposite hand, stroke along spine lightly with fingernail just adjacent to vertebrae from shoulders to coccyx	Hips and buttocks curve/turn toward stimulus side

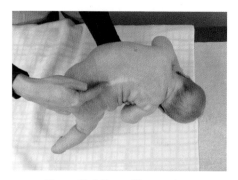

Figure **19-9** Truncal incurvation.

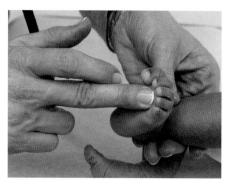

Figure **19-12** Plantar grasp.

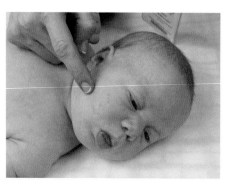

Figure **19-10** Rooting.

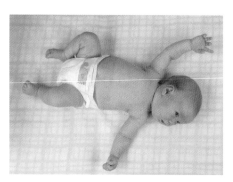

Figure **19-13** Asymmetric tonic neck reflex.

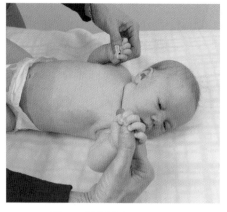

Figure **19-11** Palmar grasp.

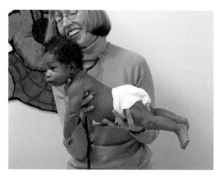

Figure **19-14** Landau reflex.

TABLE 19-4 POSTURAL REFLEXES

Reflex	How Initiated	Response
Landau	Hold infant firmly suspended in prone position with examiner's hand supporting abdomen and head; legs should extend over hand	Infant should lift head, extend spine/lower extremities
Parachute	Hold infant prone and firmly supported; slowly lower infant toward flat surface	Infants should try to protect themselves by extending arms/legs
Lateral forward	Suspend infant in prone position with arms/legs extended, support with both hands over flat surface	Infant will lift head and extend spine along horizontal plane
Positive support	Hold infant upright and firmly supported under arms while over exam table; touch infant's feet to surface	Infant should extend legs and bear some weight

areas of the body with a cotton swab when the eyes are closed. The child should be able to identify the spot by pointing to the area of the body. Pain sensation can be tested similarly in the verbal child by touching the body with the sharp and dull ends of a reflex hammer. Temperature and vibration are sensations not usually elicited in the child, but vibration can be tested with a tuning fork on different areas of the body. Discrimination sensation can be assessed in the verbal child using the following tests:

- **Stereognosis:** The ability to recognize an object by its feel. With eyes closed, ask the verbal child to identify small familiar objects placed in the palm, such as a key or a coin. If you are not testing expressive language, have the child point to the correct object when eyes are open. Children with cerebral palsy are generally unable to identify the object.
- **Graphesthesia:** The ability to identify shapes traced on the palm. Young verbal children are usually tested with shapes and older children with numbers. May be repeated in each palm to ensure accuracy in testing. Children with spatial and

proprioceptive dysfunction will not be able to discriminate shapes or numbers.
- **Two-point discrimination:** A test of spatial discrimination of the body. With the child's eyes closed, touch lightly on the skin with two points in close proximity on the body, and then follow with touching the child with one point. Ask whether the child felt one or two points. Children under 5 years of age may have difficulty comparing touch points.

Loss of sensation can reflect impairment in the peripheral nervous system, the spinal column, brainstem, or the cerebral cortex. Dysfunction of the lower motor neurons can cause the verbal child to have image confusion.

Cranial Nerves

Results of cranial nerve testing will be diminished in infants if they are drowsy, crying, or satiated after feeding, and in toddlers if they are irritable or fearful during physical examination. Cooperative preschoolers and school-age children usually delight in this activity if testing of cranial nerves is made into a game (Table 19-5 and Box 19-2).

TABLE 19-5 CRANIAL NERVE TESTING IN THE NEWBORN AND INFANT

Cranial Nerve	Test	Response
Cranial nerve I, olfactory	Pass strong-smelling substance (e.g., cloves, peppermint, anise oil) under nose (not often tested in newborns)	Observe for startle response, grimace, sniffing
Cranial nerve II, optic	Light source/ophthalmoscope on medium/large aperture	Pupils constrict in response to light, able to fix on object and follow for 60 to 90 degrees
Cranial nerve III, oculomotor	Elicit pupillary response to test optic nerve by shining pen light toward pupil	Evaluate shape, size, symmetry, spontaneous movements of pupil
Cranial nerve IV, trochlear Cranial nerve VI, abducent	"Doll's eye" maneuver—rotate head from side to side, observe eyes moving away from direction of rotation	Eyes should deviate left when turning head right; if eyes remain fixed or do not track in opposite direction, suspect brainstem dysfunction
Cranial nerve V, trigeminal	Touch infant's cheek area Test jaw muscles by placing gloved finger in infant's mouth	Infant turns cheek toward touch stimulus Infant should bite down on gloved finger and begin sucking
Cranial nerve VII, facial	Observe infant's face for symmetry of facial movements and observe when crying	Asymmetrical nasolabial folds/asymmetrical facial expression may indicate nerve palsy
Cranial nerve VIII, acoustic	With infant lying supine, ring bell sharply within a few inches of infant's ears	Observe for response to sound stimulus, such as mild startle/blink reflex NOTE: Auditory-evoked response required in many states evaluates acoustic nerve function and has replaced rough assessment of acoustic nerve and acoustic blink response to loud clap
Cranial nerve IX, glossopharyngeal	Use tongue blade to apply pressure on mid-tongue area to overcome tongue thrust	Elicit gag reflex; observe tongue movement, strength

TABLE 19-5 CRANIAL NERVE TESTING IN THE NEWBORN AND INFANT—CONT'D

Cranial Nerve	Test	Response
Cranial nerve X, vagus	Observe infant while crying	Evaluate pitch of cry and assess for hoarseness, stridor; normal cry is loud and angry; shrill, penetrating cry indicates intracranial hemorrhage; whiny, high-pitched cry indicates central nervous system dysfunction
Cranial nerve XI, accessory	With infant lying supine, turn infant's head to one side	Infant should work to bring head to midline
Cranial nerve XII, hypoglossal	Observe infant when feeding	Sucking, swallowing should be efficient, coordinated

Data from Thureen PJ, Deacon J, O'Neill P et al: *Assessment and care of the well newborn,* Philadelphia, 1999, Saunders.

Box **19-2** Cranial Nerve Testing in Preschool to School-Age Child

Cranial nerve II, optic
- Allen picture cards, tumbling E, or Snellen chart for visual acuity testing

Cranial nerves III, oculomotor; IV, trochlear; VI, abducens
- Use ophthalmoscope or light source to test direct and consensual pupillary response to light
- With examiner's hand under chin, have child follow toy, light source, or index finger through six cardinal fields of gaze to test eye movement

Cranial nerve V, trigeminal
- Observe child chewing and swallowing to test normal jaw strength
- Touch facial area with cotton swab and observe child move away from stimulus

Cranial nerve VII, facial
- Ask child to smile, frown, and puff cheeks, observe for symmetrical facial expressions

Cranial nerve VIII, acoustic
- Have child repeat words whispered from behind
- Perform audiometric testing to evaluate range of hearing

Cranial nerves IX, glossopharyngeal; X, vagus
- Observe tongue strength and movement and elicit gag reflex with tongue blade

Cranial nerves XI, accessory; XII, hypoglossal
- Have child stick tongue out and shrug shoulders

Deep Tendon Reflexes

The reflex arc of the deep tendon reflexes is a complex function of the musculoskeletal and nervous systems and requires an intact sensory neuron, a functional synapse in the spinal cord, an intact motor neuron, a functional neuromuscular junction, and a competent muscle (Table 19-6) (Figures 19-15 through 19-21).

When performing deep tendon reflexes (DTR) bilaterally, grade the response in the health record as follows:

- 4+: Brisk, hyperactive
- 3+: Active, brisker than normal
- 2+: Normal response
- 1+: Diminished response, low normal
- 0: No response

TABLE 19-6 DEEP TENDON AND SUPERFICIAL REFLEXES

Reflex	Test	Response
Deep Tendon Reflexes		
Biceps reflex	With examiner's thumb pressed against biceps tendon in antecubital space, support arm with palm prone; tap thumb briskly; tendon should respond by tightening	Flexion of forearm
Triceps reflex	Hold arm in flexed position slightly forward toward chest with forearm dangling downward, tap directly behind elbow on triceps tendon	Contraction of triceps and elbow should extend slightly
Brachioradialis reflex	Support child's forearm with palm resting down; tap briskly on radius about 2 inches above wrist	Flexion of elbow and pronation of forearm
Patellar reflex	Palpate patellar tendon just below patella and tap briskly with leg dangling; having child lock fingers and pull hard in outward direction can help elicit reflex	Contraction of quadriceps and extension of knee
Achilles tendon reflex	Support foot with ankle slightly flexed and leg relaxed, tap above heel; vary degree of flexion of foot to assist in eliciting reflex	Observe plantar flexion
Clonus	In infant, knee should be slightly flexed with infant in supine position; apply pressure to sole of foot to bring ankle into dorsiflexion	In newborn, rapid tonic-clonic movement of 4 to 5 beats is normal response; beyond newborn period, no rhythmic movements are expected
Superficial Reflexes		
Plantar reflex	Stroke sole of foot from heel to ball of foot curving medially with flat object	Movement of toes
Abdominal reflex	Stroke briskly above and below umbilicus	Abdominal muscles contract and umbilicus deviates toward the stimulus
Cremasteric reflex	In male, lightly scratch upper inner thigh	Testicle will elevate slightly on stimulated side
Anal reflex	Gently stroke anal area to test sphincter tone	Quick contraction of sphincter

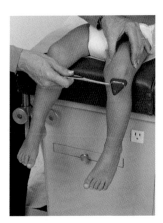

Figure **19-15** Patellar reflex.

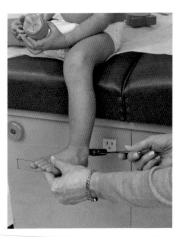

Figure **19-16** Achilles tendon reflex.

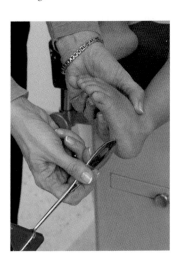

Figure **19-17** Plantar reflex.

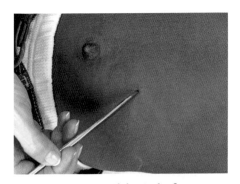

Figure **19-18** Abdominal reflex.

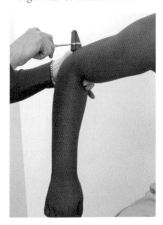

Figure **19-19** Triceps reflex.

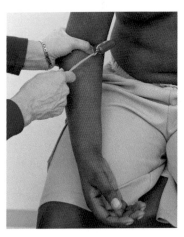

Figure **19-20** Biceps reflex.

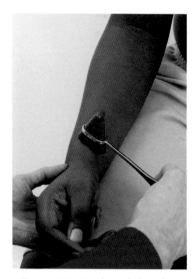

Figure **19-21** Brachioradialis reflex.

Evaluation of Cerebellar Function

Assessment of cerebellar function evaluates balance and coordination. The following tests can be presented as games, which are fun for the school-age child and are effective in assessing cerebellar function:

- **Finger-to-nose test**: With eyes closed, have child touch nose with first finger of one hand then with first finger of the other hand. Then, with eyes open, have child touch nose with first finger and then touch examiner's finger held about 18 inches in front of the child. Repeat with both hands. Then increase speed of movements with examiner's finger changing position. Consistent failure of child to point at the finger indicates dysfunction in spatial perception and coordination.

- **Finger-to-thumb test**: Using one hand, ask the child to touch each finger to the thumb in rapid succession. Repeat with both hands. Coordination can further be tested by asking child to pat knees with the palm of the hand then back of the hand in rapid succession.

Pediatric Pearls

Findings of *motor overflow,* noted when one hand performs a motor task and the other hand mirrors the movement or when mirroring movements of the lower extremities occur, indicate a lag in the normal progression of fine motor development, which may impact the child's learning.

Simple tests to evaluate cerebellar function in the preschooler:

- **Romberg test:** Assesses for balance and equilibrium. This test can be performed in the cooperative preschool child. Ask the child to stand erect with eyes closed and hands touching the sides. Observe the child's balance for several seconds while monitoring the child closely. Lesions in the cerebellum can cause the child to stagger or fall.

- **Tandem walking:** Assesses balance and coordination. Ask the child in the prekindergarten physical exam to walk heel to toe in a straight line. This is a higher order skill often not accomplished until the child is 6 years of age.

- **Hopping in place and heel-toe walking:** Tests cerebellar and intact motor function and spatial sense.

Evaluation of Cerebral Function

In the developing child, cerebral function is more challenging to assess than in adults. Assessing general cerebral function requires evaluating the level of consciousness, mood and affect, thought, memory, judgment, and communication. In the child with head trauma, the basic components of the initial neurological examination include (1) assessment of level of consciousness, (2) brainstem function, (3) pupil reactivity, and (4) motor function. Determining the level of consciousness using an adapted Glasgow Coma Scale (GCS) Score

TABLE 19-7 PEDIATRIC ADAPTATION OF THE GLASGOW COMA SCALE

EYE OPENING

Birth to 1 Year Old	> 1 Year Old	Score
Spontaneously	Spontaneously	4
To loud noise	To verbal command	3
To pain	To pain	2
No response	No response	1

MOTOR RESPONSE

Birth to 1 Year Old	> 1 Year Old	Score
Spontaneous responses	Obeys	6
Localizes pain	Localizes pain	5
Withdrawal to pain	Withdrawal to pain	4
Involuntary flexion	Involuntary flexion	3
Involuntary extension	Involuntary extension	2
No response	No response	1

VERBAL RESPONSE

Birth to 2 Years Old	2 to 5 Years Old	> 5 Years Old	Score
Cries as response, vocalizes	Purposeful words	Oriented and responds	5
Cries	Incoherent words	Disoriented and converses	4
Inappropriate crying	Cries or screams	Inappropriate words	3
Grunts	Grunts	Incomprehensible words	2
No response	No response	No response	1

SEVERITY OF INJURY*

Mild head injury	13-15	
Moderate head injury	9-12	
Severe head injury	<8	

Modified from Barkin RM, Rosen P: *Emergency pediatrics: a guide to ambulatory care,* ed 6, St Louis, 2003, Mosby.
*Calculate total score for age by assessing eye opening, best motor response, and verbal response and assigning a score for each area. Total Glasgow Coma Scale score indicates severity of the head injury.

is an appropriate assessment in the verbal child (Table 19-7). The adapted GCS assesses three major areas: eye opening, which relates to arousal and alertness; verbal ability, which relates to content and mentation; and motor ability, which reflects mentation as well as the functional integrity of the major central nervous system (CNS) pathways. A modified GCS for infants assesses the ability of eye opening (spontaneous, to speech, to pain, none), verbal (coos and babbles appropriately, irritable cries inconsolable, cries or screams persistently to pain, grunts or moans to pain, none), and motor (normal spontaneous movements, withdraws to touch, withdraws to pain, abnormal flexion, abnormal extension, none).

ABNORMAL CONDITIONS

Cerebral Palsy

An alteration in muscular tone is the general description of cerebral palsy, designated as either hypotonic, spastic, or athetoid, causing repetitive involuntary movement. This condition denotes a prenatal or early neonatal hypoxic insult to the developing brain and remains static or unchanged over time. The clinical manifestations, however, change as the central nervous system matures and myelinates. Thus a child who was hypotonic as a newborn may later develop spasticity. The degree is categorized by the limbs affected: hemiparesis—one side; quadriparesis—all four limbs; monoparesis—one limb; or paraparesis—both lower extremities. *Static encephalopathy* is another term for this condition.

Down Syndrome

Infants with Down syndrome have characteristic facies that include upward slanting palpebral fissures, and inner epicanthal folds; simian crease, brachydactyly, abnormal shortening of fingers and toes with wide-spaced first and second toes; hypotonia and macroglossia; and mental retardation. This syndrome occurs in approximately 1/1250 births. The infant is at increased risk for a multitude of medical problems including congenital cardiac defects, duodenal atresia, leukemia, thyroid dysfunction, visual and hearing defects, and obesity. Prompt referral will maximize functioning and provide the parents with a source of expert information and support.

Hypotonia

Hypotonia is a decrease in the normal resting tension in the muscle: it can present in any muscle group and at any age depending on the underlying etiology. It most commonly presents in the newborn period as a floppy infant and can be suspected by observing the infant at rest. When supine, little flexion is seen in the extremities, so arms are often straight at the infant's side and hips are abducted with lower extremities flat on the exam table. Infants with hypotonia will feel limp or floppy to the examiner. When placed in ventral suspension, the infant's head and extremities will hang or drape over the examiner's hand with little attempt to maintain the horizontal position. Hypotonia should be distinguished from decreased strength (paresis) by noting that the hypotonic infant can still actively move all extremities through normal range of motion. Although spontaneous movements may be less frequent, they are present.

Hypotonia can be caused by lesions in the central or peripheral nervous system. Infants and children with a central nervous system etiology often will have history of clues such as prenatal insult (infection, toxin, drug exposure), neonatal hypoxia or seizures, microcephaly or macrocephaly, and preservation of deep tendon reflexes. Those infants and children with a peripheral nervous system etiology often have a family history of muscular or nerve disease and on physical examination will have a loss of deep tendon reflexes.

CHARTING

A Healthy Toddler

Neurological: Alert, active, follows simple directions; gait, balance, and coordination normal for age, DTRs intact +2 bilaterally, muscle strength equal and symmetrical, cranial nerves—not tested today, Denver II normal for age.

DTR, Deep tendon reflexes.

REFERENCES

1. Porth CM: *Pathophysiology: concepts of altered health states,* Philadelphia, 2004, Lippincott.
2. Jarvis C: *Pocket companion for physical examination and health assessment,* ed 4, Philadelphia, 2004, Saunders.
3. Shore R: *Rethinking the brain,* New York, 1997, Families and Work Institute.

COMPREHENSIVE AND SYMPTOM-FOCUSED ASSESSMENT

CHAPTER 20

PEDIATRIC HEALTH VISIT CHARTING

Karen G. Duderstadt

RECORDING THE HEALTHCARE VISIT

Comprehensive assessment of the child or adolescent and accurate charting in the medical record are the hallmarks of professional clinical practice. Documentation of the thorough physical examination in the medical record is as important to the pediatric health visit as the comprehensive assessment, and it is the legal responsibility of every healthcare provider to accurately record all aspects of the healthcare visit. This chapter contains sample charting forms for the comprehensive well child visit, the symptom-focused visit, and the preparticipation sports physical visit to assist the pediatric healthcare provider.

COMPREHENSIVE WELL CHILD VISIT

The comprehensive well child visit is composed of subjective data, which includes all components of the health history, objective data from the physical examination including vital signs and laboratory screening, assessment and/or list of health conditions, anticipatory guidance for activities of daily living, a plan for each health condition, and follow-up with the child and family. Figure 20-1 presents a sample form for charting the comprehensive well child visit. Figure 20-2 presents a form for ongoing or continuity well child care.

SYMPTOM-FOCUSED VISIT

The components of the system-focused visit are the same as the comprehensive well child visit—subjective, objective, assessment, plan, and follow-up. However, the provider gathers information most relevant to a presenting problem or a particular health condition, and conducts a focused physical examination. Figure 20-3 presents a sample form for charting the system-focused visit.

PREPARTICIPATION SPORTS PHYSICAL VISIT

The preparticipation sports physical visit is the opportunity for the pediatric health provider to match the athlete to the appropriate type and level of sport, and to help prevent injury to the young athlete. The sports physical is often the healthy adolescent's only regular contact with the healthcare provider; therefore, the encounter should incorporate regular health maintenance, a confidential psychosocial screening, and a thorough physical examination, including cardiac and musculoskeletal evaluation. Figure 20-4 is a sample charting form for the preparticipation sports physical visit.

SUBJECTIVE DATA

Informant: _____ Relationship to patient: self / parent / other (Circle one)

Verify family contact information

Address: _____

Daytime Tel: _____ Evening Tel: _____ Cell Tel: _____

I. HEALTH HISTORY

A. Present Concern(s):_____

B. Child Profile
   Birth date: _____ Age: _____ Birthplace: _____
   (month/day/year)

Date of last well child visit: _____

Previous health care provider: _____ Tel: _____

Past Medical History:

Prenatal: _____

Birth & neonatal history: _____

Childhood conditions: _____

Chronic conditions: _____

Hospitalizations: _____

Unintentional injuries: _____

Intentional injuries: _____

Allergies: _____

Current medications: _____

Immunizations: _____

Lab tests—lead/hgb/hct/STI* screen: _____

Sexual History: _____

Activities of Daily Living

Nutrition/feeding: _____

Elimination: _____

Sleep: _____

Dentition/dental care: _____

School

Daycare? Yes / No   If yes, what hours/length?_____

After-school programs/care? Yes / No If yes, what hours/length?_____

Sports/Interests/Activities: _____

Safety: _____

Development

Personal-social: _____

Language: _____

Fine motor: _____

Figure 20-1 Comprehensive well child visit—initial visit form.

Gross motor: _____

Sexual development: _____

Temperament type (practitioner observation): _____

            As noted by parent? _____

Discipline method: _____

Health habits (TV/Screen hrs/day): _____

Adolescent HEADSSSVG* Assessment: _____

_____

C. Family Profile/Social History

Genetic Family History:

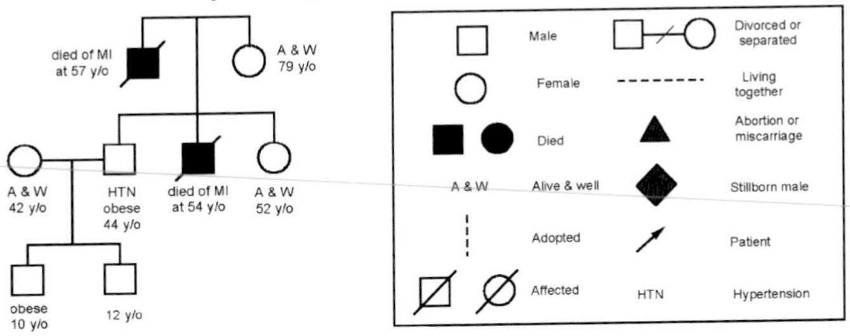

Age and Health Status of Members:

Familial health conditions: _____

Current health risks (HTN*, diabetes, obesity): _____

Parental employment _____

Home situation: _____

Cultural Assessment

Support system: _____

Environmental health history: _____

D. Review of Systems: _____

OBJECTIVE DATA

II. PHYSICAL EXAMINATION

Height: _____ Weight: _____ Temperature: _____

Respiration: _____ Heart Rate: _____ Blood Pressure: _____

H.C.: _____ BMI*: _____

General Appearance and Parent-Child Interaction

Skin: _____

Head: _____ Face: _____

Eyes: _____ Ears: _____

Nose: _____ Mouth/Throat: _____ Neck: _____

Chest and Lungs: _____ Breast: _____

Heart: _____ Abdomen: _____

Genitalia: _____ Rectum/Anus: _____

Musculoskeletal: _____ Neurological (CNs,* DTRs*): _____

Figure **20-1** Cont'd

Continued

III. DEVELOPMENTAL TESTS: _____

IV. LABORATORY TESTS: _____

ASSESSMENT
V. HEALTH ASSESSMENT & ACUTE/CHRONIC HEALTH CONDITIONS
Plan
#1 Health Maintenance

Immunization: _____

Nutrition: _____

Growth & Development: _____

Safety: _____

Follow-up: _____

Problem list
Problem #2: _____

Diagnostic/Consultation

Therapeutic: _____

Patient Education: _____

Follow-up: _____

Problem #3: _____

Diagnostic/Consultation: _____

Therapeutic: _____

Patient Education: _____

Follow-up: _____

Provider Signature: _____ Date: _____

*STIs, Sexually transmitted infections; HEADSSSVG for preadolescent & adolescent (Home, Environment/school, Activities—sports, Drug use/exposure, Sexual activity, Safety, Suicidal ideation/depression, Violence witnessed, Gang activity/exposure); HTN, hypertension; BMI, body mass index; CNs, cranial nerves; DTRs, deep tendon reflexes.

Figure **20-1** Cont'd

SUBJECTIVE DATA

Informant: _____ **Relationship to patient:** self / parent / other (Circle one)

Verify family contact information

Address: _____

Daytime Tel: _____ Evening Tel: _____ Cell Tel: _____

I. HEALTH HISTORY

  A. Present Concern(s): _____

  B. Child Profile (since last visit)

    Past Medical History:

      Illness or injury since last visit: _____

      Current medications: _____

      Allergies: _____

      Immunizations: _____

      Lab tests—lead/hgb/hct/STI* screen: _____

    Sexual History/Sexual Debut: _____

    Activities of Daily Living

      Nutrition/feeding: _____

      Elimination: _____

      Sleep: _____

      Dentition/dental care: _____

    Safety Practices: _____

    Changes in Daycare/School/After-School Care: _____

    Sports/Physical Activity: _____

    Developmental History: _____

      Health habits (TV/Screen hrs/day): _____

      Discipline method: _____

    Adolescent HEADSSSVG Assessment:* _____

  C. Family Profile/Social History (since last visit)

    Parental employment: _____

    Home situation: _____

    Support system: _____

  D. Review of Systems: _____

OBJECTIVE DATA

II. PHYSICAL EXAMINATION

  Height: _____ Weight: _____ H.C.:_____ BMI: _____Temperature: _____

  Respiration: _____ Heart Rate: _____ Blood Pressure: _____

Figure 20-2 Well-child continuity visit form.

Continued

General Appearance and Parent-Child Interaction

Skin: _____

Head: _____ Face: _____

Eyes: _____ Ears: _____

Nose: _____ Mouth/Throat: _____ Neck: _____

Chest and Lungs: _____ Breast: _____

Heart: _____ Abdomen: _____

Genitalia: _____ Rectum/Anus: _____

Musculoskeletal: _____ Neurological (CNs,* DTRs*): _____

III. Developmental Tests: _____

IV. Laboratory Tests: _____

ASSESSMENT

V. Health Assessment & Acute/Chronic Health Conditions

Plan: *#1 Health Maintenance*

Immunization: _____

Nutrition: _____

Growth & Development: _____

Dental Care: _____

Safety: _____

Follow-up: _____

Problem list

Problem #2: _____

Diagnostic/Consultation: _____

Therapeutic: _____

Patient Education: _____

Follow-up: _____

Problem #3: _____

Diagnostic/Consultation: _____

Therapeutic: _____

Patient Education: _____

Follow-up: _____

Provider Signature: _____ Date: _____

*STIs, Sexually transmitted infections; *HEADSSSVG* for preadolescent & adolescent (Home, Environment/school, Activities—sports, Drug use/exposure, Sexual activity, Safety, Suicidal ideation/depression, Violence witnessed, Gang activity/exposure); *HTN*, hypertension; *BMI*, body mass index; *CNs*, cranial nerves; *DTRs*, deep tendon reflexes.

Figure **20-2** Cont'd

SUBJECTIVE DATA

Informant: _____ **Relationship to patient:** self / parent / other (Circle one)

Verify child's age: _____

Verify phone: Daytime Tel: _____ Evening Tel: _____ Cell Tel: _____

I. HEALTH HISTORY

  A. **Present Concern(s):** _____

_____

  B. **History of Present Illness**

    Home management/medications (dosage, time, date):_____

    Exposures: _____

    Pertinent family medical history: _____

  C. **Relevant Past Medical History:** _____

  D. **Relevant Review of Systems:** _____

OBJECTIVE DATA

II. PHYSICAL EXAMINATION

Height: ____ Weight: ___ Temperature: ___Respiration: ____ Heart Rate: ____ BP: ____

  General Appearance and Parent-Child Interaction

    Skin: _____ Face: _____

    Head: _____ Eyes: _____ Ears: _____

    Nose: _____ Mouth/Throat: _____ Neck: _____

    Chest & Lungs: _____ Breast: _____ Heart: _____

    Abdomen: _____ Genitalia: _____Rectum/Anus: _____

    Musculoskeletal: _____ Neurological (CNs,* DTRs*): _____Lab Tests: ____

III. ASSESSMENT: _____

IV. PLAN

#1 Health Maintenance: next well child visit: _____ Immunization update: _____

Problem list: *Problem #2:* _____

    Diagnostic/Consultation: _____

    Therapeutic: _____

    Patient Education: _____

    Follow-up: _____

  *Problem #3:*_____

    Diagnostic/Consultation: _____

    Therapeutic: _____

    Patient Education: _____

    Follow-up: _____

Provider Signature: _____ Date: _____

*CNs, Cranial nerves; *DTRs,* deep tendon reflexes.

Figure **20-3** Symptom-focused visit form.

Preparticipation Physical Evaluation

HISTORY FORM

Date of Exam _____

Name _____ Sex_____ Age_____ Date of birth_____

Grade_____ School_____ Sport(s)_____

Address_____ Phone_____

Personal Physician _____

In case of emergency, contact:

Name _____ Relationship_____ Phone (H)_____ Phone(W)_____

Explain "Yes" answers below.
Circle questions you don't know the answers to.

	Yes	No
1. Has a doctor ever denied or restricted your participation in sports for any reason?	☐	☐
2. Do you have an ongoing medical condition (like diabetes or asthma)?	☐	☐
3. Are you currently taking any prescription or nonprescription (over-the-counter) medicines or pills?	☐	☐
4. Do you have allergies to medicines, pollens, foods, or stinging insects?	☐	☐
5. Have you ever passed out or nearly passed out DURING exercise?	☐	☐
6. Have you ever passed out or nearly passed out AFTER exercise?	☐	☐
7. Have you ever had discomfort, pain, or pressure in your chest during exercise?	☐	☐
8. Does your heart race or skip beats during exercise?	☐	☐

9. Has a doctor ever told you that you have (check all that apply):
☐ High blood pressure   ☐ A heart murmur
☐ High cholesterol   ☐ A heart infection

	Yes	No
10. Has a doctor ever ordered a test for your heart? (for example: ECG, echocardiogram)	☐	☐
11. Has anyone in your family died for no apparent reason?	☐	☐
12. Does anyone in your family have a heart problem?	☐	☐
13. Has any family member or relative died of heart problems or of sudden death before age 50?	☐	☐
14. Does anyone in your family have Marfan syndrome?	☐	☐
15. Have you ever spent the night in a hospital?	☐	☐
16. Have you ever had surgery?	☐	☐
17. Have you ever had an injury, like a sprain, muscle or ligament tear, or tendinitis, that caused you to miss a practice or game? If yes, circle affected area below:	☐	☐
18. Have you had any broken or fractured bones or dislocated joints? If yes, circle below:	☐	☐
19. Have you had a bone or joint injury that required x-rays, MRI, CT, surgery, injections, rehabilitation, physical therapy, a brace, a cast, or crutches? If yes, circle below:	☐	☐

Head	Neck	Shoulder	Upper Arm	Elbow	Forearm	Hand/ Fingers	Chest
Upper Back	Lower Back	Hip	Thigh	Knee	Calf/ Shin	Ankle	Foot/ Toes

	Yes	No
20. Have you ever had a stress fracture?	☐	☐
21. Have you been told that you have or have you had an x-ray for atlantoaxial (neck) instability?	☐	☐
22. Do you regularly use a brace or assistive device?	☐	☐
23. Has a doctor ever told you that you have asthma or allergies?	☐	☐

	Yes	No
24. Do you cough, wheeze, or have difficulty breathing during or after exercise?	☐	☐
25. Is there anyone in your family who has asthma?	☐	☐
26. Have you ever used an inhaler or taken asthma medicine?	☐	☐
27. Were you born without or are you missing a kidney, an eye, a testicle, or any other organ?	☐	☐
28. Have you had infectious mononucleosis (mono) within the last month?	☐	☐
29. Do you have any rashes, pressure sores, or other skin problems?	☐	☐
30. Have you had a herpes skin infection?	☐	☐
31. Have you ever had a head injury or concussion?	☐	☐
32. Have you been hit in the head and been confused or lost your memory?	☐	☐
33. Have you ever had a seizure?	☐	☐
34. Do you have headaches with exercise?	☐	☐
35. Have you ever had numbness, tingling, or weakness in your arms or legs after being hit or falling?	☐	☐
36. Have you ever been unable to move your arms or legs after being hit or falling?	☐	☐
37. When exercising in the heat, do you have severe muscle cramps or become ill?	☐	☐
38. Has a doctor told you that you or someone in your family has sickle cell trait or sickle cell disease?	☐	☐
39. Have you had any problems with your eyes or vision?	☐	☐
40. Do you wear glasses or contact lenses?	☐	☐
41. Do you wear protective eyewear, such as goggles or a face shield?	☐	☐
42. Are you happy with your weight?	☐	☐
43. Are you trying to gain or lose weight?	☐	☐
44. Has anyone recommended you change your weight or eating habits?	☐	☐
45. Do you limit or carefully control what you eat?	☐	☐
46. Do you have any concerns that you would like to discuss with a doctor?	☐	☐

FEMALES ONLY

	Yes	No
47. Have you ever had a menstrual period?	☐	☐

48. How old were you when you had your first menstrual period? _____
49. How many periods have you had in the last 12 months?_____

Explain "Yes" answers here: _____
_____
_____
_____
_____
_____

I hereby state that, to the best of my knowledge, my answers to the above questions are complete and correct.

Signature of Athlete_____ Signature of Parent/Guardian_____ Date_____

©2004 American Academy of Family Physicians, American Academy of Pediatrics, American College of Sports Medicine, American Medical Society for Sports Medicine, American Orthopaedic Society for Sports Medicine, and American Osteopathic Academy of Sports Medicine.

Figure **20-4** Preparticipation sports physical examination form.

Preparticipation Physical Evaluation | PHYSICAL EXAMINATION FORM

Name _____Date of Birth_____

Height_____Weight_____% Body Fat (optional)_____Pulse_____BP____ / ____ (____ / ____, ____/____)

Vision R 20/_____ L 20/_____   Corrected: Y N   Pupils: Equal _____   Unequal_____

Follow-Up Questions on More Sensitive Issues   **Yes No**
1. Do you feel stressed out or under a lot of pressure?   ❑   ❑
2. Do you ever feel so sad or hopeless that you stop doing some of your usual activities for more than a few days? ❑   ❑
3. Do you feel safe?   ❑   ❑
4. Have you ever tried cigarette smoking, even 1 or 2 puffs? Do you currently smoke?   ❑   ❑
5. During the past 30 days, did you use chewing tobacco, snuff, or dip?   ❑   ❑
6. During the past 30 days, have you had at least 1 drink of alcohol?   ❑   ❑
7. Have you ever taken steroid pills or shots without a doctor's prescription?   ❑   ❑
8. Have you ever taken any supplements to help you gain or lose weight to improve your performance?   ❑   ❑
9. Questions from the Youth Risk Behavior Survey (http://www.cdc.gov/Healthy Youth/yrbs/index.htm)
   on guns, seatbelts, unprotected sex, domestic violence, drugs, etc.   ❑   ❑
Notes: _____

	NORMAL	ABNORMAL FINDINGS	INITIALS*
MEDICAL			
Appearance			
Eyes/ears/nose/throat			
Hearing			
Lymph nodes			
Heart			
Murmurs			
Pulses			
Lungs			
Abdomen			
Genitourinary (males only)£			
Skin			
MUSCULOSKELETAL			
Neck			
Back			
Shoulder/arm			
Elbow/forearm			
Wrist/hand/fingers			
Hip/thigh			
Knee			
Leg/ankle			
Foot/toes			

*Multiple-examiner set-up only.
£Having a third party present is recommended for the genitourinary examination.

Notes: _____

Name of physician (print/type)_____Date_____

Address_____Phone_____

Signature of physician _____, MD or DO

©2004 American Academy of Family Physicians, American Academy of Pediatrics, American College of Sports Medicine, American Medical Society for Sports Medicine, American Orthopaedic Society for Sports Medicine, and American Osteopathic Academy of Sports Medicine.

Figure **20-4** Cont'd

Continued

Preparticipation Physical Evaluation

CLEARANCE FORM

Name_____Sex_____Age_____Date of birth_____

☐ Cleared without restriction
☐ Cleared, with recommendations for further evaluation or treatment for:_____
_____
_____
_____

☐ Not cleared for ☐ All sports ☐ Certain sports: _____   Reason:_____

Recommendations:_____
_____

EMERGENCY INFORMATION
Allergies _____

Other Information _____

IMMUNIZATIONS (eg, tetanus/diphtheria; measles, mumps, rubella; hepatitis A, B; influenza; poliomyelitis;
pneumococcal; meningococcal; varicella)

☐ Up to date (see attached documentation)   ☐ Not up to date (Specify) _____

Name of physician (print/type) _____Date _____

Address _____Phone _____

Signature of physician _____, MD or DO

© 2004 American Academy of Family Physicians, American Academy of Pediatrics, American College of Sports Medicine, American Medical Society for Sports Medicine, American Orthopaedic Society for Sports Medicine, and American Osteopathic Academy of Sports Medicine.

- -

Preparticipation Physical Evaluation

CLEARANCE FORM

Name_____Sex_____Age_____Date of birth_____

☐ Cleared without restriction
☐ Cleared, with recommendations for further evaluation or treatment for:_____
_____
_____
_____

☐ Not cleared for ☐ All sports ☐ Certain sports: _____   Reason:_____

Recommendations:_____
_____

EMERGENCY INFORMATION
Allergies _____

Other Information _____

IMMUNIZATIONS (eg, tetanus/diphtheria; measles, mumps, rubella; hepatitis A, B; influenza; poliomyelitis;
pneumococcal; meningococcal; varicella)

☐ Up to date (see attached documentation)   ☐ Not up to date (Specify) _____

Name of physician (print/type) _____Date _____

Address _____Phone _____

Signature of physician _____, MD or DO

© 2004 American Academy of Family Physicians, American Academy of Pediatrics, American College of Sports Medicine, American Medical Society for Sports Medicine, American Orthopaedic Society for Sports Medicine, and American Osteopathic Academy of Sports Medicine.

Figure **20-4** Cont'd

GROWTH AND BMI
CHARTS

Birth to 36 months: Boys
Length-for-age and Weight-for-age percentiles

NAME _____

RECORD# _____

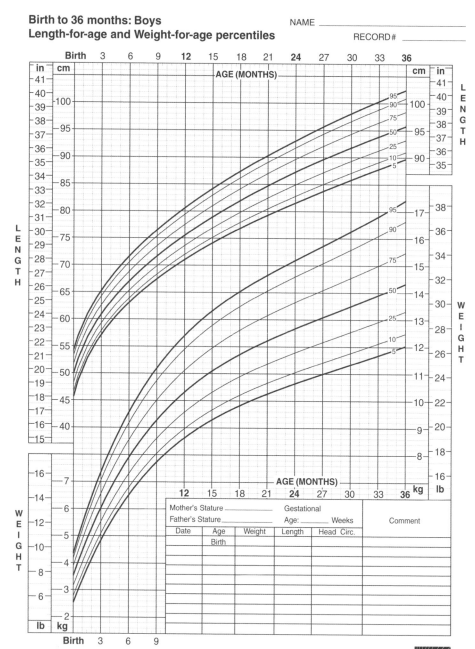

Published May 30, 2000 (modified 4/20/01).
SOURCE: Developed by the National Center for Health Statistics in collaboration with
the National Center for Chronic Disease Prevention and Health Promotion (2000).
http://www.cdc.gov/growthcharts

SAFER·HEALTHIER·PEOPLE™

Birth to 36 months: Girls
Length-for-age and Weight-for-age percentiles

NAME _____

RECORD# _____

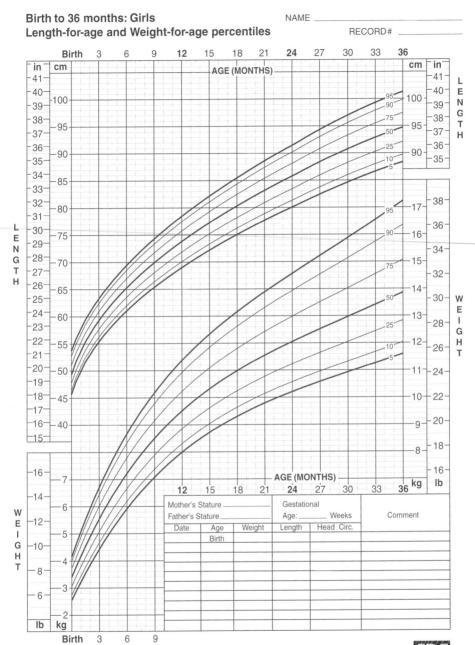

Published May 30, 2000 (modified 4/20/01).
SOURCE: Developed by the National Center for Health Statistics in collaboration with
the National Center for Chronic Disease Prevention and Health Promotion (2000).
http://www.cdc.gov/growthcharts

SAFER · HEALTHIER · PEOPLE™

Birth to 36 months: Boys
Head circumference-for-age and
Weight-for-length percentiles

NAME _____

RECORD# _____

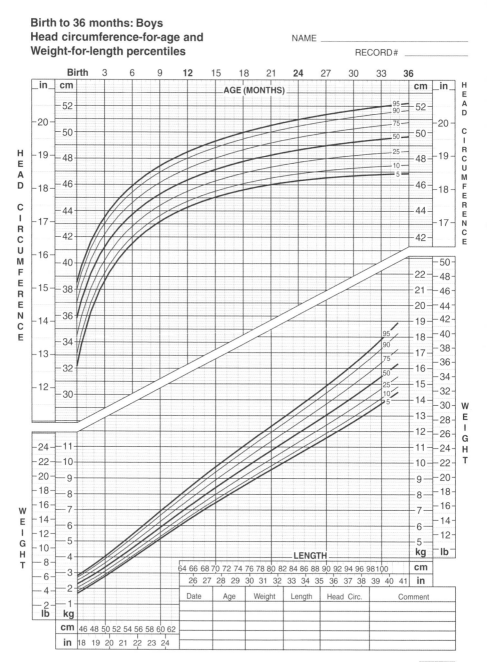

Published May 30, 2000 (modified 10/16/00).
SOURCE: Developed by the National Center for Health Statistics in collaboration with
the National Center for Chronic Disease Prevention and Health Promotion (2000).
http://www.cdc.gov/growthcharts

SAFER·HEALTHIER·PEOPLE™

Birth to 36 months: Girls
Head circumference-for-age and Weight-for-length percentiles

NAME _____

RECORD# _____

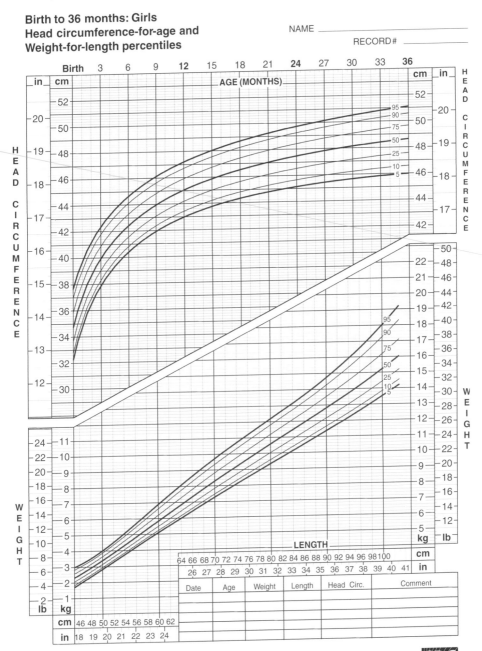

Published May 30, 2000 (modified 10/16/00).
SOURCE: Developed by the National Center for Health Statistics in collaboration with the National Center for Chronic Disease Prevention and Health Promotion (2000).
http://www.cdc.gov/growthcharts

SAFER·HEALTHIER·PEOPLE™

2 to 20 years: Boys
Stature-for-age and Weight-for-age percentiles

NAME _____

RECORD# _____

Mother's Stature		Father's Stature		
Date	Age	Weight	Stature	BMI*

*To Calculate BMI: Weight (kg) ÷ Stature (cm) ÷ Stature (cm) x 10,000
or Weight (lb) ÷ Stature (in) ÷ Stature (in) x 703

AGE (YEARS)

AGE (YEARS)

STATURE

WEIGHT

Published May 30, 2000 (modified 11/21/00).
SOURCE: Developed by the National Center for Health Statistics in collaboration with
the National Center for Chronic Disease Prevention and Health Promotion (2000).
http://www.cdc.gov/growthcharts

SAFER·HEALTHIER·PEOPLE™

2 to 20 years: Girls
Stature-for-age and Weight-for-age percentiles

NAME _____

RECORD# _____

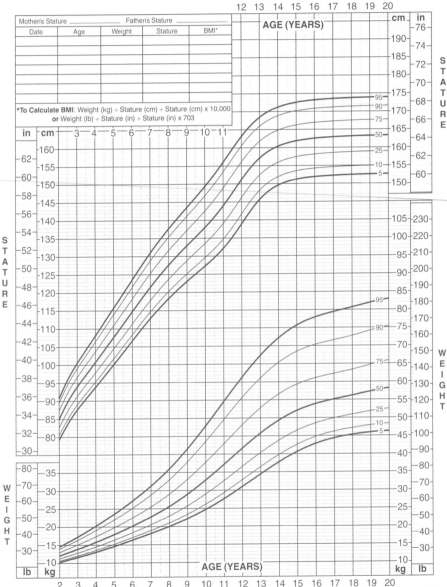

Published May 30, 2000 (modified 11/21/00).
SOURCE: Developed by the National Center for Health Statistics in collaboration with
the National Center for Chronic Disease Prevention and Health Promotion (2000).
http://www.cdc.gov/growthcharts

SAFER·HEALTHIER·PEOPLE™

2 to 20 years: Boys
Body mass index-for-age percentiles

NAME _____

RECORD# _____

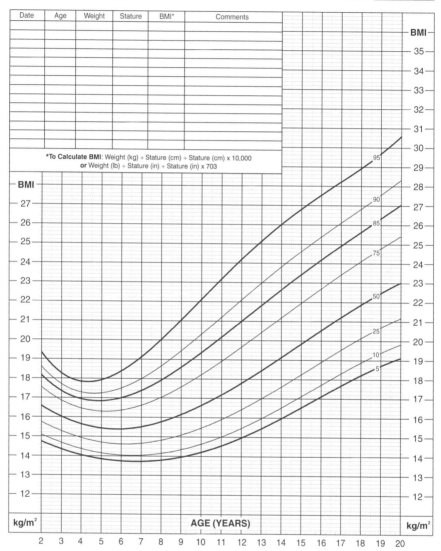

Date	Age	Weight	Stature	BMI*	Comments

*To Calculate BMI: Weight (kg) ÷ Stature (cm) ÷ Stature (cm) x 10,000
or Weight (lb) ÷ Stature (in) ÷ Stature (in) x 703

Published May 30, 2000 (modified 10/16/00).
SOURCE: Developed by the National Center for Health Statistics in collaboration with
the National Center for Chronic Disease Prevention and Health Promotion (2000).
http://www.cdc.gov/growthcharts

SAFER·HEALTHIER·PEOPLE™

2 to 20 years: Girls
Body mass index-for-age percentiles

NAME _____

RECORD# _____

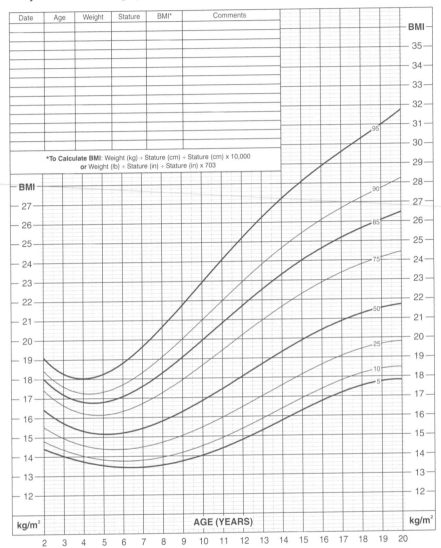

*To Calculate BMI: Weight (kg) ÷ Stature (cm) ÷ Stature (cm) x 10,000
or Weight (lb) ÷ Stature (in) ÷ Stature (in) x 703

AGE (YEARS)

Published May 30, 2000 (modified 10/16/00).
SOURCE: Developed by the National Center for Health Statistics in collaboration with
the National Center for Chronic Disease Prevention and Health Promotion (2000).
http://www.cdc.gov/growthcharts

SAFER · HEALTHIER · PEOPLE™

Weight-for-stature percentiles: Boys

NAME _____

RECORD # _____

Date	Age	Weight	Stature	Comments

STATURE

cm	80	85	90	95	100	105	110	115	120

| in | 31 | 32 | 33 | 34 | 35 | 36 | 37 | 38 | 39 | 40 | 41 | 42 | 43 | 44 | 45 | 46 | 47 |

Published May 30, 2000 (modified 10/16/00).
SOURCE: Developed by the National Center for Health Statistics in collaboration with
the National Center for Chronic Disease Prevention and Health Promotion (2000).
http://www.cdc.gov/growthcharts

SAFER · HEALTHIER · PEOPLE™

Weight-for-stature percentiles: Girls

NAME _____

RECORD# _____

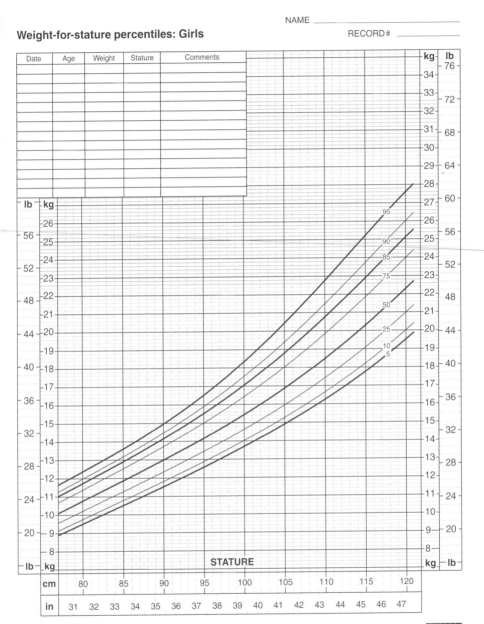

Date	Age	Weight	Stature	Comments

STATURE

cm	80	85	90	95	100	105	110	115	120
in	31	32	33	34	35	36	37	38	39	40	41	42	43	44	45	46	47

Published May 30, 2000 (modified 10/16/00).
SOURCE: Developed by the National Center for Health Statistics in collaboration with
the National Center for Chronic Disease Prevention and Health Promotion (2000).
http://www.cdc.gov/growthcharts

SAFER · HEALTHIER · PEOPLE™

FOOD PYRAMID

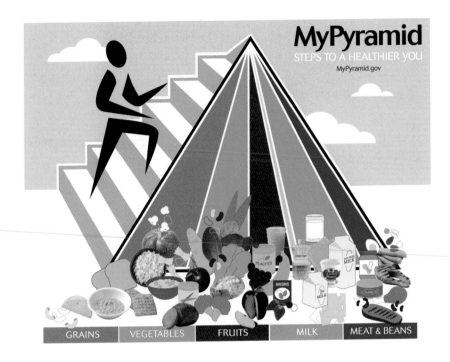

MyPyramid
STEPS TO A HEALTHIER YOU
MyPyramid.gov

| GRAINS | VEGETABLES | FRUITS | MILK | MEAT & BEANS |

GRAINS	VEGETABLES	FRUITS	MILK	MEAT & BEANS
Make half your grains whole	Vary your veggies	Focus on fruits	Get your calcium-rich foods	Go lean with protein
Eat at least 3 oz. of whole-grain cereals, breads, crackers, rice, or pasta every day	Eat more dark-green veggies like broccoli, spinach, and other dark leafy greens	Eat a variety of fruit	Go low-fat or fat-free when you choose milk, yogurt, and other milk products	Choose low-fat or lean meats and poultry
		Choose fresh, frozen, canned, or dried fruit		Bake it, broil it, or grill it
1 oz. is about 1 slice of bread, about 1 cup of breakfast cereal, or ½ cup of cooked rice, cereal, or pasta	Eat more orange vegetables like carrots and sweetpotatoes	Go easy on fruit juices	If you don't or can't consume milk, choose lactose-free products or other calcium sources such as fortified foods and beverages	Vary your protein routine -- choose more fish, beans, peas, nuts, and seeds
	Eat more dry beans and peas like pinto beans, kidney beans, and lentils			

For a 2,000-calorie diet, you need the amounts below from each food group. To find the amounts that are right for you, go to MyPyramid.gov.

| Eat 6 oz. every day | Eat 2½ cups every day | Eat 2 cups every day | Get 3 cups every day; for kids aged 2 to 8, it's 2 | Eat 5½ oz. every day |

Find your balance between food and physical activity
- Be sure to stay within your daily calorie needs.
- Be physically active for at least 30 minutes most days of the week.
- About 60 minutes a day of physical activity may be needed to prevent weight gain.
- For sustaining weight loss, at least 60 to 90 minutes a day of physical activity may be required.
- Children and teenagers should be physically active for 60 minutes every day, or most days.

Know the limits on fats, sugars, and salt (sodium)
- Make most of your fat sources from fish, nuts, and vegetable oils.
- Limit solid fats like butter, stick margarine, shortening, and lard, as well as foods that contain these.
- Check the Nutrition Facts label to keep saturated fats, *trans* fats, and sodium low.
- Choose food and beverages low in added sugars. Added sugars contribute calories with few, if any, nutrients.

MyPyramid.gov
STEPS TO A HEALTHIER YOU

U.S. Department of Agriculture
Center for Nutrition Policy and Promotion
April 2005
CNPP-15

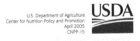

USDA

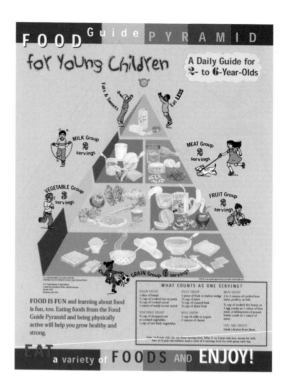

PLAN FOR YOUR YOUNG CHILD... The Pyramid Way

Use this chart to get an idea of the foods your child eats over a week. Pencil in the foods eaten each day and pencil in the corresponding triangular shape. (For example, if a slice of toast is eaten at breakfast, write in "toast" and fill in one Grain group pyramid.) The number of pyramids shown for each food group is the number of servings to be eaten each day. At the end of the week, if you see only a few blank pyramids...keep up the good work. If you notice several blank pyramids, offer foods from the missing food groups in the days to come.

	SUNDAY	MONDAY	TUESDAY	WEDNESDAY	THURSDAY	FRIDAY	SATURDAY
Milk	△△	△△	△△	△△	△△	△△	△△
Meat	△△	△△	△△	△△	△△	△△	△△
Vegetable	△△△	△△△	△△△	△△△	△△△	△△△	△△△
Fruit	△△	△△	△△	△△	△△	△△	△△
Grain	△△△	△△△	△△△	△△△	△△△	△△△	△△△
	△△△	△△△	△△△	△△△	△△△	△△△	△△△
Breakfast							
Snack							
Lunch							
Snack							
Dinner							

DENVER II DEVELOPMENTAL SCREENING TOOL

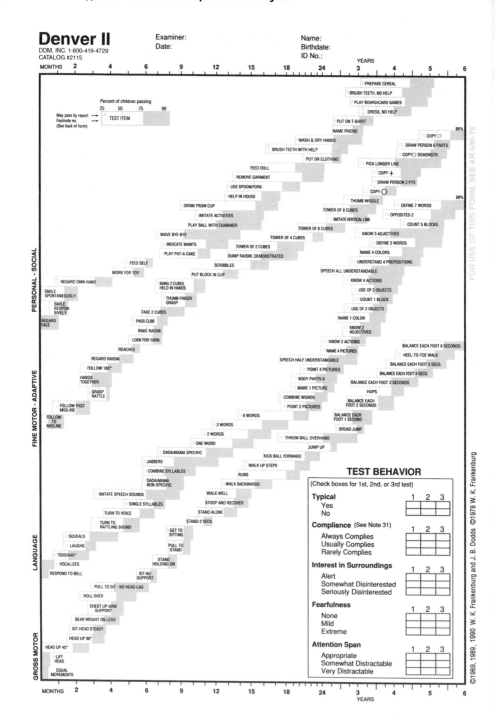

DIRECTIONS FOR ADMINISTRATION

1. Try to get child to smile by smiling, talking or waving. Do not touch him/her.
2. Child must stare at hand several seconds.
3. Parent may help guide toothbrush and put toothpaste on brush.
4. Child does not have to be able to tie shoes or button/zip in the back.
5. Move yarn slowly in an arc from one side to the other, about 8" above child's face.
6. Pass if child grasps rattle when it is touched to the backs or tips of fingers.
7. Pass if child tries to see where yarn went. Yarn should be dropped quickly from sight from tester's hand without arm movement.
8. Child must transfer cube from hand to hand without help of body, mouth, or table.
9. Pass if child picks up raisin with any part of thumb and finger.
10. Line can vary only 30 degrees or less from tester's line. |/
11. Make a fist with thumb pointing upward and wiggle only the thumb. Pass if child imitates and does not move any fingers other than the thumb.

12. Pass any enclosed form. Fail continuous round motions.

13. Which line is longer? (Not bigger.) Turn paper upside down and repeat. (pass 3 of 3 or 5 of 6)

14. Pass any lines crossing near midpoint.

15. Have child copy first. If failed, demonstrate.

When giving items 12, 14, and 15, do not name the forms. Do not demonstrate 12 and 14.

16. When scoring, each pair (2 arms, 2 legs, etc.) counts as one part.
17. Place one cube in cup and shake gently near child's ear, but out of sight. Repeat for other ear.
18. Point to picture and have child name it. (No credit is given for sounds only.)
    If less than 4 pictures are named correctly, have child point to picture as each is named by tester.

19. Using doll, tell child: Show me the nose, eyes, ears, mouth, hands, feet, tummy, hair. Pass 6 of 8.
20. Using pictures, ask child: Which one flies?... says meow?... talks?... barks?... gallops? Pass 2 of 5, 4 of 5.
21. Ask child: What do you do when you are cold?... tired?... hungry? Pass 2 of 3, 3 of 3.
22. Ask child: What do you do with a cup? What is a chair used for? What is a pencil used for? Action words must be included in answers.
23. Pass if child correctly places <u>and</u> says how many blocks are on paper. (1, 5).
24. Tell child: Put block **on** table; **under** table; **in front of** me, **behind** me. Pass 4 of 4. (Do not help child by pointing, moving head or eyes.)
25. Ask child: What is a ball?... lake?... desk?... house?... banana?... curtain?... fence?... ceiling? Pass if defined in terms of use, shape, what it is made of, or general category (such as banana is fruit, not just yellow). Pass 5 of 8, 7 of 8.
26. Ask child: If a horse is big, a mouse is __? If fire is hot, ice is __? If the sun shines during the day, the moon shines during the __? Pass 2 of 3.
27. Child may use wall or rail only, not person. May not crawl.
28. Child must throw ball overhand 3 feet to within arm's reach of tester.
29. Child must perform standing broad jump over width of test sheet (8 1/2 inches).
30. Tell child to walk forward, ⊂◯⊃⊂◯⊃⊂◯⊃→ heel within 1 inch of toe. Tester may demonstrate. Child must walk 4 consecutive steps.
31. In the second year, half of normal children are non-compliant.

OBSERVATIONS:

PEDIATRIC SYMPTOM CHECKLIST

PEDIATRIC SYMPTOM CHECKLIST

Please mark under the heading that best fits your child:

	NEVER	SOMETIMES	OFTEN
1. Complains of aches or pains	☐	☐	☐
2. Spends more time alone	☐	☐	☐
3. Tires easily, little energy	☐	☐	☐
4. Fidgety, unable to sit still	☐	☐	☐
5. Has trouble with a teacher	☐	☐	☐
6. Less interested in school	☐	☐	☐
7. Acts as if driven by a motor	☐	☐	☐
8. Daydreams too much	☐	☐	☐
9. Distracted easily	☐	☐	☐
10. Is afraid of new situations	☐	☐	☐
11. Feels sad, unhappy	☐	☐	☐
12. Is irritable, angry	☐	☐	☐
13. Feels hopeless	☐	☐	☐
14. Has trouble concentrating	☐	☐	☐
15. Less interest in friends	☐	☐	☐
16. Fights with other children	☐	☐	☐
17. Absent from school	☐	☐	☐
18. School grades dropping	☐	☐	☐
19. Is down on him or herself	☐	☐	☐
20. Visits doctor with doctor finding nothing wrong	☐	☐	☐
21. Has trouble sleeping	☐	☐	☐
22. Worries a lot	☐	☐	☐
23. Wants to be with you more than before	☐	☐	☐
24. Feels he or she is bad	☐	☐	☐
25. Takes unnecessary risks	☐	☐	☐
26. Gets hurt frequently	☐	☐	☐
27. Seems to be having less fun	☐	☐	☐
28. Acts younger than children his or her age	☐	☐	☐
29. Does not listen to rules	☐	☐	☐
30. Does not show feelings	☐	☐	☐
31. Does not understand other people's feelings	☐	☐	☐
32. Teases others	☐	☐	☐
33. Blames others for his or her troubles	☐	☐	☐
34. Takes things that do not belong to him or her	☐	☐	☐
35. Refuses to share	☐	☐	☐

Procedures and Scoring criteria for the Pediatric Symptom's Checklist (PSC)

For children 4 and 5 years of age, responses to items 5,6,17, and 18 are not counted due to their emphasis on school issues which may not be relevant.

A value of 0 is assigned to "never," 1 to "sometimes," and 2 to "often." Add these values to obain a score for the entire test.

The presence of significant behavioral or emotional difficulties is suggested when children ages 4–5 years receive 24 or more points, and when children 6–16 years receive 28 or more points.

To determine what kinds of mental health problems are present, determine the three factor scores on the PSC:

PSC Attention Subscale consists of these five items.

4. Fidgety, unable to sit still

8. Daydream Too Much

9. Distracted Easily

14. Has Trouble Concentrating

7. Acts As If Driven By Motor

Children who receive 7 or more points on these five items need a work up for attention deficit hyperactivity disorder. The American Academy of Pediatrics recently revised its recommendations on how to diagnosis ADHD, and the article is in the May 2000 issue of *Pediatrics*—a must read.

PSC Internalizing Subscale consists of these five items:

11. Feel Sad

13. Feel Hopeless

19. Is Down On Self

22. Worries A Lot

27. Seem To Have Less Fun

It is a screen for depression and anxiety. Children who receive 5 or more points on these five items need to be referred for counseling and may eventually need to be considered for anti-depressives, anxiolytics etc.

PSC Externalizing Factor consists of these seven items:

16. Fights With Other Children

29. Does Not Listen To Rules

31. Does Not Understand Others Feelings

32. Teases Others

33. Blames Others for his troubles

35. Refuse To Share

34. Take things that do not belong to him or her

It is a screen for conduct disorder, oppositional defiant disorder, rage disorder, etc. Children who receive 7 or more points on these seven items need behavioral intervention.

PSC Developmental/Academic Screening (33)

If a child fails the whole test, also refer for academic/developmental assessment. Children with mental health problems almost invariably have academic problems, and children with developmental or academic problems are at high risk of mental health problems.

Parents whose children pass the PSC but endorse numerous items should benefit from in-office counseling. If this has been tried and not found to be successful, such families should be referred for such services as parent training classes and behavior intervention programs.

Those with academic failure and difficulties (whose parents endorse items about poor school performance, absence from school, etc.), whether or not the PSC is passed, should be referred for intellectual and educational testing.

Gardner W. *et al.* The PSC-17: A brief pediatric symptom checklist psychosocial problem subscales: A report from PROS and ASPN. *Ambulatory Child Health*. 1999;5:225-236

Pediatric Laboratory Values: Common Laboratory Tests

Test/Specimen	Age/Sex/Reference	Normal Range (Conventional Units)	
Acetaminophen			
Serum or plasma	Therapeutic concentration	10-30 mcg/mL	
	Toxic concentration	>200 mcg/mL	
Antistreptolysin O titer (ASO)			
Serum	Toddler, 2-4 years	<160 Todd units/mL	
	School-age child	170-330 Todd units/mL	
Base excess			
Whole blood	Newborn	(-10)-(-2) mEq/L	
	Infant	(-7)-(-1) mEq/L	
	Toddler, 2-4 years	(-4)-$(+2)$ mEq/L	
	School-age child and older	(-3)-$(+3)$ mEq/L	
Bicarbonate, (HCO_3)			
Serum	Arterial	21-28 mEq/L	
	Venous	22-29 mEq/L	
Bilirubin, total			
Serum	Cord	Premature: <2 mg/dL	Full term: <2 mg/dL
	0-1 day	Premature: <8 mg/dL	Full term: <6 mg/dL
	1-2 days	Premature: <12 mg/dL	Full term: <8 mg/dL
	2-5 days	Premature: <16 mg/dL	Full term: <12 mg/dL
	>5 days	Premature: <20 mg/dL	Full term: <10 mg/dL

Continued

Test/Specimen	Age/Sex/Reference	Normal Range (Conventional Units)
Bilirubin, direct (conjugated)		
Serum		0-0.2 mg/dL
Bleeding time (Blood from skin puncture)		
Ivy	Normal	2-7 minutes
	Borderline	7-11 minutes
Simplate (G-D)		2.75-8 minutes
Blood volume		
Whole blood	Male	52-83 mL/kg
	Female	50-75 mL/kg
C-reactive protein (CRP)		
Serum	Cord	52-1300 ng/mL
	2-12 years	67-1800 ng/mL
Calcium, total		
Serum	Cord	9-11.5 mg/dL
	Newborn, 3-24 hours	9-10.6 mg/dL
	24-48 hours	7-12 mg/dL
	4-7 days	9-10.9 mg/dL
	Toddler, 2-4 years	8.8-10.8 mg/dL
	School-age child and older	8.4-10.2 mg/dL
Carbon dioxide, total (tCO_2)		
Serum or plasma	Cord	14-22 mEq/L
	Premature (1 week)	14-27 mEq/L
	Newborn	13-22 mEq/L
	Infant; toddler, 2-4 years	20-28 mEq/L
	School-age child or older	23-30 mEq/L
Cerebrospinal fluid (CSF)		
Pressure		70-180 mm water
Volume	Child	60-100 mL
	Adult	100-160 mL
Chloride		
Serum or	Cord	96-104 mEq/L
plasma	Newborn	97-110 mEq/L
	Child and older	98-106 mEq/L
Sweat	Normal (homozygote)	<40 mEq/L
	Marginal (e.g., asthma, Addison disease, malnutrition)	45-60 mmol/L
	Cystic fibrosis	>60 mmol/L

Test/Specimen	Age/Sex/Reference	Normal Range (Conventional Units)
Cholesterol, total		
Serum or plasma	Acceptable	<170 mg/dL
	Borderline	170-199 mg/dL
	High	≥ 200 mg/dL
Clotting time (Lee-White)		
Whole blood		5-8 minutes (glass tubes)
		5-15 minutes (room temperature)
		30 minutes (silicone tube)
Creatine kinase (CK, CPK)		
Serum	Cord blood	70-380 units/L
	5-8 hours	214-1175 units/L
	24-33 hours	130-1200 units/L
	72-100 hours	87-725 units/L
	Adult	5-130 units/L
Creatinine		
Serum	Cord	0.6-1.2 mg/dL
	Newborn	0.3-1 mg/dL
	Infant	0.2-0.4 mg/dL
	Child	0.3-0.7 mg/dL
	Adolescent	0.5-1 mg/dL
	Adult: Male	0.6-1.2 mg/dL
	Adult: Female	0.5-1.1 mg/dL
Urine, 24 hours	Premature	8.1-15 mg/kg/24 hours
	Full term	10.4-19.7 mg/kg/24 hours
	1.5-7 years	10-15 mg/kg/24 hours
	7-15 years	5.2-41 mg/kg/24 hours
Digoxin		
Serum, plasma; collect at least 12 hours after dose	Therapeutic concentration	
	CHF	0.8-1.5 ng/mL
	Arrhythmias	1.5-2 ng/mL
	Toxic concentration	
	Child	>2.5 ng/mL
	Adult	>3 ng/mL
Eosinophil count		
Whole blood, capillary blood		50-250 cells/mm^3 (mcL)

Continued

Test/Specimen	Age/Sex/Reference	Normal Range (Conventional Units)
Erythrocyte (RBC) count		
Whole blood	Cord	3.9-5.5 million/mm^3
	1-3 days	4.0-6.6 million/mm^3
	1 week	3.9-6.3 million/mm^3
	2 week	3.6-6.2 million/mm^3
	1 month	3-5.4 million/mm^3
	2 months	2.7-4.9 million/mm^3
	3-6 months	3.1-4.5 million/mm^3
	0.5-2 years	3.7-5.3 million/mm^3
	2-6 years	3.9-5.3 million/mm^3
	6-12 years	4-5.2 million/mm^3
	12-18 years: Male	4.5-5.3 million/mm^3
	12-18 years: Female	4.1-5.1 million/mm^3
Erythrocyte sedimentation rate (ESR) (Whole blood)		
Westergren	Child	0-10 mm/hour
(modified)	<50 years: Male	0-15 mm/hour
	<50 years: Female	0-20 mm/hour
Wintrobe	Child	0-13 mm/hour
	Adult: Male	0-9 mm/hour
	Adult: Female	0-20 mm/hour
Glucose		
Serum		
	Cord	45-96 mg/dL
	Newborn, 1 day	40-60 mg/dL
	Newborn, >1day	50-90 mg/dL
	Toddler, 2-4 years	60-100 mg/dL
	School-age child and older	70-105 mg/dL
Whole blood	Adult	65-95 mg/dL
Urine		
(Quantitative)		<0.5 gm/day
(Qualitative)		Negative

Glucose tolerance test (GTT), oral Serum

DOSAGES		NORMAL	DIABETIC
Adult: 75 gm	Fasting	70-105 mg/dL	≥ 126 mg/dL
Child: 1.75 gm/kg of	60 minutes	120-170 mg/dL	≥ 200 mg/dL
ideal weight up to	90 minutes	100-140 mg/dL	≥ 200 mg/dL
max of 75 gm	120 minutes	70-120 mg/dl	≥ 200 mg/dL

Test/Specimen	Age/Sex/Reference	Normal Range (Conventional Units)
Growth hormone (hGH, somatropin)		
Plasma	1 day	5-53 ng/mL
	1 week	5-27 ng/mL
	1-12 months	2-10 mg/mL
	Fasting child/adult	<0.7-6 ng/mL
Hematocrit (HCT, Hct)		
Whole blood	1 day (cap)	48%-69%
	2 day	48%-75%
	3 day	44%-72%
	2 months	28%-42%
	6-12 years	35%-45%
	12-18 years: Male	37%-49%
	12-18 years: Female	36%-46%
Hemoglobin (hb)		
Whole blood	1-3 days (cap)	14.5-22.5 gm/dL
	2 months	9-14 gm/dL
	6-12 years	11.5-15.5 gm/dL
	12-18 years: Male	13-16 gm/dL
	12-18 years: Female	12-16 gm/dL
Immunoglobulin A (IgA)		
Serum	Cord blood	1.4-3.6 mg/dL
	1-3 months	1.3-53 mg/dL
	4-6 months	4.4-84 mg/dL
	7 months-1 year	11-106 mg/dL
	2-5 years	14-159 mg/dL
	6-10 years	33-236 mg/dL
	Adult	70-312 mg/dL
Immunoglobulin G (IgG)		
Serum	Cord blood	636-1606 mg/dL
	1 month	251-906 mg/dL
	2-4 months	176-601 mg/dL
	5-12 months	172-1069 mg/dL
	1-5 years	345-1236 mg/dL
	6-10 years	608-1572 mg/dL
	Adult	639-1349 mg/dL

Continued

Test/Specimen	Age/Sex/Reference	Normal Range (Conventional Units)
Immunoglobulin M (IgM)		
Serum	Cord blood	6.3-25 mg/dL
	1-4 months	17-105 mg/dL
	5-9 months	33-126 mg/dL
	10 months-1 year	41-173 mg/dL
	2-8 years	43-207 mg/dL
	9-10 years	52-242 mg/dL
	Adult	56-352 mg/dL
Iron		
Serum	Newborn	100-250 mcg/dL
	Infant	40-100 mcg/dL
	Toddler, 2-4 years	50-120 mcg/dL
	School-age child and older: Male	65-170 mcg/dL
	School-age child and older: Female	50-170 mcg/dL
	Intoxicated child	280-2550 mcg/dL
	Fatally poisoned child	>1800 mcg/dL
Iron-binding capacity, total (TIBC)		
Serum	Infant	100-400 mcg/dL
	Child and older	250-400 mcg/dL
Lead		
Whole blood	Child	<10 mcg/L
Urine, 24 hours		<80 mcg/L
Leukocyte count (WBC count)		$\times$ **1000 cells/mm^3 (mcL)**
Whole blood	Birth	9-30
	24 hours	9.4-34
	1 month	5-19.5
	1-3 years	6-17.5
	4-7 years	5.5-15.5
	8-13 years	4.5-13.5
	Adult	4.5-11
CSF	Newborn	0-20 mononuclear
		0-10 polymorphonuclear
		0-800 RBC
	Neonate	0-5 mononuclear
		0-10 polymorphonuclear
		0-50 RBC
	Infant and older	0-5 mononuclear

Test/Specimen	Age/Sex/Reference		Normal Range (Conventional Units)
Leukocyte differential count			
Whole blood	Myelocytes	0%	0 cells/mm³ (mcL)
	Neutrophils—"bands"	3%-5%	150-400 cells/
	Neutrophils—"segs"		mm³ (mcL)
	Lymphocytes	54%-62%	3000-5800
			cells/mm³ (mcL)
	Monocytes	25%-33%	1500-3000 cells/
	Eosinophils		mm³ (mcL)
	Basophils	3%-7%	285-500 cells/
			mm³ (mcL)
		1%-3%	50-250 cells/
			mm³ (mcL)
		0-0.75%	15-50 cells/
			mm³ (mcL)
Mean corpuscular hemoglobin (MCH)			
Whole blood	Birth	31-37 pg/cell	
	1-3 days (cap)	31-37 pg/cell	
	1 week-1 month	28-40 pg/cell	
	2 months	26-34 pg/cell	
	3-6 months	25-35 pg/cell	
	0.5-2 years	23-31 pg/cell	
	2-6 years	24-30 pg/cell	
	6-12 years	25-33 pg/cell	
	12-18 years	25-35 pg/cell	
	18-49 years	26-34 pg/cell	
Mean corpuscular hemoglobin concentration (MCHC)			
Whole blood	Birth	30%-36% Hb/cell or gm Hb/dL RBC	
	1-3 days (cap)	29%-37% Hb/cell or gm Hb/dL RBC	
	1-2 weeks	28%-38% Hb/cell or gm Hb/dL RBC	
	1-2 months	29%-37% Hb/cell or gm Hb/dL RBC	
	3 months-2 years	30%-36% Hb/cell or gm Hb/dL RBC	
	2-18 years	31%-37% Hb/cell or gm Hb/dL RBC	
	>18 years	31%-37% Hb/cell or gm Hb/dL RBC	

Continued

Test/Specimen	Age/Sex/Reference	Normal Range (Conventional Units)
Mean corpuscular volume (MCV)		
Whole blood	1-3 days (cap)	95-121 mcm^3
	0.5-2 years	70-86 mcm^3
	6-12 years	77-95 mcm^3
	12-18 years: Male	78-98 mcm^3
	12-18 years: Female	78-102 mcm^3
Oxygen, partial pressure (Po$_2$)		
Whole blood,	Birth	8-24 mm Hg
arterial	5-10 minutes	33-75 mm Hg
	30 minutes	31-85 mm Hg
	>1 hour	55-80 mm Hg
	1 day	54-95 mm Hg
	>1 day (decreased with age)	83-108 mm Hg
Oxygen saturation (SaO$_2$)		
Whole blood,	Newborn	85%-90%
arterial	Infant and older	95%-99%
Partial thromboplastin time (PTT)		
Whole blood (Na citrate)		
Nonactivated		60-85 seconds (Platelin)
Activated		25-35 seconds (differs with method)
pH		
Whole blood,	Premature	7.35-7.5
arterial	(48 hours)	
	Birth, full term	7.11-7.36
	5-10 minutes	7.09-7.3
	30 minutes	7.21-7.38
	>1 hour	7.26-7.49
	1 day	7.29-7.45
	>1 day	7.35-7.45
	Must be corrected for body temperature	
Urine, random	Newborn/neonate	5-7
	Infant and older	4.5-8 (average approx 6)
Stool		7-7.5

Test/Specimen	Age/Sex/Reference	Normal Range (Conventional Units)
Platelet count (thrombocyte count)		
Whole blood (EDTA)	Newborn (after 1 week, same as adult)	$84\text{-}478 \times 10^3/\text{mm}^3$ (mcL)
	Adult	$150\text{-}400 \times 10^3/\text{mm}^3$ (mcL)
Potassium		
Serum	Newborn	3-6 mEq/L
	Neonate and older	3.5-5 mEq/L
Plasma (heparin)		3.4-4.5 mEq/L
Urine, 24 hours		2.5-125 mEq/L varies with diet
Protein		
Serum, total	Premature	4.3-7.6 gm/dL
	Newborn	4.6-7.4 gm/dL
	1-7 years	6.1-7.9 gm/dL
	8-12 years	6.4-8.1 gm/dL
	13-19 years	6.6-8.2 gm/dL
Urine, 24 hours, total		1-14 mg/dL
		50-80 mg/day (at rest)
		<250 mg/day after intense exercise
CSF total		Lumbar: 8-32 mg/dL
Prothrombin time (PT)		
One-stage (Quick)		
Whole blood (Na citrate)	In general	11-15 seconds (varies with type of thromboplastin)
	Newborn	Prolonged by 2-3 seconds
Two-stage modified (Ware and Seegers)		
Whole blood (Na citrate)		18-22 seconds
RBC count, see Erythrocyte count.		
Red blood cell volume		
Whole blood	Male	20-36 mL/kg
	Female	19-31 mL/kg

Continued

Test/Specimen	Age/Sex/Reference	Normal Range (Conventional Units)
Reticulocyte count		
Whole blood	Adult	0.5%-1.5% of erythrocytes or 25,000-75,000/mm^3 (mcL)
Capillary	1 day	0.4%-6%
	7 days	<0.1%-1.3%
	1-4 weeks	<0.1%-1.2%
	5-6 weeks	<0.1%-2.4%
	7-8 weeks	0.1%-2.9%
	9-10 weeks	<0.1%-2.6%
	11-12 weeks	0.1%-2.3%
Salicylates		
Serum, plasma	Therapeutic concentration	15-30 mg/dL
	Toxic concentration	>30 mg/dL

Sedimentation rate: see Erythrocyte sedimentation rate.

Test/Specimen	Age/Sex/Reference	Normal Range (Conventional Units)
Sodium		
Serum or plasma	Newborn	134-146 mEq/L
	Infant	139-146 mEq/L
	Child	138-145 mEq/L
	Thereafter	136-146 mEq/L
Urine, 24 hours		40-220 mEq/L (diet dependent)
Sweat	Normal	<40 mEq/L
	Indeterminate	45-60 mEq/L
	Cystic fibrosis	>60 mEq/L
Specific gravity		
Urine, random	Adult	1.002-1.030
	After 12 hours fluid restriction	>1.025
Urine, 24 hours		1.015-1.025
Thrombin time		
Whole blood (Na citrate)		Control time ± 2 seconds when control is 9-13 seconds

Test/Specimen	Age/Sex/Reference	Normal Range (Conventional Units)	
Thyroxine, total (T$_3$)			
Serum	Cord	8-13 mcg/dL	
	Newborn	11.5-24 (lower in low-birth-weight infants)	
	Neonate	9-18 mcg/dL	
	Infant	7-15 mcg/dL	
	1-5 years	7.3-15 mcg/dL	
	5-10 years	6.4-13.3 mcg/dL	
	>10 years	5-12 mcg/dL	
	Newborn screen (filter paper)	6.2-22 mcg/dL	
Triglycerides (TG)			
Serum, after ≥12 hours fasting		**Male**	**Female**
	Cord blood	10-98 mg/dL	10-98 mg/dL
	0-5 years	30-86 mg/dL	32-99 mg/dL
	6-11 years	31-108 mg/dL	35-114 mg/dL
	12-15 years	36-138 mg/dL	41-138 mg/dL
	16-19 years	40-163 mg/dL	40-128 mg/dL
Urea nitrogen			
Serum or plasma	Cord	21-40 mg/dL	
	Premature (1 week)	3-25 mg/dL	
	Newborn	3-12 mg/dL	
	Infant/child	5-18 mg/dL	
	Thereafter	7-18 mg/dL	
Urine volume			
Urine, 24 hours	Newborn	50-300 mL/day	
	Infant	350-550 mL/day	
	Child	500-1000 mL/day	
	Adolescent	700-1400 mL/day	
	School-age child and older: Male	800-1800 mL/day	
	School-age child and older: Female	600-1600 mL/day (varies with intake and other factors)	

WBC, *see* Leukocyte count

Data from Hockenberry MJ: *Wong's essentials of pediatric nursing,* ed 7, St Louis, 2005, Mosby; Behrman RE, Kliegman RM, Jenson HB: *Nelson textbook of pediatrics,* ed 17, Philadelphia, 2004, Saunders; and McMilan A et al, editors: *Oski's pediatrics: principles and practice,* ed 3, Philadelphia, 1999, Lippincott Williams & Wilkins.

ENGLISH-TO-SPANISH VOCABULARY AND PHRASES

ANATOMY

Abdomen	El abdomen Ehl ab-**doh**-mehn	Body	El cuerpo Ehl **kwehr**-poh
Ankle	El tobillo Ehl toh-**bee**-yhoh	Bone	El hueso Ehl **weh**-soh
Anus	El ano Ehl **ah**-noh	Brain	El cerebro Ehl seh-**reh**-broh
Appendix	El apéndice Ehl ah-**pehn**-dee-seh	Breasts	Los senos Lohs **seh**-nohs
Arm	El brazo Ehl **brah**-soh	Buttock	La nalga La **nahl**-gah
Artery	La arteria Lah ahr-**teh**-ree-ah	Calf	La pantorilla Lah pahn-toh-**ree**-yhah
Axilla	La axila Lah ag-**see**-lah	Cervix	El cuello uterino Ehl **kweh**-yoh oo-teh-**ree**-noh
Back	La espalda Lah ehs-**pahl**-dah	Cheek	La mejilla Lah meh-**hee**-yhah
Bladder	La vejiga Lah beh-**hee**-gah	Chest	El pecho Ehl **peh**-choh

ANATOMY—CONT'D

English	Spanish		English	Spanish
Chin	El mentón Ehl mehn-**tohn**		Forehead	La frente Lah **frehn**-teh
Clavicle	La clavícula Lah klah-**vee**-koo-lah		Foreskin	El prepucio Ehl preh-**poo**-see-oh
Ear	El oído /La oreja Ehl oh-**ee**-doh /Lah oh- **reh**-ha		Gallbladder	La vesícula biliar Lah beh-**see**-koo-lah bee-lee-**ahr**
Elbow	El codo Ehl **koh**-doh		Gingiva/gums	Las encías Lahs ehn-**see**-ahs
Eye	El ojo Ehl **oh**-hoh		Groin	La ingle Lah **een**-gleh
Eyebrow	La ceja Lah **seh**-hah		Hair	El pelo/El cabello Ehl **peh**-loh/Ehl kah- **beh**-yoh
Eyelash	La pestaña Lah pehs-**tah**-nyah		Hand	La mano Lah **mah**-noh
Eyelid	El párpado Ehl **pahr**-pah-doh		Head	La cabeza Lah kah-**beh**-sah
Face	La cara Lah **kah**-rah		Heart	El corazón Ehl koh-rah-**sohn**
Finger	El dedo Ehl **deh**-doh		Heel	El talón Ehl tah-**lohn**
Fingernail	La uña Lah **oo**-nyah		Hip	La cadera Lah kah-**deh**-rah
Foot	El pie Ehl **pee**-eh		Intestines	Los intestinos Lohs **een**-tehs-**tee**-nohs
Fontanel	La mollera/La fontanela Lah moh-**yeh**-rah/lah fohn- tah-**neh**-lah		Joint	La articulación Lah ahr-tee-koo-lah- see-**ohn**
Forearm	El antebrazo Ehl ahn-teh-**brah**-soh		Kidney	El riñón Ehl ree-**nyohn**

Continued

ANATOMY—CONT'D

Knee	La rodilla Lah roh-**dee**-yhah	Nose	La nariz Lah nah-**rees**
Knuckle	El nudillo Ehl noo-**dee**-yoh	Ovary	El ovario Ehl oh-**bah**-ree-oh
Larynx	La laringe Lah lah-**reen**-heh	Pancreas	El páncreas Ehl **pahn**-kreh-ahs
Leg	La pierna Lah pee-**ehr**-nah	Pelvis	La pelvis Lah **pehl**-bees
Lips	Los labios Lohs **lah**-bee-ohs	Penis	El pene Ehl **peh**-neh
Liver	El hígado Ehl **ee**-gah-doh	Prostate	La próstata Lah **prohs**-tah-tah
Lung	El pulmón Ehl pool-**mohn**	Pupil	La pupila Lah poo-**pee**-lah
Lymph node	El ganglio linfático Ehl **gahn**-glee-oh leen-**fah**-tee-koh	Rectum	El recto Ehl **reg**-toh
Mandible	La mandíbula Lah mahn-**dee**-boo-lah	Rib	La costilla Lah kohs-**tee**-yah
Mouth	La boca Lah **boh**-kah	Scalp	El cuero cabelludo Ehl **kweh**-roh kah-beh-**yuh**-doh
Muscle	El músculo Ehl **moos**-koo-loh	Scapula	La escápula Lah ehs-**kah**-poo-lah
Navel	El ombligo Ehl ohm-**blee**-goh	Scrotum	El escroto Ehl ehs-**kroh**-toh
Neck	El cuello Ehl **kweh**-yoh	Shoulder	El hombro Ehl **ohm**-broh
Nerve	El nervio Ehl **nehr**-bee-oh	Skin	La piel Lah pee-**ehl**
Nipple	El pezón Ehl peh-**sohn**	Skull	El cráneo Ehl **krah**-neh-oh

ANATOMY—CONT'D

Spine	El espinazo Ehl ehs-pee-**nah**-soh	Tonsils	Las anginas Lahs ahn-**hee**-nahs
Spleen	El bazo Ehl **bah**-soh	Tooth	El diente Ehl dee-**ehn**-teh
Sternum	El esternón Ehl ehs-tehr-**nohn**	Trachea	La tráquea Lah **trah**-keh-ah
Stomach	El estómago Ehl ehs-**toh**-mah-goh	Tubes	Los tubos Lohs **too**-bohs
Tendon	El tendón Ehl tehn-**dohn**	Umbilical cord	El cordón umbilical Ehl kohr-**dohn** oom- bee-lee-**kahl**
Testicles	Los testículos Lohs tehs-**tee**-koo-lohs	Urethra	La uretra Lah oo-**reh**-trah
Thigh	El muslo Ehl **moos**-loh	Uterus	El útero/La matriz Ehl **oo**-teh-roh/Lah mah-**trees**
Thorax	El tórax Ehl **toh**-raks	Uvula	La campanilla Lah kahm-pah-**nee**-yah
Throat	La garganta Lah gahr-**gahn**-tah	Vagina	La vagina Lah bah-**hee**-nah
Thumb	El pulgar Ehl pool-**gahr**	Vein	La vena Lah **beh**-nah
Thymus	El timo Ehl **tee**-moh	Vocal cords	Las cuerdas vocales Lahs **kwehr**-dahs boh-**kah**-lehs
Thyroid	La tiroides Lah tee-roh-ee-dehs	Waist	La cintura Lah seen-**too**-rah
Toes	Los dedos de los pies Lohs **deh**-dohs deh lohs **pee**-ehs	Wrist	La muñeca Lah moo-**nyeh**-kah
Tongue	La lengua Lah **lehn**-gwah		

Continued

MISCELLANEOUS TERMS

Appointment	Cita **See**-tah		Bruise	Moretón Moh-reh-**tohn**
Pill	Píldora/pastilla **Peel**-doh-rah/pahs-**tee**-yhah		Fever	Fiebre Fee-**eh**-breh
To admit	Internar Een-tehr-**nahr**		Dizzy	Mareada (o) Mah-reh-**ah**-dah (oh)
Tablet	Tableta Tah-**bleh**-tah		Feces	Heces **Eh**-sehs
To discharge	Dar de alta Dahr deh **ahl**-tah		Dizziness	Mareos Mah-**reh**-ohs
Capsule	Cápsula **Kap**-soo-lah		Phlegm	Flema **Fleh**-mah
Blood	Sangre **Sahn**-greh		Numb	Entumido (a) Ehn-too-**mee**-doh (ah)
Injection	Inyección Een-jeg-see-**ohn**		Mucus	Mocosidad Moh-koh-see-**dahd**
Urine	Orina Oh-**ree**-nah		Fracture	Fractura Frag-**too**-rah
Ointment	Pomada Poh-**mah**-dah		Sweat	Sudor Soo-**dohr**
Saliva	Saliva Sah-**lee**-bah		Sprain	Torcedura Tohr-seh-**doo**-rah
Lotion	Loción Loh-see-**ohn**		Tears	Lágrimas **Lah**-gree-mahs
Blood clot	Coágulo de sangre Koh-**ah**-goo-loh deh **sahn**- greh		Faint	Desmayo Dehs-**mah**-yhoh
Swollen	Hinchado Een-**chah**-doh		Discharge	Deshecho Dehs-**eh**-choh
Vomit	Vómito **Boh**-mee-toh		Pain	Dolor Doh-**lohr**

MISCELLANEOUS TERMS—CONT'D

Burning	Ardor Ahr-**dohr**		Rash	Salpullido Sahl-poo-**yee**-doh
Itching	Comezón Koh-meh-**sohn**		Blisters	Ampollas Ahm-**poh**-yahs
Cramps	Calambres Kah-**lahm**-brehs		Scratch	Rascar Rahs-**kahr**
Chills	Escalofríos Ehs-kah-loh-**free**-ohs		Burn	Quemadura Keh-mah-**doo**-rah

PAIN

Pain	Dolor Doh-**lohr**
Where does he/she have the pain?	¿Dónde tiene el dolor? **Dohn**-deh tee-**eh**-neh ehl doh-**lohr?**
When did the pain start?	¿Cuándo empezó el dolor? **Kwahn**-doh ehm-peh-**soh** ehl doh-**lohr?**
Where did the pain start?	¿Dónde empezó el dolor? **Dohn**-deh ehm-peh-**soh** ehl doh-**lohr?**
Does the pain go to another place?	¿Le va el dolor a otro lugar? Leh bah ehl doh-**lohr** ah **oh**-troh loo-**gahr?**
Point to where the pain goes.	Apunte a dónde le va el dolor. Ah-**poon**-teh ah **dohn**-deh leh bah ehl doh-**lohr.**
How long does the pain last?	¿Cuánto tiempo le dura el dolor? **Kwahn**-toh tee-**ehm**-poh leh **doo**-rah ehl doh-**lohr?**
seconds	segundos seh-**goon**-dohs
minutes	minutos mee-**noo**-tohs
hours	horas **oh**-rahs
constant	constante kohns-**tahn**-teh
Does the pain come and go?	¿Le va y viene el dolor? Leh **bah** ee bee-**eh**-neh ehl doh-**lohr?**
Is the pain constant?	¿Es el dolor constante? Ehs ehl doh-**lohr** kohns-**tahn**-teh?

Continued

PAIN—CONT'D

What is the pain like?	¿Cómo es el dolor? Koh-moh ehs ehl doh-**lohr?**
Acute	Agudo Ah-**goo**-doh
Severe	Severo/fuerte Seh-**beh**-roh/**fwehr**-teh
Like a knife	Como cuchillo Koh-moh koo-**chee**-yoh
Soreness	Adolorido Ah-doh-loh-**ree**-doh
Burning	Quemante Keh-**mahn**-teh
Pressure	Opresivo Oh-preh-**see**-boh
Like cramps	Como calambres **Koh**-moh kah-**lahm**-brehs
Has he/she had this type of pain before?	¿Ha tenido él/ella este tipo de dolor antes? Ah teh-**nee**-doh ehl/**eh**-yah **ehs**-teh **tee**-poh deh doh-**lohr ahn**-tehs?
What things cause the pain?	¿Qué cosas le causan el dolor? Keh **koh**-sahs leh kah-oo-sahn ehl doh-**lohr?**
Running	Correr Koh-**rher**
Walking	Caminar Kah-mee-**nahr**
Bending	Agacharse Ah-gah-**char**-seh
Breathing	Respirar Rehs-pee-**rahr**
Eating	Comer Koh-**mehr**
Coughing	Toser Toh-**sehr**

PAIN—CONT'D

What makes the pain better?	¿Qué le mejora el dolor? Keh leh meh-**hoh**-rah ehl doh-**lohr?**
Nothing	Nada **Nah**-dah
Tylenol	Tylenol **Tay**-leh-nohl
Sleeping	Dormir Dohr-**meehr**
Does he/she have fever?	¿Tiene fiebre? Tee-**eh**-neh fee-**eh**-breh?
Does he/she have vomiting?	¿Tiene vómito? Tee-**eh**-neh **boh**-mee-toh?
Did he/she fall?	¿Se cayó? Seh kah-**yoh?**
Did someone hit him/her?	¿Alguien le pegó? **Ahl**-gee-ehn leh peh-**goh?**
Does he/she have trouble breathing?	¿Tiene problemas para respirar? Tee-**eh**-neh proh-**bleh**-mahs pah-rah rehs-pee-**rahr?**
Is the pain . . .	¿Es el dolor . . . Ehs ehl doh-**lohr** . . .
the same	igual ee-**gwahl**
better	mejor meh-**hohr**
worse	peor peh-**ohr**
. . . since it started?	. . . desde que empezó? . . . dehs-deh **keh** ehm-peh-**soh?**
Has he/she taken something for the pain?	¿Ha tomado algo para el dolor? Ah toh-**mah**-doh **ahl**-goh pah-rah ehl doh-**lohr?**
Tylenol	Tylenol **Tay**-leh-nohl
Aspirin	Aspirina Ahs-pee-**ree**-nah
Ibuprofen	Ibuprofen Ee-boo-**proh**-fehn

ADDITIONAL RESOURCES AVAILABLE ONLINE

Development

Ages and Stages Questionnaires (ASQ)
www.brookespublishing.com/store/books/bricker-asq

Developmental Behavioral Pediatrics Online
www.dbpeds.org

Family Psychosocial Screening
www.fpnotebook.com/PED52.htm

48 Months/4 Year Questionnaire
http://ruccs.rutgers.edu/~karin/PERINATAL/asq-sampleforms.pdf *

Growth Charts for Boys and Girls with Down Syndrome
www.ndss.org/content.cfm?fuseaction=InfoRes.HlthArticle&article=603

Parents' Evaluation of Developmental Status (PEDS)
www.forepath.org

Recommended Dietary Fluoride Supplement Schedule
www.cdc.gov/OralHealth/factsheets/fl-supplements.htm

---

*This link requires Adobe Acrobat Reader.

Recommended 2005 Childhood & Adolescent Immunization Schedule
www.cdc.gov/nip/recs/child-schedule.htm

Professional Resources

American Academy of Pediatric Dentistry
www.aapd.org

American Academy of Pediatrics
www.aap.org

American Academy of Pediatrics: Pediatric Research in Office Settings (PROS)
www.aap.org/pros

National Association of Pediatric Nurse Practitioners (NAPNAP)
www.napnap.org

Society of Pediatric Nurses
www.pedsnurses.org

Parent/Patient Information

Parents as Teachers (national center)
www.parentsasteachers.org

Virtual Children's Hospital (University of Iowa)
www.vh.org/pediatric

INDEX

C

Calcaneus, 234
Calcification, dental, 155
Candidiasis, 165, 166, 215, 216, 227
Capitate bones, 234
Caput succedaneum, 105
Carboplatin, 152
Cardiac apex position, 81
Cardiac catheterization, 83
Cardiothoracic ratios, 81
Cardiovascular system
    anatomy and physiology of, 71-75
    diagnostic procedures for, 80-83
    physical assessment of, 75-80
    sports participation and, 248, 252-253
    symptoms of, 83-87
Carditis, 248
Caries, 166-167
Carpal bones, 234
Cartilage, 112, 138
Cataracts, 128
Cat-scratch fever, 120
Cecum, 175
Central cyanosis, 76-77, 97
Cephalhematomas, 105
Cephalocaudal growth, 11
Cerebellums, 262, 276
Cerebral cortex, 260, 262, 268
Cerebral palsy, 249, 263, 278
Cerebrospinal fluid, 262
Cerebrums, 260-261, 276-277
Cerumen, 140, 148
Cervical chains, 116
Cervical lymphadenitis, 120
Cervical nodes, 117, 118
Cervix, 224, 225, 226, 229
Chests, 15, 84, 87, 90, 95-96. *See also*
    Respiratory system
Cheyne-stokes breathing, 97
Chlamydia trachomatis, 215, 223
Choana, 158
Choanal atresia, 158
Choledochal cysts, 173, 186

Cholesteatomas, 140, 151
Chordee, 194
Choroid, 123-124
Ciliary bodies, 123
Ciliary muscles, 121-122
Circumcision, 200, 228
Circumduction, 238
Cisplatin, 152
Clavicles, 239
Clearance forms, 290
Cleft palates, 155
Clitoris, 214, 227, 229
Clonus, 268, 274
Clubbing, 77
Clubfoot, 255
Coarctation of aortas, 19, 77
Cocaine, 263
Coccyx, 233
Coil closures, 83
Collecting vessels, 113
Colobomas, 127-128
Colons, 171, 175
Color vision, 132, 134
Colposcopies, 213
Columella, 157
Comedones, 64
Conductive hearing loss, 151-152
Condyloid joints, 238
Confidentiality, 41
Congenital hearing loss, 152
Congenital heart disease, 72-75, 83, 248
Congestive heart failure, 74, 77
Conjunctivitis, 122, 134
Consolidations, 98
Contextual healthcare, 3
Continuous murmurs, 80
Corneal light reflexes, 128-129
Corona glandis, 190
Corpus callosum, 261
Corpus cavernosa, 190
Cortex, 260, 262, 268
Corticosteroids, 205, 250
Costochondritis, 87
Cover-uncover tests, 129-130, 133

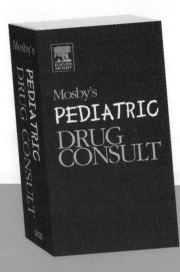